Please note the information contained within this document is for educational and entertainment purposes only. All effort has been executed to present accurate, up to date, reliable, complete information. No warranties of any kind are declared or implied. Readers acknowledge that the author is not engaged in the rendering of legal, financial, medical, or professional advice. The content within this book has been derived from various sources. Please consult a licensed professional before attempting any techniques outlined in this book. By reading this document, the reader agrees that under no circumstances is the author responsible for any losses, direct or indirect, that are incurred as a result of the use of the information contained within this document, including, but not limited to, errors, omissions, or inaccuracies.

CONTENTS

INTRODUCTION

About the Oster Toaster Oven
What Does It Do?

I know what you're thinking...isn't a toaster oven just a miniature oven? In some ways, yes, but the features and benefits of the Oster Convection Toaster Oven really set it apart from conventional ovens as well as other toaster ovens. The Oster Toaster Oven features advanced digital controls allowing you maximum flexibility and accuracy, but it also harnesses the power of convection cooking for faster, more even cooking. And because it features a large cooking space, you are able to cook a wide variety of different dishes without having to turn on your regular oven.

What Does It NOT Do?

The Oster Toaster Oven is a marvel of functionality. From convection cooking to perfect defrosting, it does so many things. But there are a few things it can't do. The Oster Toaster Oven will not take the place of your microwave because it will not heat up food as quickly. It does, however, heat up much faster than a conventional oven. You are also somewhat limited by the size of the Oster Toaster Oven. While it does feature a large cooking compartment, you will not be able to cook a twenty-pound turkey in it. Other than these few limitations, the Oster Toaster Oven can handle most of your cooking needs.

Who Is It Good For?

Because the Oster Toaster Oven is so versatile and easy to use, it is good for practically anyone. Families who want the flexibility to cook small meals and snacks will love how simple it is to use. And if you happen to be cooking large meals for holidays, like Thanksgiving, the Oster Toaster Oven is a great way to free up space in your regular oven, or keep things warm until dinnertime. The Oster Toaster Oven is also perfect for college students and singles who often need to cook quick meals for one. Instead of preheating your large regular oven, the Oster Toaster Oven heats in seconds and is specifically designed to handle small meals. It also allows you to easily defrost items, saving you time.

Perfect for the Whole Family

The Oster Toaster Oven is a great alternative to a conventional oven because it offers greater flexibility, so everyone in the family can use it. Because you often only need to make small meals or snacks, your regular oven can be inefficient. First of all, a regular oven takes time to heat up. The Oster Toaster Oven, on the other hand, heats up in just a fraction of the time so you can get cooking right away. The Oster Toaster Oven's easy-to-use digital controls also take a lot of the guesswork out of cooking. You don't have to be a professional chef to easily make meals that are sure to please. The Oster Toaster Oven is also perfect for those times when the family is making a really big meal and there just isn't enough space in the regular oven.

Who Is It NOT Good For?

While the Oster Toaster Oven is perfect for nearly any situation, if you have limited space in your kitchen and do not need another cooking appliance, the Oster Toaster Oven may not be for you. Also, if your family prefers to only make large meals, the small size of the Oster Toaster Oven may not be large enough to meet your needs.

A Few Cautions

As with any cooking appliance with a heating element, you will want to exercise caution when operating the Oster Toaster Oven. Always make sure the oven is placed on a stable and level surface and that children are properly supervised while using it. When removing items from the oven, always be sure to wear oven mitts and use the side handles to move the oven when hot.

When opening the door to the oven, make sure your face is a safe distance, as the oven will be very hot after cooking. Before cleaning the trays or inner surfaces of the oven, make sure it has fully cooled after cooking. And of course, make sure to turn the oven off as soon as you have finished cooking.

Health Benefits

One of the main issues facing families these days is overconsuming processed foods and fast food, which are often high in fat, sugars, and preservatives. One of the best ways to deal with this is to learn to cook healthy meals at home, but the problem is that cooking at home can be time consuming and it involves a lot of equipment. That's where your Oster Toaster Oven comes in. Because it is so easy to use and clean, cooking at home is no longer a hassle. The Oster Toaster Oven features easy-to-use controls and convection cooking, so even a beginner can become an expert home chef in no time. Once you've gotten the hang of how it works, the whole family will want to join in the fun of cooking fast, easy, and most importantly, healthy meals.

A Brief History of Toaster Ovens

Believe it or not, the toaster oven actually predates the pop-up toaster by about nine years. The first toaster oven was produced in 1910 by the Westinghouse Company as a way to incorporate most of the functions of a traditional oven, but in a much smaller package. The pop up toaster we're all familiar with didn't come along until 1919. Over the years, features were added to toaster ovens to give them more flexibility and function. Most notably, we saw toaster ovens designed with settings for different types of food. Eventually, features like convection were added and allowed users to cook virtually anything in their toaster ovens... as long as it was small enough.

How to use the Oster Toaster Oven

Setting Up Your Toaster Oven

Your toaster oven really couldn't be easier to use. The front door allows you access to the racks, which slide in and out for you to easily reach your food before, during, and after cooking.

Once you have removed the toaster oven from the box, place it on a level surface near a grounded power outlet. Plug the toaster oven in and remove the trays from the oven. Before using, make sure to thoroughly clean the trays with soap and water. You are now set up and ready to start using your Oster Toaster Oven.

Learning the controls

The great thing about the Oster Toaster Oven is that all of the controls are labeled for easy use. You don't have to bother with confusing dials. Let's take a look at how the Oster Toaster Oven works.

1 Temperature Control Knob: This controls the oven temperature. Simply turn clockwise to set the oven to any temperature between 0°F to 450°F.

2 Function Selector Knob: This controls HOW the temperature you selected above is achieved. Depending on which function you select (Warm, Broil, Bake, Toast, Turbo), and which temperature you've selected, the oven will turn on/off its heating elements and air circulation. Refer to the recipe for which function mode to select.

3 Timer Control Knob with Bell Signal: This knob is basically an "on" button with a timer built-in. The oven will turn off when the timer runs out and you'll hear its bell go "ding!".

4 Removeable Crumb Tray: This tray is at the bottom, under the heating elements. It pulls out for easy cleaning.

5 Baking Pan & Cookie Sheet: Use this for baking.

6 Removeable Wire Rack: Use this for broiling and grilling. You can place it in two positions to get closer or further from the above heating elements.

Tempered Glass Door: For easy viewing of food. The cooking process

The Oster Toaster Oven is one of the most advanced toaster ovens on the planet due to its digital controls and user-friendly design. But perhaps the best feature of the Oster Toaster Oven is its ability to cook using convection. Unlike regular baking, convection produces the most even heat possible by circulating the heated air. It's perfect for many different types of cooking that require food to be evenly cooked throughout. It's also a great way to ensure amazing results when baking.

From the moment you choose your cooking program, the Oster Toaster Oven begins heating quickly. A great feature of this oven is that is preheats so quickly. And unlike many competing toaster ovens, the Oster allows you to cook up to 450°F, which allows you to cook many foods you would not be able to cook in other toaster ovens. When you're finished cooking, the timer will go off and the oven will automatically turn itself off. That's not just a great way to save energy, it's also an important safety feature. After the oven has had a chance to cool, you can clean it using a damp cloth or sponge to remove any spatter that may have occurred during the cooking process.

Workarounds

We've already explored many of the things your Oster Toaster Oven can do, so now let's talk a little about problem solving. When you're cooking in a conventional oven, it is pretty common to line your baking sheets with aluminum foil. It's a great way to keep those baking trays from getting dirty, and that's pretty helpful after your meal. But using aluminum foil in the Oster Toaster Oven is not a good idea because using aluminum foil in the Oster Toaster Oven can cause the oven to get too hot - sometimes over 500°F, and a toaster oven, unlike your conventional oven, isn't designed to safely work at such a high temperature. To combat this problem and still have a way to line the trays of your toaster oven, try using parchment paper. It will keep food from sticking to the trays, and you can just throw it out after cooking.

You may have noticed that the Oster Toaster Oven features a large cooking space inside the oven. As a result, you can cook more efficiently by cooking on several levels at once. While only one cooking rack is included with the oven, you can purchase additional racks. Just make sure to purchase racks in the correct size.

Often, you will see packaged foods with a different temperature recommendation for cooking food in toaster ovens. However, because the Oster Toaster Oven cooks almost exactly like a regular oven, it is usually not necessary to use the recommended toaster oven temperature setting. Doing this may actually cause your food to come out overcooked. We suggest that you reduce all toaster oven temperature recommendations by twenty-five degrees to avoid overcooking.

APPETIZERS AND SIDE DISHES

1. Eggplant Cakes With Yogurt

Servings:4
Cooking Time: 20 Minutes
Ingredients:

- 1 ½ cups flour
- 1 tsp cinnamon
- 3 eggs
- 2 tsp baking powder
- 2 tbsp sugar
- 1 cup milk
- 2 tbsp butter, melted
- 1 tbsp yogurt
- 1 eggplant, chopped
- Pinch of salt
- 2 tbsp cream cheese

Directions:

1. Preheat on AirFry function to 350 F. In a bowl, whisk the eggs along with the sugar, salt, cinnamon, cream cheese, flour, and baking powder. In another bowl, combine all of the liquid ingredients. Gently combine the dry and liquid mixtures; stir in eggplant.
2. Line muffin tins and pour the batter in. Press Start and AirFry for 12 minutes. Check with a toothpick: if it doesn't come up clean, cook them for an additional 2 to 3 minutes. Serve chilled.

2. Air Fry Garlic Baby Potatoes

Servings: 4
Cooking Time: 20 Minutes
Ingredients:

- 1 lb baby potatoes, cut into quarters
- 1/2 tsp granulated garlic
- 1 tbsp olive oil
- 1/2 tsp dried parsley
- 1/4 tsp salt

Directions:

1. Fit the oven with the rack in position 2.
2. In a mixing bowl, toss baby potatoes with oil, garlic, parsley, and salt.
3. Transfer potatoes in air fryer basket then place air fryer basket in baking pan.
4. Place a baking pan on the oven rack. Set to air fry at 350 F for 20 minutes.
5. Serve and enjoy.
- **Nutrition Info:** Calories 97 Fat 3.6 g Carbohydrates 14.4 g Sugar 0.1 g Protein 3 g Cholesterol 0 mg

3. Salty Carrot Chips

Servings:2
Cooking Time: 20 Minutes
Ingredients:

- 3 large carrots, washed and peeled
- Salt to taste

Directions:

1. Using a mandolin slicer, cut the carrots very thinly heightwise. Season with salt to taste. Place in the frying basket and spray them lightly with cooking spray. Select AirFry function, adjust the temperature to 380 F, and press Start. Cook for 14-16 minutes until crispy.

4. Cheesy Broccoli Rice

Servings: 8
Cooking Time: 20 Minutes
Ingredients:

- 1 1/2 cups cooked brown rice
- 1 garlic clove, chopped
- 16 oz frozen broccoli florets
- 1 large onion, chopped
- 1 tbsp butter
- 3 tbsp parmesan cheese, grated
- 10.5 oz condensed cheddar cheese soup
- 1/3 cup almond milk

Directions:

1. Fit the oven with the rack in position
2. Heat butter in a 10-inch pan over medium heat.
3. Add onion and cook until tender.
4. Add garlic and broccoli in the pan and cook until broccoli is tender.
5. Stir in rice, soup, and milk and cook until hot.
6. Stir in cheese and pour broccoli mixture into the greased baking dish.
7. Set to bake at 350 F for 25 minutes. After 5 minutes place the baking dish in the preheated oven.
8. Serve and enjoy.
- **Nutrition Info:** Calories 244 Fat 8.3 g Carbohydrates 35.4 g Sugar 2.7 g Protein 6 g Cholesterol 14 mg

5. Spicy And Sweet Nuts

Servings: 4 Cups
Cooking Time: 15 Minutes
Ingredients:

- 1 pound (454 g) walnut halves and pieces
- ½ cup granulated sugar
- 3 tablespoons vegetable oil
- 1 teaspoon cayenne pepper
- ½ teaspoon fine salt

Directions:

1. Soak the walnuts in a large bowl with boiling water for a minute or two. Drain the walnuts. Stir in the sugar, oil and cayenne pepper to coat well. Spread the walnuts in a single layer in the baking pan.
2. Slide the baking pan into Rack Position 1, select Convection Bake, set temperature to 325ºF (163ºC) and set time to 15 minutes.

3. After 7 or 8 minutes, remove from the oven. Stir the nuts. Return the pan to the oven and continue cooking, check frequently.
4. When cooking is complete, the walnuts should be dark golden brown. Remove from the oven. Sprinkle the nuts with the salt and let cool. Serve warm.

6. Party Macaroni Quiche With Greek Yogurt

Servings: 4
Cooking Time: 30 Minutes
Ingredients:
- 8 tbsp leftover macaroni with cheese
- Extra cheese for serving
- Pastry as much needed for forming 4 shells
- Salt and black pepper to taste
- 1 tsp garlic puree
- 2 tbsp Greek yogurt
- 2 whole eggs
- 12 oz milk

Directions:
1. Preheat on Air Fry function to 360 F. Roll the pastry to form 4 shells. Place them in the Air Fryer pan.
2. In a bowl, mix leftover macaroni with cheese, yogurt, eggs, milk, and garlic puree. Spoon this mixture into the pastry shells. Top with the cheese evenly. Cook for 20 minutes.

7. Crunchy Cheese Twists

Servings: 8
Cooking Time: 45 Minutes
Ingredients:
- 2 cups cauliflower florets, steamed
- 1 egg
- 3 ½ oz oats
- 1 red onion, diced
- 1 tsp mustard
- 5 oz cheddar cheese, shredded
- Salt and black pepper to taste

Directions:
1. Preheat on Air Fry function to 350 F. Place the oats in a food processor and pulse until they are the consistency of breadcrumbs.
2. Place the cauliflower florets in a large bowl. Add in the rest of the ingredients and mix to combine. Take a little bit of the mixture and twist it into a straw.
3. Place onto a lined baking tray and repeat the process with the rest of the mixture. Cook for 10 minutes, turn over, and cook for an additional 10 minutes. Serve.

8. Green Bean Casserole(3)

Servings: 4
Cooking Time: 20 Minutes
Ingredients:
- 1 lb. fresh green beans, edges trimmed
- ½ oz. pork rinds, finely ground
- 1 oz. full-fat cream cheese
- ½ cup heavy whipping cream.
- ¼ cup diced yellow onion
- ½ cup chopped white mushrooms
- ½ cup chicken broth
- 4 tbsp. unsalted butter.
- ¼ tsp. xanthan gum

Directions:
1. In a medium skillet over medium heat, melt the butter. Sauté the onion and mushrooms until they become soft and fragrant, about 3–5 minutes.
2. Add the heavy whipping cream, cream cheese and broth to the pan. Whisk until smooth. Bring to a boil and then reduce to a simmer. Sprinkle the xanthan gum into the pan and remove from heat
3. Chop the green beans into 2-inch pieces and place into a 4-cup round baking dish. Pour the sauce mixture over them and stir until coated. Top the dish with ground pork rinds. Place into the air fryer basket
4. Adjust the temperature to 320 Degrees F and set the timer for 15 minutes. Top will be golden and green beans fork tender when fully cooked. Serve warm.
- **Nutrition Info:** Calories: 267; Protein: 6g; Fiber: 2g; Fat: 24g; Carbs: 7g

9. Easy Crunchy Garlic Croutons

Servings: 4
Cooking Time: 20 Minutes
Ingredients:
- 2 cups bread, cubed
- 2 tbsp butter, melted
- Garlic salt and black pepper to taste

Directions:
1. In a bowl, toss the bread cubes with butter, garlic salt, and pepper until well-coated. Place the cubes in the Air Fryer basket and fit in the baking tray. Cook in the oven for 12 minutes at 380 F on Air Fry function or until golden brown and crispy.

10. Rosemary & Thyme Roasted Fingerling Potatoes

Servings: 4
Cooking Time: 25 Minutes
Ingredients:
- 1 small bag baby fingerling potatoes
- 3 tablespoons olive oil
- Salt and pepper to taste
- 2 teaspoons rosemary
- 2 teaspoons thyme

Directions:
1. Start by preheating the toaster oven to 400°F.

2. Toss potatoes in olive oil and place on a baking sheet.
3. Pierce each potato to prevent overexpansion.
4. Sprinkle salt, pepper, rosemary, and thyme over the potatoes.
5. Roast for 25 minutes.
- **Nutrition Info:** Calories: 123, Sodium: 3 mg, Dietary Fiber: 1.2 g, Total Fat: 10.7 g, Total Carbs: 7.5 g, Protein: 0.9 g.

11. Herby Carrot Cookies

Servings:6
Cooking Time: 30 Minutes
Ingredients:
- 6 carrots, sliced
- Salt and black pepper to taste
- 1 tbsp parsley
- ½ cup oats
- 1 whole egg, beaten
- 1 tbsp thyme

Directions:
1. Preheat on Air Fryer function to 360 F. In a saucepan over medium heat, add carrots and cover with water. Cook for 10 minutes until tender. Remove to a plate. Season with salt, pepper, and parsley and mash using a fork.
2. Add in egg, oats, and thyme as you continue mashing to mix well. Form the batter into cookie shapes. Place in the frying basket and press Start. Cook for 15 minutes until edges are browned.

12. Homemade Prosciutto Wrapped Cheese Sticks

Servings: 6
Cooking Time: 50 Minutes
Ingredients:
- 1 lb cheddar cheese
- 12 slices of prosciutto
- 1 cup flour
- 2 eggs, beaten
- 4 tbsp olive oil
- 1 cup breadcrumbs

Directions:
1. Cut the cheese into 6 equal sticks. Wrap each piece with 2 prosciutto slices. Place them in the freezer just enough to set. Preheat on Air Fry function to 390 F. Dip the croquettes into flour first, then in eggs, and coat with breadcrumbs. Drizzle the basket with oil and fit in the baking tray. Cook for 10 minutes or until golden. Serve.

13. Crispy Eggplant Slices

Servings: 4
Cooking Time: 8 Minutes
Ingredients:

- 1 medium eggplant, peeled and cut into ½-inch round slices
- Salt, as required
- ½ cup all-purpose flour
- 2 eggs, beaten
- 1 cup Italian-style breadcrumbs
- ¼ cup olive oil

Directions:
1. In a colander, add the eggplant slices and sprinkle with salt. Set aside for about 45 minutes.
2. With paper towels, pat dry the eggplant slices.
3. In a shallow dish, place the flour.
4. Crack the eggs in a second dish and beat well.
5. In a third dish, mix together the oil, and breadcrumbs.
6. Coat each eggplant slice with flour, then dip into beaten eggs and finally, coat with the breadcrumbs mixture.
7. Press "Power Button" of Air Fry Oven and turn the dial to select the "Air Fry" mode.
8. Press the Time button and again turn the dial to set the cooking time to 8 minutes.
9. Now push the Temp button and rotate the dial to set the temperature at 390 degrees F.
10. Press "Start/Pause" button to start.
11. When the unit beeps to show that it is preheated, open the lid.
12. Arrange the eggplant slices in "Air Fry Basket" and insert in the oven.
13. Serve warm.
- **Nutrition Info:** Calories 332 Total Fat 16.6 g Saturated Fat 2.8 g Cholesterol 82 mg Sodium 270 mg Total Carbs 38.3 g Fiber 5.7 g Sugar 5.3 g Protein 9.1 g

14. Ham & Pineapple Tortilla Pizzas

Servings:2
Cooking Time: 15 Minutes
Ingredients:
- 2 tortillas
- 8 ham slices
- 8 mozzarella cheese slices
- 8 thin pineapple slices
- 2 tbsp tomato sauce
- 1 tsp dried parsley

Directions:
1. Preheat on Pizza function to 330 F. Spread the tomato sauce onto the tortillas. Arrange 4 ham slices on each tortilla. Top with pineapple and mozzarella slices and sprinkle with parsley. Place in the oven and press Start. Cook for 10 minutes and serve.

15. Simple Chicken Breasts

Servings: 4
Cooking Time: 30 Minutes

Ingredients:
- 4 boneless, skinless chicken breasts
- 1 tsp salt and black pepper
- 1 tsp garlic powder

Directions:
1. Spray the breasts and the Air Fryer basket with cooking spray. Rub chicken with salt, garlic powder, and black pepper. Arrange the breasts on the basket. Fit in the baking pan and cook for 20 minutes at 360 F on Bake function until nice and crispy. Serve warm.

16. Holiday Pumpkin Wedges

Servings: 3
Cooking Time: 30 Minutes
Ingredients:
- ½ pumpkin, washed and cut into wedges
- 1 tbsp paprika
- 1 whole lime, squeezed
- 1 cup paleo dressing
- 1 tbsp balsamic vinegar
- Salt and black pepper to taste
- 1 tsp turmeric

Directions:
1. Preheat on Air Fry function to 360 F. Place the pumpkin wedges in your Air Fryer baking tray and cook for 20 minutes. In a bowl, mix lime juice, vinegar, turmeric, salt, pepper and paprika to form a marinade. Pour the marinade over pumpkin and cook for 5 more minutes.

17. Vegetable & Walnut Stuffed Ham Rolls

Servings:4
Cooking Time: 15 Minutes
Ingredients:
- 1 carrot, chopped
- 4 large ham slices
- ¼ cup walnuts, finely chopped
- 1 zucchini, chopped
- 1 garlic clove, minced
- 2 tbsp olive oil
- 1 tbsp ginger powder
- 2 tbsp fresh basil leaves, chopped
- Salt and black pepper to taste

Directions:
1. Heat olive oil in a pan over medium heat and sauté zucchini, carrot, garlic, and ginger for 5-6 minutes until tender. Stir in basil, walnuts, and salt.
2. Divide the mixture between ham slices and then fold one side above the filling and roll in. Transfer to a baking tray. Select Bake function, adjust the temperature to 360 F, and press Start. Bake the rolls for 8 minutes.

18. Lime Pumpkin Wedges

Servings:4

Cooking Time: 30 Minutes
Ingredients:
- 1 lb pumpkin, cut into wedges
- 1 tbsp paprika
- 1 whole lime, squeezed
- 1 cup paleo dressing
- 1 tbsp balsamic vinegar
- Salt and black pepper to taste
- 1 tsp turmeric

Directions:
1. Preheat on AirFry function to 360 F. Add the pumpkin wedges in a baking tray and press Start. Cook for 20 minutes. In a bowl, mix lime juice, vinegar, turmeric, salt, pepper, and paprika. Pour the mixture over pumpkin and cook for 5 more minutes. Serve.

19. Easy Cheesy Stuffed Mushrooms

Servings: 4
Cooking Time: 15 Minutes
Ingredients:
- Nonstick cooking spray
- 1/3 cup cream cheese, soft
- 1 tbsp. parmesan cheese, grated
- ¼ tsp garlic salt
- 2 tbsp. spinach, thaw, press dry & chop
- 8 oz. mushrooms, rinsed & stems removed
- 1 tbsp. panko bread crumbs

Directions:
1. Lightly spray baking sheet with cooking spray.
2. In a medium bowl, combine cream cheese, parmesan, salt, and spinach, mix well.
3. Place mushrooms on baking sheet and fill with cheese mixture. Sprinkle bread crumbs over top.
4. Set oven to bake on 350°F for 20 minutes. After 5 minutes, place baking pan in position 2 of the oven and cook mushrooms 15 minutes until tops are lightly browned. Serve hot.
- **Nutrition Info:** Calories 121, Total Fat 7g, Saturated Fat 4g, Total Carbs 8g, Net Carbs 7g, Protein 4g, Sugar 2g, Fiber 1g, Sodium 168mg, Potassium 225mg, Phosphorus 86mg

20. Cheesy Jalapeño Poppers

Servings: 8
Cooking Time: 15 Minutes
Ingredients:
- 6 ounces (170 g) cream cheese, at room temperature
- 4 ounces (113 g) shredded Cheddar cheese
- 1 teaspoon chili powder
- 12 large jalapeño peppers, deseeded and sliced in half lengthwise
- 2 slices cooked bacon, chopped

- ¼ cup panko bread crumbs
- 1 tablespoon butter, melted

Directions:
1. In a medium bowl, whisk together the cream cheese, Cheddar cheese and chili powder. Spoon the cheese mixture into the jalapeño halves and arrange them in the baking pan.
2. In a small bowl, stir together the bacon, bread crumbs and butter. Sprinkle the mixture over the jalapeño halves.
3. Slide the baking pan into Rack Position 1, select Convection Bake, set temperature to 375ºF (190ºC) and set time to 15 minutes.
4. When cooking is complete, remove from the oven. Let the poppers cool for 5 minutes before serving.

21. Yogurt Masala Cashew

Servings: 2
Cooking Time: 25 Minutes
Ingredients:
- 8 oz Greek yogurt
- 2 tbsp mango powder
- 8¾ oz cashew nuts
- Salt and black pepper to taste
- 1 tsp coriander powder
- ½ tsp masala powder
- ½ tsp black pepper powder

Directions:
1. Preheat on Air Fry function to 350 F. In a bowl, mix all powders, salt, and pepper. Add in cashews and toss to coat thoroughly. Place the cashews in your Air Fryer baking pan and cook for 15 minutes, shaking every 5 minutes. Serve.

22. Beef Enchilada Dip

Servings: 8
Cooking Time: 10 Minutes
Ingredients:
- 2 lbs. ground beef
- ½ onion, chopped fine
- 2 cloves garlic, chopped fine
- 2 cups enchilada sauce
- 2 cups Monterrey Jack cheese, grated
- 2 tbsp. sour cream

Directions:
1. Place rack in position
2. Heat a large skillet over med-high heat. Add beef and cook until it starts to brown. Drain off fat.
3. Stir in onion and garlic and cook until tender, about 3 minutes. Stir in enchilada sauce and transfer mixture to a small casserole dish and top with cheese.
4. Set oven to convection bake on 325°F for 10 minutes. After 5 minutes, add casserole to

the oven and bake 3-5 minutes until cheese is melted and mixture is heated through.
5. Serve warm topped with sour cream.
- **Nutrition Info:** Calories 414, Total Fat 22g, Saturated Fat 10g, Total Carbs 15g, Net Carbs 11g, Protein 39g, Sugar 8g, Fiber 4g, Sodium 1155mg, Potassium 635mg, Phosphorus 385mg

23. Bbq Full Chicken

Servings:3
Cooking Time: 50 Minutes
Ingredients:
- 1 (3,5 pounds) whole chicken, cut into pieces
- 1 tsp salt
- 1 tsp smoked paprika
- 1 tsp garlic powder
- 1 cup BBQ sauce

Directions:
1. Mix salt, paprika, and garlic and coat chicken pieces. Place them skin-side down in the toaster oven. Select Bake function, adjust the temperature to 400 F, and press Start. Cook for around 25 minutes until slightly golden.
2. Remove to a plate and brush with some barbecue sauce. Return the chicken to the oven, skin-side up and bake for 15-20 more minutes. Serve with the remaining barbecue sauce.

24. Cheesy Squash Casserole

Servings: 6
Cooking Time: 30 Minutes
Ingredients:
- 2 lbs yellow summer squash, cut into chunks
- 1/2 cup liquid egg substitute
- 3/4 cup cheddar cheese, shredded
- 1/4 cup mayonnaise
- 1/4 tsp salt

Directions:
1. Fit the oven with the rack in position
2. Add squash in a saucepan then pour enough water in a saucepan to cover the squash. Bring to boil.
3. Turn heat to medium and cook for 10 minutes or until tender. Drain well.
4. In a large mixing bowl, combine together squash, egg substitute, mayonnaise, 1/2 cup cheese, and salt.
5. Transfer squash mixture into a greased baking dish.
6. Set to bake at 375 F for 35 minutes. After 5 minutes place the baking dish in the preheated oven.
7. Sprinkle remaining cheese on top.
8. Serve and enjoy.

- **Nutrition Info:** Calories 130 Fat 8.2 g Carbohydrates 7.7 g Sugar 3.5 g Protein 8 g Cholesterol 18 mg

25. Chili Corn On The Cob

Servings:4
Cooking Time: 15 Minutes
Ingredients:
- 2 tablespoon olive oil, divided
- 2 tablespoons grated Parmesan cheese
- 1 teaspoon garlic powder
- 1 teaspoon chili powder
- 1 teaspoon ground cumin
- 1 teaspoon paprika
- 1 teaspoon salt
- ¼ teaspoon cayenne pepper (optional)
- 4 ears fresh corn, shucked

Directions:
1. Grease the air fryer basket with 1 tablespoon of olive oil. Set aside.
2. Combine the Parmesan cheese, garlic powder, chili powder, cumin, paprika, salt, and cayenne pepper (if desired) in a small bowl and stir to mix well.
3. Lightly coat the ears of corn with the remaining 1 tablespoon of olive oil. Rub the cheese mixture all over the ears of corn until completely coated.
4. Arrange the ears of corn in the greased basket in a single layer.
5. Put the air fryer basket on the baking pan and slide into Rack Position 2, select Air Fry, set temperature to 400ºF (205ºC), and set time to 15 minutes.
6. Flip the ears of corn halfway through the cooking time.
7. When cooking is complete, they should be lightly browned. Remove from the oven and let them cool for 5 minutes before serving.

26. Avocado Fries

Servings: 4
Cooking Time: 20 Minutes
Ingredients:
- 1 oz. pork rinds, finely ground
- 2 medium avocados

Directions:
1. Cut each avocado in half. Remove the pit. Carefully remove the peel and then slice the flesh into ¼-inch-thick slices.
2. Place the pork rinds into a medium bowl and press each piece of avocado into the pork rinds to coat completely. Place the avocado pieces into the air fryer basket. Adjust the temperature to 350 Degrees F and set the timer for 5 minutes. Serve immediately
- **Nutrition Info:** Calories: 153; Protein: 4g; Fiber: 6g; Fat: 19g; Carbs: 9g

27. Cheddar Cheese Cauliflower Casserole

Servings: 8
Cooking Time: 35 Minutes
Ingredients:
- 4 cups cauliflower florets
- 1 1/2 cups cheddar cheese, shredded
- 1 cup sour cream
- 4 bacon slices, cooked and crumbled
- 3 green onions, chopped

Directions:
1. Fit the oven with the rack in position
2. Boil water in a large pot. Add cauliflower in boiling water and cook for 8-10 minutes or until tender. Drain well.
3. Transfer cauliflower in a large bowl.
4. Add half bacon, half green onion, 1 cup cheese, and sour cream in cauliflower bowl and mix well.
5. Transfer mixture into a greased baking dish and sprinkle with remaining cheese.
6. Set to bake at 350 F for 30 minutes. After 5 minutes place the baking dish in the preheated oven.
7. Garnish with remaining green onion and bacon.
8. Serve and enjoy.
- **Nutrition Info:** Calories 213 Fat 17.1 g Carbohydrates 4.7 g Sugar 1.5 g Protein 10.8 g Cholesterol 45 mg

28. Lemon-garlic Kale Salad

Servings: 8
Cooking Time: 10 Minutes
Ingredients:
- 2 cups sliced almonds
- 1/3 cup lemon juice
- 1 teaspoon salt
- 1-1/2 cups olive oil
- 4 cloves crushed garlic
- 12 ounces kale, stems removed

Directions:
1. Set toaster oven to toast and toast almonds for about 5 minutes.
2. Combine lemon juice and salt in a small bowl, then add olive oil and garlic; mix well and set aside.
3. Slice kale into thin ribbons; place in a bowl and sprinkle with almonds.
4. Remove garlic from dressing, then add desired amount of dressing to kale and toss.
5. Add additional dressing if necessary, and serve.
- **Nutrition Info:** Calories: 487, Sodium: 312 mg, Dietary Fiber: 3.7 g, Total Fat: 49.8 g, Total Carbs: 10.2 g, Protein: 6.5 g.

29. Crunchy Parmesan Snack Mix

Servings: 6 Cups
Cooking Time: 6 Minutes

Ingredients:
- 2 cups oyster crackers
- 2 cups Chex rice
- 1 cup sesame sticks
- $^2/_3$ cup finely grated Parmesan cheese
- 8 tablespoons unsalted butter, melted
- 1½ teaspoons granulated garlic
- ½ teaspoon kosher salt

Directions:
1. Toss together all the ingredients in a large bowl until well coated. Spread the mixture in the baking pan in an even layer.
2. Slide the baking pan into Rack Position 1, select Convection Bake, set temperature to 350ºF (180ºC) and set time to 6 minutes.
3. After 3 minutes, remove from the oven and stir the mixture. Return to the oven and continue cooking.
4. When cooking is complete, the mixture should be lightly browned and fragrant. Let cool before serving.

30. Marinara Chicken Breasts

Servings: 2
Cooking Time: 20 Minutes
Ingredients:
- 2 chicken breasts, ½ inch thick
- 1 egg, beaten
- ½ cup breadcrumbs
- A pinch of salt and black pepper
- 2 tbsp marinara sauce
- 2 tbsp Grana Padano cheese, grated
- 2 slices mozzarella cheese

Directions:
1. Dip the breasts into the egg, then into the crumbs, and arrange on the Air fryer baking sheet. Cook for 6-8 minutes at 400 F on Air Fry function. Turn over and drizzle with marinara sauce, Grana Padano and mozzarella cheeses. Cook for 5 more minutes. Serve.

31. Bacon Wrapped Asparagus

Servings: 4
Cooking Time: 4
Ingredients:
- 20 spears asparagus
- 4 bacon slices
- 1 tbsp olive oil
- 1 tbsp sesame oil
- 1 tbsp brown sugar
- 1 garlic clove, crushed

Directions:
1. Preheat on Air Fry function to 380 F. In a bowl, mix the oils, sugar, and crushed garlic. Separate the asparagus into 4 bunches (5 spears in 1 bunch) and wrap each bunch with a bacon slice. Coat the bunches with the oil mixture. Place them in your Air Fryer

basket and fit in the baking tray. Cook for 8 minutes, shaling once. Serve warm.

32. Tasty Carrot Chips

Servings: 2
Cooking Time: 20 Minutes
Ingredients:
- 3 large carrots, washed and peeled
- Salt to taste

Directions:
1. Using a mandolin slicer, slice the carrots very thinly heightwise. Put the carrot strips in a bowl and season with salt. Grease the fryer basket lightly with cooking spray, and add the carrot strips. Fit in the baking tray and cook in the at 350 F for 10 minutes on Air Fry function, stirring once halfway through. Serve warm.

33. Air-fried Herb Mushrooms

Servings: 2
Cooking Time: 25 Minutes
Ingredients:
- 1 lbs mushrooms, wash, dry, and cut into quarter
- 1 tbsp white vermouth
- 1 tsp herb de Provence
- 1/4 tsp garlic powder
- 1/2 tbsp olive oil

Directions:
1. Fit the oven with the rack in position 2.
2. Add all ingredients to the bowl and toss well.
3. Transfer mushrooms in the air fryer basket then place the air fryer basket in the baking pan.
4. Place a baking pan on the oven rack. Set to air fry at 350 F for 25 minutes.
5. Serve and enjoy.
- **Nutrition Info:** Calories 99 Fat 4.5 g Carbohydrates 8.1 g Sugar 4 g Protein 7.9 g Cholesterol 0 mg

34. Spicy Broccoli With Hot Sauce

Servings:6
Cooking Time: 14 Minutes
Ingredients:
- Broccoli:
- 1 medium-sized head broccoli, cut into florets
- 1½ tablespoons olive oil
- 1 teaspoon shallot powder
- 1 teaspoon porcini powder
- ½ teaspoon freshly grated lemon zest
- ½ teaspoon hot paprika
- ½ teaspoon granulated garlic
- $^1/_3$ teaspoon fine sea salt
- $^1/_3$ teaspoon celery seeds
- Hot Sauce:

- ½ cup tomato sauce
- 1 tablespoon balsamic vinegar
- ½ teaspoon ground allspice

Directions:
1. In a mixing bowl, combine all the ingredients for the broccoli and toss to coat. Transfer the broccoli to the air fryer basket.
2. Put the air fryer basket on the baking pan and slide into Rack Position 2, select Air Fry, set temperature to 360ºF (182ºC), and set time to 14 minutes.
3. Meanwhile, make the hot sauce by whisking together the tomato sauce, balsamic vinegar, and allspice in a small bowl.
4. When cooking is complete, remove the broccoli from the oven and serve with the hot sauce.

35. Parmesan Zucchini Rounds

Servings: 4
Cooking Time: 20 Minutes
Ingredients:
- 4 zucchinis; sliced
- 1 ½ cups parmesan; grated
- ¼ cup parsley; chopped.
- 1 egg; whisked
- 1 egg white; whisked
- ½ tsp. garlic powder
- Cooking spray

Directions:
1. Take a bowl and mix the egg with egg whites, parmesan, parsley and garlic powder and whisk.
2. Dredge each zucchini slice in this mix, place them all in your air fryer's basket, grease them with cooking spray and cook at 370°F for 20 minutes
3. Divide between plates and serve as a side dish.
- **Nutrition Info:** Calories: 183; Fat: 6g; Fiber: 2g; Carbs: 3g; Protein: 8g

36. Coriander Artichokes(2)

Servings: 4
Cooking Time: 20 Minutes
Ingredients:
- 12 oz. artichoke hearts
- 1 tbsp. lemon juice
- 1 tsp. coriander, ground
- ½ tsp. cumin seeds
- ½ tsp. olive oil
- Salt and black pepper to taste.

Directions:
1. In a pan that fits your air fryer, mix all the ingredients, toss, introduce the pan in the fryer and cook at 370°F for 15 minutes
2. Divide the mix between plates and serve as a side dish.

- **Nutrition Info:** Calories: 200; Fat: 7g; Fiber: 2g; Carbs: 5g; Protein: 8g

37. Bread Sticks

Servings: 6
Cooking Time: 6 Minutes
Ingredients:
- 1 egg 1/8 teaspoon ground cinnamon
- Pinch of ground nutmeg Pinch of ground cloves
- Salt, to taste
- 2 bread slices
- 1 tablespoon butter, softened
- Nonstick cooking spray
- 1 tablespoon icing sugar

Directions:
1. In a bowl, add the eggs, cinnamon, nutmeg, cloves and salt and beat until well combined.
2. Spread the butter over both sides of the slices evenly.
3. Cut each bread slice into strips.
4. Dip bread strips into egg mixture evenly.
5. Press "Power Button" of Air Fry Oven and turn the dial to select the "Air Fry" mode.
6. Press the Time button and again turn the dial to set the cooking time to 6 minutes.
7. Now push the Temp button and rotate the dial to set the temperature at 355 degrees F.
8. Press "Start/Pause" button to start.
9. When the unit beeps to show that it is preheated, open the lid.
10. Arrange the breadsticks in "Air Fry Basket" and insert in the oven.
11. After 2 minutes of cooking, spray the both sides of the bread strips with cooking spray.
12. Serve immediately with the topping of icing sugar.
- **Nutrition Info:** Calories 41 Total Fat 2.8 g Saturated Fat 1.5 g Cholesterol 32 mg Sodium 72 mg Total Carbs 3 g Fiber 0.1 g Sugar 1.5 g Protein 1.2 g

38. Green Bean Casserole(1)

Servings: 4
Cooking Time: 20 Minutes
Ingredients:
- 1 lb. fresh green beans, edges trimmed
- ½ oz. pork rinds, finely ground
- 1 oz. full-fat cream cheese
- ½ cup heavy whipping cream.
- ¼ cup diced yellow onion
- ½ cup chopped white mushrooms
- ½ cup chicken broth
- 4 tbsp. unsalted butter.
- ¼ tsp. xanthan gum

Directions:
1. In a medium skillet over medium heat, melt the butter. Sauté the onion and mushrooms

until they become soft and fragrant, about 3–5 minutes.
2. Add the heavy whipping cream, cream cheese and broth to the pan. Whisk until smooth. Bring to a boil and then reduce to a simmer. Sprinkle the xanthan gum into the pan and remove from heat
3. Chop the green beans into 2-inch pieces and place into a 4-cup round baking dish. Pour the sauce mixture over them and stir until coated. Top the dish with ground pork rinds. Place into the air fryer basket
4. Adjust the temperature to 320 Degrees F and set the timer for 15 minutes. Top will be golden and green beans fork tender when fully cooked. Serve warm.
- **Nutrition Info:** Calories: 267; Protein: 3.6g; Fiber: 3.2g; Fat: 23.4g; Carbs: 9.7g

39. Air Fried Green Tomatoes(1)

Servings: 4
Cooking Time: 20 Minutes
Ingredients:
- 2 medium green tomatoes
- ⅓ cup grated Parmesan cheese.
- ¼ cup blanched finely ground almond flour.
- 1 large egg.

Directions:
1. Slice tomatoes into ½-inch-thick slices. Take a medium bowl, whisk the egg. Take a large bowl, mix the almond flour and Parmesan.
2. Dip each tomato slice into the egg, then dredge in the almond flour mixture. Place the slices into the air fryer basket
3. Adjust the temperature to 400 Degrees F and set the timer for 7 minutes. Flip the slices halfway through the cooking time. Serve immediately
- **Nutrition Info:** Calories: 106; Protein: 6.2g; Fiber: 1.4g; Fat: 6.7g; Carbs: 5.9g

40. Air Fryer Chicken Breasts

Servings:4
Cooking Time: 30 Minutes
Ingredients:
- 4 chicken breasts
- 1 tbsp olive oil
- Salt and black pepper to taste
- 1 tsp garlic powder

Directions:
1. Brush the breasts with olive oil and season with salt, garlic powder, and black pepper. Arrange the breasts on the frying basket. Select AirFry function, adjust the temperature to 380 F, and press Start. Cook for 20 minutes until nice and crispy. Serve warm.

41. Roasted Tomatoes

Servings: 4
Cooking Time: 20 Minutes
Ingredients:
- 4 tomatoes; halved
- ½ cup parmesan; grated
- 1 tbsp. basil; chopped.
- ½ tsp. onion powder
- ½ tsp. oregano; dried
- ½ tsp. smoked paprika
- ½ tsp. garlic powder
- Cooking spray

Directions:
1. Take a bowl and mix all the ingredients except the cooking spray and the parmesan.
2. Arrange the tomatoes in your air fryer's pan, sprinkle the parmesan on top and grease with cooking spray
3. Cook at 370°F for 15 minutes, divide between plates and serve.
- **Nutrition Info:** Calories: 200; Fat: 7g; Fiber: 2g; Carbs: 4g; Protein: 6g

42. Sausage Mushroom Caps(2)

Servings: 2
Cooking Time: 20 Minutes
Ingredients:
- ½ lb. Italian sausage
- 6 large Portobello mushroom caps
- ¼ cup grated Parmesan cheese.
- ¼ cup chopped onion
- 2 tbsp. blanched finely ground almond flour
- 1 tsp. minced fresh garlic

Directions:
1. Use a spoon to hollow out each mushroom cap, reserving scrapings.
2. In a medium skillet over medium heat, brown the sausage about 10 minutes or until fully cooked and no pink remains. Drain and then add reserved mushroom scrapings, onion, almond flour, Parmesan and garlic.
3. Gently fold ingredients together and continue cooking an additional minute, then remove from heat
4. Evenly spoon the mixture into mushroom caps and place the caps into a 6-inch round pan. Place pan into the air fryer basket
5. Adjust the temperature to 375 Degrees F and set the timer for 8 minutes. When finished cooking, the tops will be browned and bubbling. Serve warm.
- **Nutrition Info:** Calories: 404; Protein: 24.3g; Fiber: 4.5g; Fat: 25.8g; Carbs: 18.2g

43. Cabbage And Radishes Mix

Servings: 4
Cooking Time: 20 Minutes
Ingredients:

- 6 cups green cabbage; shredded
- ½ cup celery leaves; chopped.
- ¼ cup green onions; chopped.
- 6 radishes; sliced
- 3 tbsp. olive oil
- 2 tbsp. balsamic vinegar
- ½ tsp. hot paprika
- 1 tsp. lemon juice

Directions:
1. In your air fryer's pan, combine all the ingredients and toss well.
2. Introduce the pan in the fryer and cook at 380°F for 15 minutes. Divide between plates and serve as a side dish
- **Nutrition Info:** Calories: 130; Fat: 4g; Fiber: 3g; Carbs: 4g; Protein: 7g

44. Butternut Squash Croquettes

Servings:4
Cooking Time: 17 Minutes
Ingredients:
- $^1/_3$ butternut squash, peeled and grated
- $^1/_3$ cup all-purpose flour
- 2 eggs, whisked
- 4 cloves garlic, minced
- 1½ tablespoons olive oil
- 1 teaspoon fine sea salt
- $^1/_3$ teaspoon freshly ground black pepper, or more to taste
- $^1/_3$ teaspoon dried sage
- A pinch of ground allspice

Directions:
1. Line the air fryer basket with parchment paper. Set aside.
2. In a mixing bowl, stir together all the ingredients until well combined.
3. Make the squash croquettes: Use a small cookie scoop to drop tablespoonfuls of the squash mixture onto a lightly floured surface and shape into balls with your hands. Transfer them to the basket.
4. Put the air fryer basket on the baking pan and slide into Rack Position 2, select Air Fry, set temperature to 345ºF (174ºC), and set time to 17 minutes.
5. When cooking is complete, the squash croquettes should be golden brown. Remove from the oven to a plate and serve warm.

45. Baked Cauliflower & Mushrooms

Servings: 6
Cooking Time: 20 Minutes
Ingredients:
- 1 lb mushrooms, cleaned
- 8 garlic cloves, peeled
- 2 cups cherry tomatoes
- 2 cups cauliflower florets
- 1 tbsp fresh parsley, chopped

- 1 tbsp Italian seasoning
- 2 tbsp olive oil
- Pepper
- Salt

Directions:
1. Fit the oven with the rack in position
2. Add cauliflower, mushrooms, Italian seasoning, olive oil, garlic, cherry tomatoes, pepper, and salt into the mixing bowl and toss well.
3. Transfer cauliflower and mushroom mixture on a baking pan.
4. Set to bake at 400 F for 25 minutes. After 5 minutes place the baking pan in the preheated oven.
5. Garnish with parsley and serve.
- **Nutrition Info:** Calories 89 Fat 5.8 g Carbohydrates 8.2 g Sugar 3.9 g Protein 3.8 g Cholesterol 2 mg

46. Jicama Fries(2)

Servings: 4
Cooking Time: 20 Minutes
Ingredients:
- 1 small jicama; peeled.
- ¼ tsp. onion powder.
- ¾tsp. chili powder
- ¼ tsp. ground black pepper
- ¼ tsp. garlic powder.

Directions:
1. Cut jicama into matchstick-sized pieces.
2. Place pieces into a small bowl and sprinkle with remaining ingredients. Place the fries into the air fryer basket
3. Adjust the temperature to 350 Degrees F and set the timer for 20 minutes. Toss the basket two or three times during cooking. Serve warm.
- **Nutrition Info:** Calories: 37; Protein: 0.8g; Fiber: 4.7g; Fat: 0.1g; Carbs: 8.7g

47. Thyme & Carrot Cookies

Servings: 8
Cooking Time: 30 Minutes
Ingredients:
- 6 carrots, sliced
- Salt and black pepper to taste
- 1 tbsp parsley
- 1 ¼ oz oats
- 1 whole egg, beaten
- 1 tbsp thyme

Directions:
1. Preheat on Air Fryer function to 360 F. In a saucepan, add carrots and cover with hot water. Cook over medium heat for 10 minutes until tender. Remove to a plate. Season with salt, pepper, and parsley and mash using a fork. Add the beaten egg, oats,

and thyme as you continue mashing to mix well.

2. Form the batter into cookie shapes. Place in your Air Fryer baking tray and cook for 15 minutes until edges are browned. Serve chilled.

48. Lemon-thyme Bruschetta

Servings: 10
Cooking Time: 7 Minutes
Ingredients:
- 1 baguette
- 8 ounces ricotta cheese
- 1 lemon
- Salt
- Freshly cracked black pepper
- Honey
- 8 sprigs fresh thyme

Directions:
1. Start by preheating toaster oven to 425°F.
2. Thinly slice baguette, and zest lemon.
3. Mix ricotta and lemon zest together and season with salt and pepper.
4. Toast the baguette slices for 7 minutes or until they start to brown.
5. Spread ricotta mix over slices.
6. Drizzle with honey and top with thyme, then serve.
- **Nutrition Info:** Calories: 60, Sodium: 71 mg, Dietary Fiber: 0.6 g, Total Fat: 2.0 g, Total Carbs: 7.6 g, Protein: 3.5 g.

49. Bread Cheese Sticks

Servings:6
Cooking Time: 5 Minutes
Ingredients:
- 6 (6 oz) bread cheese
- 2 tbsp butter, melted
- 2 cups panko crumbs

Directions:
1. With a knife, cut the cheese into equal-sized sticks. Brush each stick with butter and dip into the panko crumbs. Arrange the sticks in a single layer on the basket tray. Select AirFry function, adjust the temperature to 390 F, and press Start. Cook for 10-12 minutes. Serve warm.

50. Air Fried Mac & Cheese

Servings: 1
Cooking Time: 15 Minutes
Ingredients:
- 1 cup cooked macaroni
- 1 cup grated cheddar cheese
- ½ cup warm milk
- 1 tbsp Parmesan cheese
- Salt and black pepper to taste

Directions:

1. Preheat on Air Fry function to 350 F. Add the macaroni to Air Fryer baking pan. Stir in the cheddar cheese and milk. Season with salt and pepper. Place the dish in the toaster oven and cook for 10 minutes. Sprinkle with Parmesan cheese and serve.

51. Cheesy Sticks With Thai Sauce

Servings: 4
Cooking Time: 20 Minutes + Freezing Time
Ingredients:
- 12 mozzarella string cheese
- 2 cups breadcrumbs
- 3 eggs
- 1 cup sweet Thai sauce
- 4 tbsp skimmed milk

Directions:
1. Pour the crumbs in a bowl. Crack the eggs into another bowl and beat with the milk. One after the other, dip each cheese sticks in the egg mixture, in the crumbs, then egg mixture again and then in the crumbs back. Place the cheese sticks in a cookie sheet and freeze for 2 hours.
2. Preheat on Air Fry function to 380 F. Arrange the sticks in the frying basket without overcrowding. Fit in the baking tray and cook for 8 minutes, flipping them halfway through cooking until browned. Serve with the Thai sauce.

52. Pineapple And Cauliflower Rice

Servings: 6
Cooking Time: 20 Minutes
Ingredients:
- 2 cups rice
- 1 cauliflower, separated into florets and chopped
- 4 cups water
- ½ pineapple, peeled and chopped
- Salt and ground black pepper, to taste
- 2 teaspoons extra virgin olive oil

Directions:
1. In the Instant Pot, mix the rice with the pineapple, cauliflower, water, oil, salt and pepper, mix, cover and cook 2 minutes in manual mode.
2. Release the pressure naturally for 10 minutes, uncover the Instant Pot, mix with a fork, add more salt and pepper, divide between the plates and serve.
- **Nutrition Info:** Calories: 100, Fat: 2.7, Fiber: 2.9, Carbohydrate: 12, Proteins: 4.9

53. Baked Cauliflower & Tomatoes

Servings: 4
Cooking Time: 20 Minutes
Ingredients:
- 4 cups cauliflower florets

- 1 tbsp capers, drained
- 3 tbsp olive oil
- 1/2 cup cherry tomatoes, halved
- 2 tbsp fresh parsley, chopped
- 2 garlic cloves, sliced
- Pepper
- Salt

Directions:
1. Fit the oven with the rack in position
2. In a bowl, toss together cherry tomatoes, cauliflower, oil, garlic, capers, pepper, and salt and spread in baking pan.
3. Set to bake at 450 F for 25 minutes. After 5 minutes place the baking pan in the preheated oven.
4. Garnish with parsley and serve.
- **Nutrition Info:** Calories 123 Fat 10.7 g Carbohydrates 6.9 g Sugar 3 g Protein 2.4 g Cholesterol 0 mg

54. Baked Ratatouille

Servings: 6
Cooking Time: 55 Minutes
Ingredients:
- 1 large eggplant, steamed and sliced
- 1/4 tsp dried thyme
- 2 bell pepper, sliced
- 4 tomatoes, sliced
- 2 tbsp olive oil
- 4 medium zucchini, sliced
- 1 tsp dried basil
- 1/2 tsp dried oregano

Directions:
1. Fit the oven with the rack in position
2. Add all vegetable slices to a large bowl and season with salt and drizzle with oil.
3. Layer vegetable slices into the greased baking dish.
4. Set to bake at 400 F for 60 minutes. After 5 minutes place the baking dish in the preheated oven.
5. Sprinkle with dried herbs.
6. Serve and enjoy.
- **Nutrition Info:** Calories 108 Fat 5.3 g Carbohydrates 15.2 g Sugar 8.7 g Protein 3.5 g Cholesterol 0 mg

55. Cheesy Broccoli Gratin

Servings:2
Cooking Time: 14 Minutes
Ingredients:
- $^1/_3$ cup fat-free milk
- 1 tablespoon all-purpose or gluten-free flour
- ½ tablespoon olive oil
- ½ teaspoon ground sage
- ¼ teaspoon kosher salt
- ⅛ teaspoon freshly ground black pepper
- 2 cups roughly chopped broccoli florets

- 6 tablespoons shredded Cheddar cheese
- 2 tablespoons panko bread crumbs
- 1 tablespoon grated Parmesan cheese
- Olive oil spray

Directions:
1. Spritz the baking pan with olive oil spray.
2. Mix the milk, flour, olive oil, sage, salt, and pepper in a medium bowl and whisk to combine. Stir in the broccoli florets, Cheddar cheese, bread crumbs, and Parmesan cheese and toss to coat.
3. Pour the broccoli mixture into the prepared baking pan.
4. Slide the baking pan into Rack Position 1, select Convection Bake, set temperature to 330ºF (166ºC), and set time to 14 minutes.
5. When cooking is complete, the top should be golden brown and the broccoli should be tender. Remove from the oven and serve immediately.

56. Buttered Corn

Servings: 2
Cooking Time: 20 Minutes
Ingredients:
- 2 corn on the cob
- Salt and freshly ground black pepper, as needed
- 2 tablespoons butter, softened and divided

Directions:
1. Sprinkle the cobs evenly with salt and black pepper.
2. Then, rub with 1 tablespoon of butter.
3. With 1 piece of foil, wrap each cob.
4. Press "Power Button" of Air Fry Oven and turn the dial to select the "Air Fry" mode.
5. Press the Time button and again turn the dial to set the cooking time to 20 minutes.
6. Now push the Temp button and rotate the dial to set the temperature at 320 degrees F.
7. Press "Start/Pause" button to start.
8. When the unit beeps to show that it is preheated, open the lid.
9. Arrange the cobs in "Air Fry Basket" and insert in the oven.
10. Serve warm.
- **Nutrition Info:** Calories 186 Total Fat 12.2 g Saturated Fat 7.4 g Cholesterol 31 mg Sodium 163 mg Total Carbs 20.1 g Fiber 2.5 g Sugar 3.2g Protein 2.9 g

57. Cabbage & Carrot Canapes With Amul Cheese

Servings:2
Cooking Time: 15 Minutes
Ingredients:
- 1 whole cabbage, cut in rounds
- 1 cube Amul cheese
- ½ carrot, cubed

- ¼ onion, cubed
- ¼ bell pepper, cubed
- 1 tbsp fresh basil, chopped

Directions:
1. Preheat on AirFry function to 360 F. In a bowl, mix onion, carrot, bell pepper, and cheese. Toss to coat everything evenly. Add cabbage to the frying basket. Top with the veggie mixture and place in the oven. Press Start and cook for 8 minutes. Serve topped with basil.

58. Amul Cheesy Cabbage Canapes

Servings: 2
Cooking Time: 15 Minutes
Ingredients:
- 1 whole cabbage, washed and cut in rounds
- 1 cube Amul cheese
- ½ carrot, cubed
- ¼ onion, cubed
- ¼ red bell pepper, cubed
- 1 tsp fresh basil, chopped

Directions:
1. Preheat on Air Fry function to 360 F. Using a bowl, mix onion, carrot, bell pepper, and cheese. Toss to coat everything evenly. Add cabbage rounds to the Air fryer baking pan.
2. Top with the veggie mixture and cook for 8 minutes. Garnish with basil and serve.

59. Cheese & Rice Stuffed Mushrooms

Servings:4
Cooking Time: 20 Minutes
Ingredients:
- 1 pound Swiss brown mushrooms
- 2 tbsp olive oil
- 1 cup cooked brown rice
- 1 cup Grana Padano cheese, grated
- 1 tsp dried mixed herbs
- Salt and black pepper to taste

Directions:
1. Brush the mushrooms with oil and arrange them on the frying basket. In a bowl, mix rice, Grana Padano cheese, herbs, salt, and pepper. Stuff the mushrooms with the mixture. Select Bake function, adjust the temperature to 360 F, and press Start. Bake for 14 minutes until the mushrooms are golden and the cheese is melted. Serve warm.

60. Tasty Butternut Squash

Servings: 4
Cooking Time: 15 Minutes
Ingredients:
- 4 cups butternut squash, cut into 1-inch pieces
- 1 tbsp brown sugar
- 2 tbsp olive oil

- 1 tsp Chinese 5 spice powder

Directions:
1. Fit the oven with the rack in position 2.
2. Toss squash into the bowl with remaining ingredients.
3. Transfer squash in the air fryer basket then places the air fryer basket in the baking pan.
4. Place a baking pan on the oven rack. Set to air fry at 400 F for 15 minutes.
5. Serve and enjoy.
- **Nutrition Info:** Calories 132 Fat 7.1 g Carbohydrates 18.6 g Sugar 5.3 g Protein 1.4 g Cholesterol 0 mg

61. Buffalo Quesadillas

Servings: 8
Cooking Time: 5 Minutes
Ingredients:
- Nonstick cooking spray
- 2 cups chicken, cooked & chopped fine
- ½ cup Buffalo wing sauce
- 2 cups Monterey Jack cheese, grated
- ½ cup green onions, sliced thin
- 8 flour tortillas, 8-inch diameter
- ¼ cup blue cheese dressing

Directions:
1. Lightly spray the baking pan with cooking spray.
2. In a medium bowl, add chicken and wing sauce and toss to coat.
3. Place tortillas, one at a time on work surface. Spread ¼ of the chicken mixture over tortilla and sprinkle with cheese and onion. Top with a second tortilla and place on the baking pan.
4. Set oven to broil on 400°F for 8 minutes. After 5 minutes place baking pan in position 2. Cook quesadillas 2-3 minutes per side until toasted and cheese has melted. Repeat with remaining ingredients.
5. Cut quesadillas in wedges and serve with blue cheese dressing or other dipping sauce.
- **Nutrition Info:** Calories 376, Total Fat 20g, Saturated Fat 8g, Total Carbs 27g, Net Carbs 26g, Protein 22g, Sugar 2g, Fiber 2g, Sodium 685mg, Potassium 201mg, Phosphorus 301mg

62. Artichoke Hearts And Tarragon

Servings: 4
Cooking Time: 20 Minutes
Ingredients:
- 12 oz. artichoke hearts
- 2 tbsp. tarragon; chopped.
- 4 tbsp. butter; melted
- Juice of ½ lemon
- Salt and black pepper to taste.

Directions:

1. Take a bowl and mix all the ingredients, toss, transfer the artichokes to your air fryer's basket and cook at 370°F for 15 minutes

2. Divide between plates and serve as a side dish.
- **Nutrition Info:** Calories: 200; Fat: 7g; Fiber: 2g; Carbs: 3g; Protein: 7g

BREAKFAST RECIPES

63. Balsamic Chicken With Spinach & Kale

Servings:1
Cooking Time: 20 Minutes
Ingredients:
- ½ cup baby spinach
- ½ cup romaine lettuce, shredded
- 3 large kale leaves, chopped
- 1 chicken breast, cut into cubes
- 2 tbsp olive oil
- 1 tsp balsamic vinegar
- 1 garlic clove, minced
- Salt and black pepper to taste

Directions:
1. Place the chicken, some olive oil, garlic, salt, and pepper in a bowl; toss to combine. Put on a lined baking dish and cook in the for 14 minutes at 390F on Bake function.
2. Meanwhile, place the greens in a large bowl. Add the remaining olive oil and balsamic vinegar. Season with salt and pepper and toss to combine. Top with the sliced chicken and serve.

64. Berry Breakfast Oatmeal

Servings: 4
Cooking Time: 20 Minutes
Ingredients:
- 1 egg
- 2 cups old fashioned oats
- 1 cup blueberries
- 1/4 cup maple syrup
- 1 1/2 cups milk
- 1/2 cup blackberries
- 1/2 cup strawberries, sliced
- 1 1/2 tsp baking powder
- 1/2 tsp salt

Directions:
1. Fit the oven with the rack in position
2. In a bowl, mix together oats, salt, and baking powder.
3. Add vanilla, egg, maple syrup, and milk and stir well. Add berries and fold well.
4. Pour mixture into the greased baking dish.
5. Set to bake at 375 F for 25 minutes. After 5 minutes place the baking dish in the preheated oven.
6. Serve and enjoy.
- **Nutrition Info:** Calories 461 Fat 8.4 g Carbohydrates 80.7 g Sugar 23.4 g Protein 15 g Cholesterol 48 mg

65. Easy Cheesy Breakfast Casserole

Servings: 8
Cooking Time: 30 Minutes
Ingredients:
- 6 eggs, lightly beaten
- 8 oz can crescent rolls
- 2 cups cheddar cheese, shredded
- 1 lb breakfast sausage, cooked

Directions:
1. Fit the oven with the rack in position
2. Spray a 9*13-inch baking dish with cooking spray and set aside.
3. Spread crescent rolls in the bottom of the prepared baking dish and top with sausage, egg, and cheese.
4. Set to bake at 350 F for 35 minutes. After 5 minutes place the baking dish in the preheated oven.
5. Serve and enjoy.
- **Nutrition Info:** Calories 465 Fat 34.6 g Carbohydrates 11.8 g Sugar 2.4 g Protein 24.2 g Cholesterol 200 mg

66. Air Fried French Toast

Servings: 4
Cooking Time: 6 Minutes
Ingredients:
- 2 slices of sourdough bread
- 3 eggs
- 1 tablespoon of margarine
- 1 tsp. of liquid vanilla
- 3 tsp.s of honey
- 2 tablespoons of Greek yogurt Berries

Directions:
1. Preheat the air fryer to 356°F.
2. Pour the vanilla in the eggs and whisk to mix. Spread the margarine on all sides of the bread and soak in the eggs to absorb.
3. Put the bread into the air fryer basket and cook for 3 minutes Turn the bread over and cook for another 3 minutes.
4. Transfer to a place, top with yogurt and berries with a sprinkle of honey.
- **Nutrition Info:** Calories 99 Fat 8.2 g Carbohydrates 0.2 g Sugar 0.2 g Protein 6 g Cholesterol 18 mg

67. Creamy Mushroom And Spinach Omelet

Servings: 2
Cooking Time: 10 Minutes
Ingredients:
- 4 eggs, lightly beaten
- 2 tbsp heavy cream
- 2 cups spinach, chopped
- 1 cup mushrooms, chopped
- 3 oz feta cheese, crumbled
- 1 tbsp fresh parsley, chopped
- Salt and black pepper to taste

Directions:
1. Spray a baking pan with cooking spray. In a bowl, whisk eggs and heavy cream until

combined. Stir in spinach, mushrooms, feta, salt, and pepper.
2. Pour into the basket tray and cook in your for 6-10 minutes at 350 F on Bake function until golden and set. Sprinkle with parsley, cut into wedges, and serve.

68. Easy French-style Apple Cake

Servings:6
Cooking Time: 25 Minutes
Ingredients:
- 2 ¾ oz flour
- 5 tbsp sugar
- 1 ¼ oz butter
- 3 tbsp cinnamon
- 2 whole apple, sliced

Directions:
1. Preheat on Bake function to 360 F. In a bowl, mix 3 tbsp sugar, butter, and flour; form pastry using the batter. Roll out the pastry on a floured surface and transfer it to the basket.
2. Arrange the apple slices atop. Cover apples with sugar and cinnamon and press Start. Cook cook for 20 minutes. Sprinkle with powdered sugar and mint and serve.

69. Egg And Avocado Burrito

Servings:4
Cooking Time: 4 Minutes
Ingredients:
- 4 low-sodium whole-wheat flour tortillas
- Filling:
- 1 hard-boiled egg, chopped
- 2 hard-boiled egg whites, chopped
- 1 ripe avocado, peeled, pitted, and chopped
- 1 red bell pepper, chopped
- 1 (1.2-ounce / 34-g) slice low-sodium, low-fat American cheese, torn into pieces
- 3 tablespoons low-sodium salsa, plus additional for serving (optional)
- Special Equipment:
- 4 toothpicks (optional), soaked in water for at least 30 minutes

Directions:
1. Make the filling: Combine the egg, egg whites, avocado, red bell pepper, cheese, and salsa in a medium bowl and stir until blended.
2. Assemble the burritos: Arrange the tortillas on a clean work surface and place ¼ of the prepared filling in the middle of each tortilla, leaving about 1½-inch on each end unfilled. Fold in the opposite sides of each tortilla and roll up. Secure with toothpicks through the center, if needed.
3. Transfer the burritos to the air fryer basket.
4. Put the air fryer basket on the baking pan and slide into Rack Position 2, select Air Fry,

set temperature to 390ºF (199ºC) and set time to 4 minutes.
5. When cooking is complete, the burritos should be crisp and golden brown.
6. Allow to cool for 5 minutes and serve with salsa, if desired.

70. Cheesy Breakfast Casserole

Servings:4
Cooking Time: 16 Minutes
Ingredients:
- 6 slices bacon
- 6 eggs
- Salt and pepper, to taste
- Cooking spray
- ½ cup chopped green bell pepper
- ½ cup chopped onion
- ¾ cup shredded Cheddar cheese

Directions:
1. Place the bacon in a skillet over medium-high heat and cook each side for about 4 minutes until evenly crisp. Remove from the heat to a paper towel-lined plate to drain. Crumble it into small pieces and set aside.
2. Whisk the eggs with the salt and pepper in a medium bowl.
3. Spritz the baking pan with cooking spray.
4. Place the whisked eggs, crumbled bacon, green bell pepper, and onion in the prepared pan.
5. Slide the baking pan into Rack Position 1, select Convection Bake, set temperature to 400ºF (205ºC) and set time to 8 minutes.
6. After 6 minutes, remove the pan from the oven. Scatter the Cheddar cheese all over. Return the pan to the oven and continue to cook for another 2 minutes.
7. When cooking is complete, let sit for 5 minutes and serve on plates.

71. Golden Cod Tacos With Salsa

Servings:4
Cooking Time: 15 Minutes
Ingredients:
- 2 eggs
- 1¼ cups Mexican beer
- 1½ cups coconut flour
- 1½ cups almond flour
- ½ tablespoon chili powder
- 1 tablespoon cumin
- Salt, to taste
- 1 pound (454 g) cod fillet, slice into large pieces
- 4 toasted corn tortillas
- 4 large lettuce leaves, chopped
- ¼ cup salsa
- Cooking spray

Directions:

1. Spritz the air fryer basket with cooking spray.
2. Break the eggs in a bowl, then pour in the beer. Whisk to combine well.
3. Combine the coconut flour, almond flour, chili powder, cumin, and salt in a separate bowl. Stir to mix well.
4. Dunk the cod pieces in the egg mixture, then shake the excess off and dredge into the flour mixture to coat well. Arrange the cod in the pan.
5. Put the air fryer basket on the baking pan and slide into Rack Position 2, select Air Fry, set temperature to 375ºF (190ºC) and set time to 15 minutes.
6. Flip the cod halfway through the cooking time.
7. When cooking is complete, the cod should be golden brown.
8. Unwrap the toasted tortillas on a large plate, then divide the cod and lettuce leaves on top. Baste with salsa and wrap to serve.

72. Parmesan Asparagus

Servings:4
Cooking Time: 20 Minutes
Ingredients:
- 1 lb asparagus spears
- ¼ cup flour
- 1 cup breadcrumbs
- ½ cup Parmesan cheese, grated
- 2 eggs, beaten
- Salt and black pepper to taste

Directions:
1. Preheat on AirFry function to 370 F. Combine breadcrumbs, Parmesan cheese, salt, and pepper in a bowl. Line a baking sheet with parchment paper.
2. Dip the spears into the flour first, then into the eggs, and finally coat with the crumb mixture. Arrange them on a baking tray and press Start. Bake for 8-10 minutes. Serve warm.

73. Honey Banana Pastry With Berries

Servings: 2
Cooking Time: 15 Minutes
Ingredients:
- 3 bananas, sliced
- 3 tbsp honey
- 2 puff pastry sheets, cut into thin strips
- Fresh berries to serve

Directions:
1. Preheat on Bake function to 340 F. Place the banana slices into a baking dish. Cover with the pastry strips and top with honey. Cook for 12 minutes. Serve with berries.

74. Tortilla De Patatas With Spinach

Servings:4
Cooking Time: 25 Minutes
Ingredients:
- 3 cups potato cubes, boiled
- 2 cups spinach, chopped
- 5 eggs, lightly beaten
- ¼ cup heavy cream
- 1 cup mozzarella cheese, grated
- ½ cup fresh parsley, chopped
- Salt and black pepper to taste

Directions:
1. Preheat on Bake function to 390 F. Place the potatoes in a greased baking dish. In a bowl, whisk eggs, heavy cream, spinach, mozzarella cheese, parsley, salt, and pepper and pour over the potatoes. Press Start. Cook for 16 minutes until nice and golden. Serve warm.

75. Quick Cheddar Omelet

Servings:1
Cooking Time: 15 Minutes
Ingredients:
- 2 eggs, beaten
- 1 cup cheddar cheese, shredded
- 1 whole onion, chopped
- 2 tbsp soy sauce

Directions:
1. Preheat on AirFry function to 340 F. Drizzle soy sauce over the chopped onions. Sauté the onions ina greased pan over medium heat for 5 minutes; turn off the heat.
2. In a bowl, mix the eggs with salt and pepper. Pour the egg mixture over onions and cook in the for 6 minutes. Top with cheddar cheese and bake for 4 more minutes. Serve and enjoy!

76. Italian Sandwich

Servings:1
Cooking Time: 7 Minutes
Ingredients:
- 2 bread slices
- 4 tomato slices
- 4 mozzarella cheese slices
- 1 tbsp olive oil
- 1 tbsp fresh basil, chopped
- Salt and black pepper to taste

Directions:
1. Preheat on Toast function to 350 F. Place the bread slices in the toaster oven and toast for 5 minutes. Arrange two tomato slices on each bread slice. Season with salt and pepper.
2. Top each slice with 2 mozzarella slices. Return to the oven and cook for 1 more minute. Drizzle the caprese toasts with olive oil and top with chopped basil.

77. Cashew Granola With Cranberries

Servings:6
Cooking Time: 12 Minutes
Ingredients:

- 3 cups old-fashioned rolled oats
- 2 cups raw cashews
- 1 cup unsweetened coconut chips
- ½ cup honey
- ¼ cup vegetable oil
- $1/3$ cup packed light brown sugar
- ¼ teaspoon kosher salt
- 1 cup dried cranberries

Directions:

1. In a large bowl, stir together all the ingredients, except for the cranberries. Spread the mixture in the baking pan in an even layer.
2. Slide the baking pan into Rack Position 1, select Convection Bake, set temperature to 325ºF (163ºC) and set time to 12 minutes.
3. After 5 to 6 minutes, remove the pan and stir the granola. Return the pan to the oven and continue cooking.
4. When cooking is complete, remove the pan. Let the granola cool to room temperature. Stir in the cranberries before serving.

78. Caprese Sandwich With Sourdough Bread

Servings: 2
Cooking Time: 15 Minutes
Ingredients:

- 4 slices sourdough bread
- 2 tbsp mayonnaise
- 2 slices ham
- 2 lettuce leaves
- 1 tomato, sliced
- 2 slices mozzarella cheese
- Salt and black pepper to taste

Directions:

1. On a clean board, lay the sourdough slices and spread with mayonnaise. Top 2 of the slices with ham, lettuce, tomato, and mozzarella cheese. Season with salt and pepper.
2. Top with the remaining two slices to form two sandwiches. Spray with oil and transfer to the Air Fryer basket. Fit in the baking tray and cook for 10 minutes at 350 F on Bake function, flipping once halfway through cooking. Serve hot.

79. Salsa Verde Golden Chicken Empanadas

Servings: 12 Empanadas
Cooking Time: 12 Minutes
Ingredients:

- 1 cup boneless, skinless rotisserie chicken breast meat, chopped finely
- ¼ cup salsa verde
- $2/3$ cup shredded Cheddar cheese
- 1 teaspoon ground cumin
- 1 teaspoon ground black pepper
- 2 purchased refrigerated pie crusts, from a minimum 14.1-ounce (400 g) box
- 1 large egg
- 2 tablespoons water
- Cooking spray

Directions:

1. Spritz the air fryer basket with cooking spray. Set aside.
2. Combine the chicken meat, salsa verde, Cheddar, cumin, and black pepper in a large bowl. Stir to mix well. Set aside.
3. Unfold the pie crusts on a clean work surface, then use a large cookie cutter to cut out 3½-inch circles as much as possible.
4. Roll the remaining crusts to a ball and flatten into a circle which has the same thickness of the original crust. Cut out more 3½-inch circles until you have 12 circles in total.
5. Make the empanadas: Divide the chicken mixture in the middle of each circle, about 1½ tablespoons each. Dab the edges of the circle with water. Fold the circle in half over the filling to shape like a half-moon and press to seal, or you can press with a fork.
6. Whisk the egg with water in a small bowl.
7. Arrange the empanadas in the pan and spritz with cooking spray. Brush with whisked egg.
8. Put the air fryer basket on the baking pan and slide into Rack Position 2, select Air Fry, set temperature to 350ºF (180ºC) and set time to 12 minutes.
9. Flip the empanadas halfway through the cooking time.
10. When cooking is complete, the empanadas will be golden and crispy.
11. Serve immediately.

80. Smart Oven Breakfast Sandwich

Servings:x
Cooking Time:x
Ingredients:

- 1 large egg
- 1 slice cheese
- Salt and pepper, to taste
- 1 English muffin, split

Directions:

1. Coat a small 4-inch round metal pan with cooking oil.
2. Crack egg into prepared pan, poke yolk with a fork or toothpick, and season with salt and pepper.

3. Place pan and split English muffin in the center of the cooking rack in your toaster oven.
4. Select the TOAST setting on DARK and toast for one cycle.
5. Check the egg and muffin and remove if ready. If further cooking is needed, set for another cycle of toasting until desired level of doneness is achieved.
6. Layer egg and cheese inside English muffin and enjoy.

81. Turkey Breakfast Sausage Patties

Servings:4
Cooking Time: 10 Minutes
Ingredients:
- 1 tablespoon chopped fresh thyme
- 1 tablespoon chopped fresh sage
- 1¼ teaspoons kosher salt
- 1 teaspoon chopped fennel seeds
- ¾ teaspoon smoked paprika
- ½ teaspoon onion powder
- ½ teaspoon garlic powder
- ⅛ teaspoon crushed red pepper flakes
- ⅛ teaspoon freshly ground black pepper
- 1 pound (454 g) 93% lean ground turkey
- ½ cup finely minced sweet apple (peeled)

Directions:
1. Thoroughly combine the thyme, sage, salt, fennel seeds, paprika, onion powder, garlic powder, red pepper flakes, and black pepper in a medium bowl.
2. Add the ground turkey and apple and stir until well incorporated. Divide the mixture into 8 equal portions and shape into patties with your hands, each about ¼ inch thick and 3 inches in diameter.
3. Place the patties in the air fryer basket in a single layer.
4. Put the air fryer basket on the baking pan and slide into Rack Position 2, select Air Fry, set temperature to 400ºF (205ºC), and set time to 10 minutes.
5. Flip the patties halfway through the cooking time.
6. When cooking is complete, the patties should be nicely browned and cooked through. Remove from the oven to a plate and serve warm.

82. Green Cottage Omelet

Servings:1
Cooking Time: 20 Minutes
Ingredients:
- 3 eggs
- 3 tbsp cottage cheese
- 3 tbsp kale, chopped
- ½ tbsp fresh parsley, chopped
- Salt and black pepper to taste

- 1 tsp olive oil

Directions:
1. Beat the eggs with a pinch of salt and black pepper in a bowl. Stir in the rest of the ingredients. Drizzle a baking pan with olive oil. Pour the pan into the oven and press Start. Cook for 15 minutes on Bake function at 360 F until slightly golden and set. Serve warm.

83. Smoked Sausage Breakfast Mix

Servings: 4
Cooking Time: 30 Minutes
Ingredients:
- 1 and 1/2 pounds smoked sausage, diced and browned
- A pinch of salt and black pepper
- 1 and 1/2 cups grits
- 4 and 1/2 cups water
- 16 ounces cheddar cheese, shredded
- 1 cup milk
- ¼ tsp. garlic powder
- 1 and 1/2 tsp.s thyme, diced
- Cooking spray
- 4 eggs, whisked

Directions:
1. Put the water in a pot, bring to a boil over medium heat, add grits, stir, cover, cook for 5 minutes and take off heat.
2. Add cheese, stir until it melts and mix with milk, thyme, salt, pepper, garlic powder and eggs and whisk really well.
3. Heat up your air fryer at 300 °F, grease with cooking spray and add browned sausage.
4. Add grits mix, spread and cook for 25 minutes.
5. Divide among plates and serve for breakfast.
- **Nutrition Info:** Calories 113 Fat 8.2 g Carbohydrates 0.3 g Protein 5.4 g

84. Paprika Baked Eggs

Servings:6
Cooking Time: 10 Minutes
Ingredients:
- 6 large eggs
- 1 tsp paprika

Directions:
1. Preheat fryer to 300 F. Lay the eggs in the basket and press Start. Cook for 8 minutes on Bake function. Using tongs, dip the eggs in a bowl with icy water. Let sit for 5 minutes before peeling. Slice, sprinkle with paprika, and serve.

85. Mediterranean Spinach Frittata

Servings: 6
Cooking Time: 20 Minutes
Ingredients:
- 6 eggs

- 1/2 cup frozen spinach, drained the excess liquid
- 1/4 cup feta cheese, crumbled
- 1/4 cup olives, chopped
- 1/4 cup kalamata olives, chopped
- 1/2 cup tomatoes, diced
- 1/2 tsp garlic powder
- 1 tsp oregano
- 1/4 cup milk
- 1/2 tsp pepper
- 1/4 tsp salt

Directions:
1. Fit the oven with the rack in position
2. Spray 9-inch pie pan with cooking spray and set aside.
3. In a bowl, whisk eggs with oregano, garlic powder, milk, pepper, and salt until well combined.
4. Add olives, feta cheese, tomatoes, and spinach and mix well.
5. Pour egg mixture into the prepared pie pan.
6. Set to bake at 400 F for 25 minutes. After 5 minutes place the pie pan in the preheated oven.
7. Serve and enjoy.
- **Nutrition Info:** Calories 103 Fat 7.2 g Carbohydrates 2.9 g Sugar 1.5 g Protein 7.2 g Cholesterol 170 mg

86. Perfect Chicken Casserole

Servings: 8
Cooking Time: 30 Minutes
Ingredients:
- 8 eggs
- 1 cup mozzarella cheese, shredded
- 8 oz can crescent rolls
- 1 1/2 cups basil pesto
- 3/4 lb chicken breasts, cooked & shredded
- Pepper
- Salt

Directions:
1. Fit the oven with the rack in position
2. Spray a 9*13-inch baking dish with cooking spray and set aside.
3. In a bowl, mix shredded chicken and pesto and set aside.
4. In a separate bowl, eggs, pepper, and salt.
5. Roll out the crescent roll into the prepared baking dish. Top with shredded chicken.
6. Pour egg mixture over chicken and top with shredded mozzarella cheese.
7. Set to bake at 350 F for 35 minutes. After 5 minutes place the baking dish in the preheated oven.
8. Serve and enjoy.
- **Nutrition Info:** Calories 266 Fat 14.3 g Carbohydrates 11.7 g Sugar 2.4 g Protein 21 g Cholesterol 203 mg

87. Healthy Baked Oatmeal

Servings: 6
Cooking Time: 20 Minutes
Ingredients:
- 1 egg
- 1/3 cup dried cranberries
- 1 tsp vanilla
- 1 1/2 tsp cinnamon
- 2 tbsp butter, melted
- 1/2 cup applesauce
- 1 1/2 cups milk
- 1 tsp baking powder
- 1/3 cup light brown sugar
- 2 cups old fashioned oats
- 1/4 tsp salt

Directions:
1. Fit the oven with the rack in position
2. Grease 8*8-inch baking dish and set aside.
3. In a bowl, mix egg, vanilla, butter, applesauce, baking powder, cinnamon, brown sugar, oats, and salt.
4. Add milk and stir well.
5. Add cranberries and fold well.
6. Pour mixture into the prepared baking dish.
7. Set to bake at 350 F for 25 minutes. After 5 minutes place the baking dish in the preheated oven.
8. Serve and enjoy.
- **Nutrition Info:** Calories 330 Fat 9.3 g Carbohydrates 50.6 g Sugar 14.4 g Protein 9.7 g Cholesterol 42 mg

88. Strawberry Cheesecake Pastries

Servings: 6
Cooking Time: 20 Minutes
Ingredients:
- 1 sheet puff pastry, thawed
- ¼ cup cream cheese, soft
- 1 tbsp. strawberry jam
- 1 ½ cups strawberries, sliced
- 1 egg
- 1 tbsp. water
- 6 tsp powdered sugar, sifted

Directions:
1. Line the baking pan with parchment paper.
2. Lay the puff pastry on a cutting board and cut into 6 rectangles. Transfer to prepared pan, placing them 1-inch apart.
3. Lightly score the pastry, creating a ½-inch border, do not cut all the way through. Use a fork to prick the center.
4. In a small bowl, combine cream cheese and jam until thoroughly combined. Spoon mixture evenly into centers of the pastry and spread it within the scored area.
5. Top pastries with sliced berries.
6. In a small bowl, whisk together egg and water. Brush edges of pastry with the egg wash.

7. Set to bake at 350°F for 20 minutes. After 5 minutes, place the baking pan in position 1 and bake pastries until golden brown and puffed.
8. Remove from oven and let cool. Dust with powdered sugar before serving.
- **Nutrition Info:** Calories 205, Total Fat 13g, Saturated Fat 4g, Total Carbs 19g, Net Carbs 18g, Protein 3g, Sugar 6g, Fiber 1g, Sodium 107mg, Potassium 97mg, Phosphorus 50mg

89. Tomato-corn Frittata With Avocado Dressing

Servings:2 Or 3
Cooking Time: 20 Minutes
Ingredients:
- ½ cup cherry tomatoes, halved
- Kosher salt and freshly ground black pepper, to taste
- 6 large eggs, lightly beaten
- ½ cup fresh corn kernels
- ¼ cup milk
- 1 tablespoon finely chopped fresh dill
- ½ cup shredded Monterey Jack cheese
- Avocado Dressing:
- 1 ripe avocado, pitted and peeled
- 2 tablespoons fresh lime juice
- ¼ cup olive oil
- 1 scallion, finely chopped
- 8 fresh basil leaves, finely chopped

Directions:
1. Put the tomato halves in a colander and lightly season with salt. Set aside for 10 minutes to drain well. Pour the tomatoes into a large bowl and fold in the eggs, corn, milk, and dill. Sprinkle with salt and pepper and stir until mixed.
2. Pour the egg mixture into the baking pan.
3. Slide the baking pan into Rack Position 1, select Convection Bake, set temperature to 300ºF (150ºC) and set time to 15 minutes.
4. When done, remove the pan from the oven. Scatter the cheese on top.
5. Slide the baking pan into Rack Position 1, select Convection Bake, set temperature to 315ºF (157ºC) and set time to 5 minutes. Return the pan to the oven.
6. Meanwhile, make the avocado dressing: Mash the avocado with the lime juice in a medium bowl until smooth. Mix in the olive oil, scallion, and basil and stir until well incorporated.
7. When cooking is complete, the frittata will be puffy and set. Let the frittata cool for 5 minutes and serve alongside the avocado dressing.

90. Jalapeno Corn Egg Bake

Servings: 2

Cooking Time: 25 Minutes
Ingredients:
- 3 eggs
- 1/4 cup can corn, drained
- 1/2 cup cottage cheese
- 1 1/2 tbsp jalapeno, chopped
- 1/2 cup pepper jack cheese, shredded
- 1/8 tsp pepper
- 1/8 tsp sea salt

Directions:
1. Fit the oven with the rack in position
2. In a bowl, whisk eggs with pepper and salt.
3. Stir in corn, jalapeno, pepper jack cheese, and cottage cheese.
4. Pour egg mixture into the greased 7*5-inch baking dish.
5. Set to bake at 350 F for 30 minutes. After 5 minutes place the baking dish in the preheated oven.
6. Serve and enjoy.
- **Nutrition Info:** Calories 252 Fat 15.1 g Carbohydrates 6.7 g Sugar 1.5 g Protein 22.3 g Cholesterol 274 mg

91. Healthy Breakfast Cookies

Servings: 12
Cooking Time: 15 Minutes
Ingredients:
- 2 cups quick oats
- 1/4 cup chocolate chips
- 1 1/2 tbsp chia seeds
- 1/4 cup shredded coconut
- 1/2 cup mashed banana
- 1/4 cup applesauce
- 1/4 cup honey
- 1/2 tsp cinnamon
- 3/4 cup almond butter

Directions:
1. Fit the oven with the rack in position
2. Line baking pan with parchment paper and set aside.
3. Add all ingredients into the mixing bowl and mix until well combined.
4. Using a cookie scoop drop 12 scoops of oat mixture onto a prepared baking pan and lightly flatten the cookie.
5. Set to bake at 325 F for 20 minutes. After 5 minutes place the baking pan in the preheated oven.
6. Serve and enjoy.
- **Nutrition Info:** Calories 117 Fat 3.4 g Carbohydrates 20.1 g Sugar 9.2 g Protein 2.6 g Cholesterol 1 mg

92. Bourbon Vanilla French Toast

Servings:4
Cooking Time: 6 Minutes
Ingredients:
- 2 large eggs

- 2 tablespoons water
- $^2/_3$ cup whole or 2% milk
- 1 tablespoon butter, melted
- 2 tablespoons bourbon
- 1 teaspoon vanilla extract
- 8 (1-inch-thick) French bread slices
- Cooking spray

Directions:
1. Spray the baking pan with cooking spray.
2. Beat the eggs with the water in a shallow bowl until combined. Add the milk, melted butter, bourbon, and vanilla and stir to mix well.
3. Dredge 4 slices of bread in the batter, turning to coat both sides evenly. Transfer the bread slices to the baking pan.
4. Slide the baking pan into Rack Position 1, select Convection Bake, set temperature to 320ºF (160ºC) and set time to 6 minutes.
5. Flip the slices halfway through the cooking time.
6. When cooking is complete, the bread slices should be nicely browned.
7. Remove from the oven to a plate and serve warm.

93. Cherry Cinnamon Almond Breakfast Scones

Servings:x
Cooking Time:x
Ingredients:
- 2 cups all-purpose flour
- ½ cup chopped almonds
- ¾ cup milk
- ½ tsp cinnamon
- 2 tsp baking powder
- 3 Tbsp brown sugar
- Pinch of salt
- ½ cup cold butter
- 1½ cups dried cherries
- Zest of one lemon
- 2 Tbsp turbinado sugar

Directions:
1. Preheat oven to 375°F.
2. Combine flour, baking powder, brown sugar and salt.
3. Add cold butter, cut into small pieces, and pinch until dough becomes crumbly.
4. Add dried cherries, zest and chopped almonds to combine.
5. Add the milk and mix dough gently. Do not overwork.
6. Grease oven and spread dough uniformly.
7. Combine cinnamon and turbinado sugar and sprinkle on top.
8. Bake for about 25 minutes or until scone is cooked through.

94. Easy Egg Bites

Servings: 6
Cooking Time: 30 Minutes
Ingredients:
- 5 eggs
- 3 bacon slices, cooked & chopped
- 4 tbsp cottage cheese
- 1/2 cup cheddar cheese, shredded
- 1/4 tsp pepper
- 1/4 tsp salt

Directions:
1. Fit the oven with the rack in position
2. Spray 6-cups muffin tin with cooking spray and set aside.
3. Add all ingredients except bacon into the blender and blend for 30 seconds.
4. Pour egg mixture into the prepared muffin tin then divide cooked bacon evenly in all egg cups.
5. Set to bake at 325 F for 35 minutes. After 5 minutes place muffin tin in the preheated oven.
6. Serve and enjoy.
- **Nutrition Info:** Calories 151 Fat 10.9 g Carbohydrates 0.9 g Sugar 0.4 g Protein 11.8 g Cholesterol 158 mg

95. Fennel And Eggs Mix

Servings: 4
Cooking Time: 20 Minutes
Ingredients:
- 1 tablespoon avocado oil
- 1 yellow onion, chopped
- ½ teaspoon cumin, ground
- 1 teaspoon rosemary, dried
- 8 eggs, whisked
- 1 fennel bulb, shredded
- 1 tablespoon chives, chopped
- Salt and black pepper to the taste

Directions:
1. In a bowl, combine the onion with the eggs, fennel and the other ingredients except the oil and whisk.
2. Heat up your air fryer with the oil at 360 degrees F, add the oil, add the fennel mix, cover, cook for 20 minutes, divide between plates and serve for breakfast.
- **Nutrition Info:** calories 220, fat 11, fiber 3, carbs 4, protein 6

96. Breakfast Oatmeal Cake

Servings: 8
Cooking Time: 25 Minutes
Ingredients:
- 2 eggs
- 1 tbsp coconut oil
- 3 tbsp yogurt
- 1/2 tsp baking powder
- 1 tsp cinnamon

- 1 tsp vanilla
- 3 tbsp honey
- 1/2 tsp baking soda
- 1 apple, peel & chopped
- 1 cup oats

Directions:
1. Fit the oven with the rack in position
2. Line baking dish with parchment paper and set aside.
3. Add 3/4 cup oats and remaining ingredients into the blender and blend until smooth.
4. Add remaining oats and stir well.
5. Pour mixture into the prepared baking dish.
6. Set to bake at 350 F for 30 minutes. After 5 minutes place the baking dish in the preheated oven.
7. Slice and serve.
- **Nutrition Info:** Calories 114 Fat 3.6 g Carbohydrates 18.2 g Sugar 10 g Protein 3.2 g Cholesterol 41 mg

97. Tator Tots Casserole

Servings: 8
Cooking Time: 30 Minutes
Ingredients:
- 8 eggs
- 28 oz tator tots
- 8 oz pepper jack cheese, shredded
- 2 green onions, sliced
- 1/4 cup milk
- 1 lb breakfast sausage, cooked
- Pepper
- Salt

Directions:
1. Fit the oven with the rack in position
2. Spray 13*9-inch baking pan with cooking spray and set aside.
3. In a bowl, whisk eggs with milk, pepper, and salt.
4. Layer sausage in a prepared baking pan then pour the egg mixture and sprinkle with half shredded cheese and green onions.
5. Add tator tots on top.
6. Set to bake at 400 F for 35 minutes. After 5 minutes place the baking pan in the preheated oven.
7. Top with remaining cheese and serve.
- **Nutrition Info:** Calories 398 Fat 31.5 g Carbohydrates 2 g Sugar 0.8 g Protein 22.1 g Cholesterol 251 mg

98. Delicious Baked Eggs

Servings: 8
Cooking Time: 45 Minutes
Ingredients:
- 12 eggs
- 1/2 cup all-purpose flour
- 16 oz cottage cheese
- 16 oz cheddar cheese, shredded

- 1 tsp salt

Directions:
1. Fit the oven with the rack in position
2. Grease 9*13-inch baking pan with butter and set aside.
3. In a large bowl, whisk eggs with flour, cottage cheese, cheddar cheese, and salt.
4. Pour egg mixture into the prepared baking pan.
5. Set to bake at 350 F for 50 minutes. After 5 minutes place the baking pan in the preheated oven.
6. Serve and enjoy.
- **Nutrition Info:** Calories 402 Fat 26.5 g Carbohydrates 9.3 g Sugar 1 g Protein 31 g Cholesterol 310 mg

99. Breaded Cauliflowers In Alfredo Sauce

Servings: 4
Cooking Time: 20 Minutes
Ingredients:
- 4 cups cauliflower florets
- 1 tbsp butter, melted
- ¼ cup alfredo sauce
- 1 cup breadcrumbs
- 1 tsp sea salt

Directions:
1. Whisk the alfredo sauce along with the butter. In a shallow bowl, combine the breadcrumbs with the sea salt. Dip each cauliflower floret into the alfredo mixture first, and then coat in the crumbs. Drop the prepared florets into the Air Fryer basket. Fit in the baking tray.
2. Set the temperature of your to 380 F and cook for 15 minutes on Air Fry function. Shake the florets twice during cooking. Serve.

100. Creamy Potato Gratin With Nutmeg

Servings: 4
Cooking Time: 30 Minutes
Ingredients:
- 1 lb potatoes, peeled and sliced
- ½ cup sour cream
- ½ cup mozzarella cheese, grated
- ½ cup milk
- ½ tsp nutmeg
- Salt and black pepper to taste

Directions:
1. Preheat on Bake function to 390 F. In a bowl, combine sour cream, milk, pepper, salt, and nutmeg. Place the potato slices in the bowl with the milk mixture and stir to coat well.
2. Transfer the mixture to a baking dish and press Start. Cook for 20 minutes, then

sprinkle grated cheese on top and cook for 5 more minutes. Serve warm.

101.Brioche Breakfast Pudding

Servings: 8
Cooking Time: 45 Minutes
Ingredients:

- 1 loaf brioche bread, cut in cubes
- ½ tbsp. coconut oil, soft
- 4 cups milk
- 1 can coconut milk
- 6 eggs
- ½ cup sugar
- 2 tsp vanilla
- ¼ tsp salt
- 1 cup coconut, shredded
- ½ cup chocolate chips

Directions:

1. Place rack in position 1 of the oven. Grease an 8x11-inch baking pan with coconut oil.
2. Add the bread cubes to the pan, pressing lightly to settle.
3. In a large bowl, whisk together milk, coconut milk, eggs, sugar, vanilla, and salt until combined.
4. Stir in coconut and chocolate chips. Pour evenly over bread. Cover with plastic wrap and refrigerate 2 hours or overnight.
5. Set oven to bake on 350°F for 50 minutes. After 5 minutes, add the pudding to the oven and bake 40-45 minutes, or until top is beginning to brown and it passes the toothpick test.
6. Remove to wire rack and let cool 5-10 minutes before serving.
- **Nutrition Info:** Calories 476, Total Fat 24g, Saturated Fat 15g, Total Carbs 51g, Net Carbs 48g, Protein 14g, Sugar 30g, Fiber 3g, Sodium 398mg, Potassium 443mg, Phosphorus 288mg

102.Sausage Omelet

Servings: 2
Cooking Time: 13 Minutes
Ingredients:

- 4 eggs
- 1 bacon slice, chopped
- 2 sausages, chopped
- 1 yellow onion, chopped

Directions:

1. In a bowl, crack the eggs and beat well.
2. Add the remaining ingredients and gently, stir to combine.
3. Place the mixture into a baking pan.
4. Press "Power Button" of Air Fry Oven and turn the dial to select the "Air Fry" mode.
5. Press the Time button and again turn the dial to set the cooking time to 13 minutes.

6. Now push the Temp button and rotate the dial to set the temperature at 320 degrees F.
7. Press "Start/Pause" button to start.
8. When the unit beeps to show that it is preheated, open the lid.
9. Arrange pan over the "Wire Rack" and insert in the oven.
10. Cut into equal-sized wedges and serve hot.
- **Nutrition Info:** Calories 325 Total Fat 23.1 g Saturated Fat 7.4 g Cholesterol 368 mg Sodium 678 mg Total Carbs 6 g Fiber 1.2 g Sugar 3 g Protein 22.7 g

103.Banana Cake With Peanut Butter

Servings:2
Cooking Time: 35 Minutes
Ingredients:

- 1 cup + 1 tbsp flour
- 1 tsp baking powder
- ⅓ cup sugar
- 2 bananas, mashed
- ¼ cup vegetable oil
- 1 egg, beaten
- 1 tsp vanilla extract
- ¾ cup chopped walnuts
- ¼ tsp salt
- 2 tbsp peanut butter
- 2 tbsp sour cream

Directions:

1. Preheat on AirFry function to 330 F. In a bowl, combine flour, salt, and baking powder In another bowl, combine bananas, oil, egg, peanut butter, vanilla, sugar, and sour cream.
2. Gently mix the both mixtures. Stir in the chopped walnuts. Pour the batter into a greased baking dish and press Start. Cook for 25 minutes. Serve chilled.

104.Hearty Sweet Potato Baked Oatmeal

Servings: 6
Cooking Time: 30 Minutes
Ingredients:

- 1 egg, lightly beaten
- 1 tsp vanilla
- 1 1/2 cups milk
- 1 tsp baking powder
- 2 tbsp ground flax seed
- 1 cup sweet potato puree
- 1/4 tsp nutmeg
- 2 tsp cinnamon
- 1/3 cup maple syrup
- 2 cups old fashioned oats
- 1/4 tsp salt

Directions:

1. Fit the oven with the rack in position
2. Spray an 8-inch square baking pan with cooking spray and set aside.

3. Add all ingredients except oats into the mixing bowl and mix until well combined.
4. Add oats and stir until just combined.
5. Pour mixture into the prepared baking pan.
6. Set to bake at 350 F for 35 minutes. After 5 minutes place the baking pan in the preheated oven.
7. Serve and enjoy.
- **Nutrition Info:** Calories 355 Fat 6.3 g Carbohydrates 62.3 g Sugar 17.1 g Protein 10.9 g Cholesterol 32 mg

105. Mini Brown Rice Quiches

Servings:6
Cooking Time: 14 Minutes
Ingredients:
- 4 ounces (113 g) diced green chilies
- 3 cups cooked brown rice
- 1 cup shredded reduced-fat Cheddar cheese, divided
- ½ cup egg whites
- $^1/_3$ cup fat-free milk
- ¼ cup diced pimiento
- ½ teaspoon cumin
- 1 small eggplant, cubed
- 1 bunch fresh cilantro, finely chopped
- Cooking spray

Directions:
1. Spritz a 12-cup muffin pan with cooking spray.
2. In a large bowl, stir together all the ingredients, except for ½ cup of the cheese.
3. Scoop the mixture evenly into the muffin cups and sprinkle the remaining ½ cup of the cheese on top.
4. Put the muffin pan into Rack Position 1, select Convection Bake, set temperature to 400ºF (205ºC) and set time to 14 minutes.
5. When cooking is complete, remove from the oven and check the quiches. They should be set.
6. Carefully transfer the quiches to a platter and serve immediately.

106. Vanilla Granola

Servings:4
Cooking Time: 40 Minutes
Ingredients:
- 1 cup rolled oats
- 3 tablespoons maple syrup
- 1 tablespoon sunflower oil
- 1 tablespoon coconut sugar
- ¼ teaspoon vanilla
- ¼ teaspoon cinnamon
- ¼ teaspoon sea salt

Directions:
1. Mix together the oats, maple syrup, sunflower oil, coconut sugar, vanilla, cinnamon, and sea salt in a medium bowl

and stir to combine. Transfer the mixture to the baking pan.
2. Slide the baking pan into Rack Position 1, select Convection Bake, set temperature to 248ºF (120ºC) and set time to 40 minutes.
3. Stir the granola four times during cooking.
4. When cooking is complete, the granola will be mostly dry and lightly browned.
5. Let the granola stand for 5 to 10 minutes before serving.

107. Smart Oven Jalapeño Popper Grilled Cheese Recipe

Servings:x
Cooking Time:x
Ingredients:
- 1 medium Jalapeño
- 2 slices Whole Grain Bread
- 2 teaspoons Mayonnaise
- 1/2-ounce Shredded Mild Cheddar Cheese, (about 2 tablespoons)
- 2 teaspoons Honey
- 1-ounce Cream Cheese, softened
- 1 tablespoon Sliced Green Onions
- dash of Garlic Powder
- 1-ounce Shredded Monterey Jack Cheese, (about 1/4 cup)
- 1/4 cup Corn Flakes Cereal

Directions:
1. Cut jalapeño into 1/4-inch slices. If you want your Classic Sandwich less spicy, use a paring knife to remove the seeds and veins.
2. Adjust cooking rack to the top placement and select the BROIL setting. Place jalapeño slices on a baking sheet, and broil until they have softened and are just starting to brown, about 2 to 4 minutes. Remove pan and set aside.
3. Adjust the cooking rack to the bottom position. Place an empty sheet pan inside of the toaster oven, and preheat to 400°F on the BAKE setting.
4. Spread one side of each slice of bread with mayonnaise. Place the bread mayo-side-down on a cutting board.
5. In a small bowl, combine the cream cheese, green onion, and garlic powder. Spread each slice of bread with the mixture. Arrange jalapeño slices in an even layer on one slice and distribute the cheese evenly over both pieces of bread.
6. Carefully remove the pan and add the bread, mayo-side-down, to the pan. Return to the oven and bake until the bread is toasted and the cheese is melted and bubbly, about 6 to 7 minutes.
7. Finishing Touches

8. Drizzle the honey over the jalapeño and sprinkle with corn flakes. Immediately top with the remaining cheesy bread slice.

108.Chicken Omelet

Servings: 2
Cooking Time: 16 Minutes
Ingredients:
- 1 teaspoon butter
- 1 small yellow onion, chopped
- ½ jalapeño pepper, seeded and chopped
- 3 eggs
- Salt and ground black pepper, as required
- ¼ cup cooked chicken, shredded

Directions:
1. In a frying pan, melt the butter over medium heat and cook the onion for about 4-5 minutes.
2. Add the jalapeño pepper and cook for about 1 minute.
3. Remove from the heat and set aside to cool slightly.
4. Meanwhile, in a bowl, add the eggs, salt, and black pepper and beat well.
5. Add the onion mixture and chicken and stir to combine.
6. Place the chicken mixture into a small baking pan.
7. Press "Power Button" of Air Fry Oven and turn the dial to select the "Air Fry" mode.
8. Press the Time button and again turn the dial to set the cooking time to 6 minutes.
9. Now push the Temp button and rotate the dial to set the temperature at 355 degrees F.
10. Press "Start/Pause" button to start.
11. When the unit beeps to show that it is preheated, open the lid.
12. Arrange pan over the "Wire Rack" and insert in the oven.
13. Cut the omelet into 2 portions and serve hot.
- **Nutrition Info:** Calories 153 Total Fat 9.1 g Saturated Fat 3.4 g Cholesterol 264 mg Sodium 196 mg Total Carbs 4 g Fiber 0.9 g Sugar 2.1 g Protein 13.8 g

109.American Cheese Sandwich

Servings:1
Cooking Time: 10 Minutes
Ingredients:
- 2 tbsp butter
- 2 slices bread
- 3 American cheese slices

Directions:
1. Preheat on Bake function to 370 F. Spread 1 tsp butter on the outside of each of the bread slices. Place the cheese on the inside of one bread slice. Top with the other slice. Press Start and cook for 4 minutes. Flip the sandwich over and cook for an additional 4 minutes.

110.Glazed Strawberry Toast

Servings: 4 Toasts
Cooking Time: 8 Minutes
Ingredients:
- 4 slices bread, ½-inch thick
- 1 cup sliced strawberries
- 1 teaspoon sugar
- Cooking spray

Directions:
1. On a clean work surface, lay the bread slices and spritz one side of each slice of bread with cooking spray.
2. Place the bread slices in the air fryer basket, sprayed side down. Top with the strawberries and a sprinkle of sugar.
3. Put the air fryer basket on the baking pan and slide into Rack Position 2, select Air Fry, set temperature to 375ºF (190ºC), and set time to 8 minutes.
4. When cooking is complete, the toast should be well browned on each side. Remove from the oven to a plate and serve.

111.Amazing Strawberry Pancake

Servings:4
Cooking Time: 30 Minutes
Ingredients:
- 3 eggs, beaten
- 2 tbsp unsalted butter
- ½ cup flour
- 2 tbsp sugar, powdered
- ½ cup milk
- 1 ½ cups fresh strawberries, sliced

Directions:
1. Preheat to 330 F on Bake function. Add butter to a pan and melt over low heat. In a bowl, mix flour, milk, eggs, and vanilla. Add the mixture to the pan with melted butter.
2. Place the pan in the oven and press Start. Cook for 14-16 minutes until the pancake is fluffy and golden brown. Drizzle powdered sugar and toss sliced strawberries on top.

112.Spinach, Leek And Cheese Frittata

Servings:2
Cooking Time: 22 Minutes
Ingredients:
- 4 large eggs
- 4 ounces (113 g) baby bella mushrooms, chopped
- 1 cup (1 ounce / 28-g) baby spinach, chopped
- ½ cup (2 ounces / 57-g) shredded Cheddar cheese
- $1/_3$ cup (from 1 large) chopped leek, white part only
- ¼ cup halved grape tomatoes
- 1 tablespoon 2% milk
- ¼ teaspoon dried oregano

- ¼ teaspoon garlic powder
- ½ teaspoon kosher salt
- Freshly ground black pepper, to taste
- Cooking spray

Directions:
1. Lightly spritz the baking pan with cooking spray.
2. Whisk the eggs in a large bowl until frothy. Add the mushrooms, baby spinach, cheese, leek, tomatoes, milk, oregano, garlic powder, salt, and pepper and stir until well blended. Pour the mixture into the prepared baking pan.
3. Slide the baking pan into Rack Position 1, select Convection Bake, set temperature to 300ºF (150ºC) and set time to 22 minutes.
4. When cooked, the center will be puffed up and the top will be golden brown.
5. Let the frittata cool for 5 minutes before slicing to serve.

113.French Toast Sticks

Servings:4
Cooking Time: 12 Minutes
Ingredients:
- 3 slices low-sodium whole-wheat bread, each cut into 4 strips
- 1 tablespoon unsalted butter, melted
- 1 tablespoon 2 percent milk
- 1 tablespoon sugar
- 1 egg, beaten
- 1 egg white
- 1 cup sliced fresh strawberries
- 1 tablespoon freshly squeezed lemon juice

Directions:
1. Arrange the bread strips on a plate and drizzle with the melted butter.
2. In a bowl, whisk together the milk, sugar, egg and egg white.
3. Dredge the bread strips into the egg mixture and place on a wire rack to let the batter drip off. Arrange half the coated bread strips in the air fryer basket.
4. Put the air fryer basket on the baking pan and slide into Rack Position 2, select Air Fry, set temperature to 380ºF (193ºC) and set time to 6 minutes.
5. After 3 minutes, remove from the oven and turn the strips over. Return to the oven to continue cooking.
6. When cooking is complete, the strips should be golden brown. Repeat with the remaining strips.
7. In a small bowl, mash the strawberries with a fork and stir in the lemon juice. Serve the French toast sticks with the strawberry sauce.

114.Chicken Breakfast Muffins

Servings: 12
Cooking Time: 15 Minutes
Ingredients:
- 10 eggs
- 1/3 cup green onions, chopped
- 1 cup chicken, cooked and chopped
- 1/4 tsp pepper
- 1 tsp sea salt

Directions:
1. Fit the oven with the rack in position
2. Spray 12-cups muffin tin with cooking spray and set aside.
3. In a large bowl, whisk eggs with pepper and salt.
4. Add remaining ingredients and stir well.
5. Pour egg mixture into the greased muffin tin.
6. Set to bake at 400 F for 20 minutes, after 5 minutes, place the muffin tin in the oven.
7. Serve and enjoy.
- **Nutrition Info:** Calories 71 Fat 4 g Carbohydrates 0.5 g Sugar 0.3 g Protein 8 g Cholesterol 145 mg

115.Beans And Pork Mix

Servings: 4
Cooking Time: 20 Minutes
Ingredients:
- 1-pound pork stew meat, ground
- 1 red onion, chopped
- 1 tablespoon olive oil
- 1 cup canned kidney beans, drained and rinsed
- 1 teaspoon chili powder
- Salt and black pepper to the taste
- ¼ teaspoon cumin, ground

Directions:
1. Heat up your air fryer at 360 degrees F, add the meat and the onion and cook for 5 minutes.
2. Add the beans and the rest of the ingredients, toss and cook for 15 minutes more.
3. Divide everything into bowls and serve for breakfast.
- **Nutrition Info:** calories 203, fat 4, fiber 6, carbs 12, protein 4

116.Raspberries Maple Pancakes

Servings: 4
Cooking Time: 15 Minutes
Ingredients:
- 2 cups all-purpose flour
- 1 cup milk
- 3 eggs, beaten
- 1 tsp baking powder
- 1 cup brown sugar
- 1 ½ tsp vanilla extract

- ½ cup frozen raspberries, thawed
- 2 tbsp maple syrup
- A pinch of salt

Directions:
1. Preheat on Bake function to 400 F. In a bowl, mix the flour, baking powder, salt, milk, eggs, vanilla extract, and sugar until smooth. Stir in the raspberries. Do it gently to avoid coloring the batter.
2. Grease a pie pan with cooking spray. Drop the batter onto the pan. Make sure to leave some space between the pancakes. Cook for 10-15 minutes. Drizzle with maple syrup and serve.

117.Pumpkin And Yogurt Bread

Servings: 4
Cooking Time: 15 Minutes
Ingredients:
- 2 large eggs
- 8 tablespoons pumpkin puree
- 6 tablespoons banana flour
- 4 tablespoons plain Greek yogurt
- 6 tablespoons oats
- 4 tablespoons honey
- 2 tablespoons vanilla essence
- Pinch of ground nutmeg

Directions:
1. Preheat the Air fryer to 360 ºF and grease a loaf pan.
2. Mix together all the ingredients except oats in a bowl and beat with the hand mixer until smooth.
3. Add oats and mix until well combined.
4. Transfer the mixture into the prepared loaf pan and place in the Air fryer.
5. Cook for about 15 minutes and remove from the Air fryer.
6. Place onto a wire rack to cool and cut the bread into desired size slices to serve.
- **Nutrition Info:** Calories: 212 Cal Total Fat: 3.4 g Saturated Fat: 0 g Cholesterol: 0 mg Sodium: 49 mg Total Carbs: 36 g Fiber: 0 g Sugar: 20.5 g Protein: 6.6 g

118.Blackberries Bowls

Servings: 4
Cooking Time: 30 Minutes
Ingredients:
- 1 ½ cups coconut milk
- ½ cup coconut; shredded
- ½ cup blackberries
- 2 tsp. stevia

Directions:
1. In your air fryer's pan, mix all the ingredients, stir, cover and cook at 360°F for 15 minutes.
2. Divide into bowls and serve

- **Nutrition Info:** Calories: 171; Fat: 4g; Fiber: 2g; Carbs: 3g; Protein: 5g

119.Veggie Frittata

Servings:4
Cooking Time: 12 Minutes
Ingredients:
- ½ cup chopped red bell pepper
- $^1/_3$ cup grated carrot
- $^1/_3$ cup minced onion
- 1 teaspoon olive oil
- 1 egg
- 6 egg whites
- $^1/_3$ cup 2% milk
- 1 tablespoon shredded Parmesan cheese

Directions:
1. Mix together the red bell pepper, carrot, onion, and olive oil in the baking pan and stir to combine.
2. Slide the baking pan into Rack Position 1, select Convection Bake, set temperature to 350ºF (180ºC) and set time to 12 minutes.
3. After 3 minutes, remove the pan from the oven. Stir the vegetables. Return the pan to the oven and continue cooking.
4. Meantime, whisk together the egg, egg whites, and milk in a medium bowl until creamy.
5. After 3 minutes, remove the pan from the oven. Pour the egg mixture over the top and scatter with the Parmesan cheese. Return the pan to the oven and continue cooking for additional 6 minutes.
6. When cooking is complete, the eggs will be set and the top will be golden around the edges.
7. Allow the frittata to cool for 5 minutes before slicing and serving.

120.Feta & Tomato Tart With Olives

Servings:2
Cooking Time: 40 Minutes
Ingredients:
- 4 eggs
- ½ cup tomatoes, chopped
- 1 cup feta cheese, crumbled
- 1 tbsp fresh basil, chopped
- 1 tbsp fresh oregano, chopped
- ¼ cup Kalamata olives, pitted and chopped
- ¼ cup onions, chopped
- 2 tbsp olive oil
- ½ cup milk
- Salt and black pepper to taste

Directions:
1. Preheat on Bake function to 340 F. Brush a pie pan with olive oil. Beat the eggs along with the milk, salt, and pepper. Stir in the remaining ingredients. Pour the egg mixture

into the pan and press Start. Cook for 15-18 minutes. Serve sliced.

121.Veggies Breakfast Salad

Servings: 4
Cooking Time: 15 Minutes
Ingredients:
- 2 tablespoons olive oil
- 1 cup cherry tomatoes, halved
- 1 zucchini, cubed
- 1 eggplant, cubed
- 1 red onion, chopped
- 1 fennel bulb, shredded
- 1 cup cheddar, shredded
- 2 tablespoons chives, chopped
- Salt and black pepper to the taste
- 8 eggs, whisked

Directions:
1. Add the oil to your air fryer, heat it up at 350 degrees F, add the onion and fennel and cook for 2 minutes.
2. Add the tomatoes and the other ingredients except the cheese and toss.
3. Sprinkle the cheese on top, cook the mix for 13 minutes more, divide into bowls and serve for breakfast.
- **Nutrition Info:** calories 221, fat 8, fiber 3, carbs 4, protein 8

122.Sweet Breakfast Casserole

Servings: 4
Cooking Time: 30 Minutes
Ingredients:
- 3 tablespoons brown sugar
- 4 tablespoons margarine
- 2 tablespoons white sugar
- 1/2 tsp. cinnamon powder
- 1/2 cup flour
- For the casserole:
- 2 eggs
- 2 tablespoons white sugar
- 2 and 1/2 cups white flour
- 1 tsp. baking soda
- 1 tsp. baking powder
- 2 eggs
- 1/2 cup milk
- 2 cups margarine milk
- 4 tablespoons margarine
- Zest from 1 lemon, grated
- 1 and 2/3 cup blueberries

Directions:
1. In a bowl, mix eggs with 2 tablespoons white sugar, 2 and 1/2 cups white flour, baking powder, baking soda, 2 eggs, milk, margarine milk, 4 tablespoons margarine, lemon zest and blueberries, stir and pour into a pan that fits your air fryer.
2. In another bowls, mix 3 tablespoons brown sugar with 2 tablespoons white sugar, 4

tablespoons margarine, 1/2 cup flour and cinnamon, stir until you obtain a crumble and spread over blueberries mix.
3. Place in preheated air fryer and bake at 300 °F for 30 minutes.
4. Divide among plates and serve for breakfast.
- **Nutrition Info:** Calories 101 Fat 9.4 g Carbohydrates 0.3 g Sugar 0.2 g Protein 7 g Cholesterol 21 mg

123.Spinach And Ricotta Pockets

Servings: 8 Pockets
Cooking Time: 10 Minutes
Ingredients:
- 2 large eggs, divided
- 1 tablespoon water
- 1 cup baby spinach, roughly chopped
- ¼ cup sun-dried tomatoes, finely chopped
- 1 cup ricotta cheese
- 1 cup basil, chopped
- ¼ teaspoon red pepper flakes
- ¼ teaspoon kosher salt
- 2 refrigerated rolled pie crusts
- 2 tablespoons sesame seeds

Directions:
1. Spritz the air fryer basket with cooking spray.
2. Whisk an egg with water in a small bowl.
3. Combine the spinach, tomatoes, the other egg, ricotta cheese, basil, red pepper flakes, and salt in a large bowl. Whisk to mix well.
4. Unfold the pie crusts on a clean work surface and slice each crust into 4 wedges. Scoop up 3 tablespoons of the spinach mixture on each crust and leave ½ inch space from edges.
5. Fold the crust wedges in half to wrap the filling and press the edges with a fork to seal.
6. Arrange the wraps in the pan and spritz with cooking spray. Sprinkle with sesame seeds.
7. Put the air fryer basket on the baking pan and slide into Rack Position 2, select Air Fry, set temperature to 380ºF (193ºC) and set time to 10 minutes.
8. Flip the wraps halfway through the cooking time.
9. When cooked, the wraps will be crispy and golden.
10. Serve immediately.

124.Breakfast Sandwich

Servings: 1
Cooking Time: 7minutes
Ingredients:
- 2 Bacon Slices
- 1 Egg
- 1 English muffin Salt& Pepper to taste

Directions:

1. Beat the egg into a soufflé cup and add salt and pepper to taste.
2. Heat the air fryer to 390°F and place the soufflé cup, English muffin and bacon into the tray.
3. Cook all the ingredients for 6-10 minutes. Assemble sandwich and enjoy.

- **Nutrition Info:** Calories 113 Fat 8.2 g Carbohydrates 0.3 g Sugar 0.2 g Protein 5.4 g Cholesterol 18 mg

LUNCH RECIPES

125.Turkey And Almonds

Servings: 2
Cooking Time: 10 Minutes
Ingredients:
- 1 big turkey breast, skinless; boneless and halved
- 2 shallots; chopped
- 1/3 cup almonds; chopped
- 1 tbsp. sweet paprika
- 2 tbsp. olive oil
- Salt and black pepper to taste.

Directions:
1. In a pan that fits the air fryer, combine the turkey with all the other ingredients, toss.
2. Put the pan in the machine and cook at 370°F for 25 minutes
3. Divide everything between plates and serve.
- **Nutrition Info:** Calories: 274; Fat: 12g; Fiber: 3g; Carbs: 5g; Protein: 14g

126.Spice-roasted Almonds

Servings: 32
Cooking Time: 10 Minutes
Ingredients:
- 1 tablespoon chili powder
- 1 tablespoon olive oil
- 1/2 teaspoon salt
- 1/2 teaspoon ground cumin
- 1/2 teaspoon ground coriander
- 1/4 teaspoon ground cinnamon
- 1/4 teaspoon black pepper
- 2 cups whole almonds

Directions:
1. Start by preheating toaster oven to 350°F.
2. Mix olive oil, chili powder, coriander, cinnamon, cumin, salt, and pepper.
3. Add almonds and toss together.
4. Transfer to a baking pan and bake for 10 minutes.
- **Nutrition Info:** Calories: 39, Sodium: 37 mg, Dietary Fiber: 0.8 g, Total Fat: 3.5 g, Total Carbs: 1.4 g, Protein: 1.3 g.

127.Lamb Gyro

Servings: 4
Cooking Time: 25 Minutes
Ingredients:
- 1 pound ground lamb
- ¼ red onion, minced
- ¼ cup mint, minced
- ¼ cup parsley, minced
- 2 cloves garlic, minced
- ½ teaspoon salt
- ⅛ teaspoon rosemary
- ½ teaspoon black pepper
- 4 slices pita bread
- ¾ cup hummus
- 1 cup romaine lettuce, shredded
- ½ onion sliced
- 1 Roma tomato, diced
- ½ cucumber, skinned and thinly sliced
- 12 mint leaves, minced
- Tzatziki sauce, to taste

Directions:
1. Mix ground lamb, red onion, mint, parsley, garlic, salt, rosemary, and black pepper until fully incorporated.
2. Select the Broil function on the COSORI Air Fryer Toaster Oven, set time to 25 minutes and temperature to 450°F, then press Start/Cancel to preheat.
3. Line the food tray with parchment paper and place ground lamb on top, shaping it into a patty 1-inch-thick and 6 inches in diameter.
4. Insert the food tray at top position in the preheated air fryer toaster oven, then press Start/Cancel.
5. Remove when done and cut into thin slices.
6. Assemble each gyro starting with pita bread, then hummus, lamb meat, lettuce, onion, tomato, cucumber, and mint leaves, then drizzle with tzatziki.
7. Serve immediately.
- **Nutrition Info:** Calories: 409 kcal Total Fat: 14.6 g Saturated Fat: 0 g Cholesterol: 0 mg Sodium: 0 mg Total Carbs: 29.9 g Fiber: 0 g Sugar: 0 g Protein: 39.4 g

128.Chicken Legs With Dilled Brussels Sprouts

Servings: 2
Cooking Time: 10 Minutes
Ingredients:
- 2 chicken legs
- 1/2 teaspoon paprika
- 1/2 teaspoon kosher salt
- 1/2 teaspoon black pepper
- 1/2 pound Brussels sprouts
- 1 teaspoon dill, fresh or dried

Directions:
1. Start by preheating your Air Fryer to 370 degrees F.
2. Now, season your chicken with paprika, salt, and pepper. Transfer the chicken legs to the cooking basket. Cook for 10 minutes.
3. Flip the chicken legs and cook an additional 10 minutes. Reserve.
4. Add the Brussels sprouts to the cooking basket; sprinkle with dill. Cook at 380 degrees F for 15 minutes, shaking the basket halfway through.
5. Serve with the reserved chicken legs.

- **Nutrition Info:** 365 Calories; 21g Fat; 3g Carbs; 36g Protein; 2g Sugars; 3g Fiber

129.Skinny Black Bean Flautas

Servings: 10
Cooking Time: 25 Minutes
Ingredients:
- 2 (15-ounce) cans black beans
- 1 cup shredded cheddar
- 1 (4-ounce) can diced green chilies
- 2 teaspoons taco seasoning
- 10 (8-inch) whole wheat flour tortillas
- Olive oil

Directions:
1. Start by preheating toaster oven to 350°F.
2. Drain black beans and mash in a medium bowl with a fork.
3. Mix in cheese, chilies, and taco seasoning until all ingredients are thoroughly combined.
4. Evenly spread the mixture over each tortilla and wrap tightly.
5. Brush each side lightly with olive oil and place on a baking sheet.
6. Bake for 12 minutes, turn, and bake for another 13 minutes.
- **Nutrition Info:** Calories: 367, Sodium: 136 mg, Dietary Fiber: 14.4 g, Total Fat: 2.8 g, Total Carbs: 64.8 g, Protein: 22.6 g.

130.Roasted Garlic(2)

Servings: 12 Cloves
Cooking Time: 12 Minutes
Ingredients:
- 1 medium head garlic
- 2 tsp. avocado oil

Directions:
1. Remove any hanging excess peel from the garlic but leave the cloves covered. Cut off ¼ of the head of garlic, exposing the tips of the cloves
2. Drizzle with avocado oil. Place the garlic head into a small sheet of aluminum foil, completely enclosing it. Place it into the air fryer basket. Adjust the temperature to 400 Degrees F and set the timer for 20 minutes. If your garlic head is a bit smaller, check it after 15 minutes
3. When done, garlic should be golden brown and very soft
4. To serve, cloves should pop out and easily be spread or sliced. Store in an airtight container in the refrigerator up to 5 days.
5. You may also freeze individual cloves on a baking sheet, then store together in a freezer-safe storage bag once frozen.
- **Nutrition Info:** Calories: 11; Protein: 2g; Fiber: 1g; Fat: 7g; Carbs: 0g

131.Turmeric Mushroom(3)

Servings: 4
Cooking Time: 12 Minutes
Ingredients:
- 1 lb. brown mushrooms
- 4 garlic cloves; minced
- ¼ tsp. cinnamon powder
- 1 tsp. olive oil
- ½ tsp. turmeric powder
- Salt and black pepper to taste.

Directions:
1. In a bowl, combine all the ingredients and toss.
2. Put the mushrooms in your air fryer's basket and cook at 370°F for 15 minutes
3. Divide the mix between plates and serve as a side dish.
- **Nutrition Info:** Calories: 208; Fat: 7g; Fiber: 3g; Carbs: 5g; Protein: 7g

132.Cheese-stuffed Meatballs

Servings: 4
Cooking Time: 10 Minutes
Ingredients:
- ⅓ cup soft bread crumbs
- 3 tablespoons milk
- 1 tablespoon ketchup
- 1 egg
- ½ teaspoon dried marjoram
- Pinch salt
- Freshly ground black pepper
- 1-pound 95 percent lean ground beef
- 20 ½-inch cubes of cheese
- Olive oil for misting

Directions:
1. Preparing the ingredients. In a large bowl, combine the bread crumbs, milk, ketchup, egg, marjoram, salt, and pepper, and mix well. Add the ground beef and mix gently but thoroughly with your hands. Form the mixture into 20 meatballs. Shape each meatball around a cheese cube. Mist the meatballs with olive oil and put into the instant crisp air fryer basket.
2. Air frying. Close air fryer lid. Bake for 10 to 13 minutes or until the meatballs register 165°f on a meat thermometer.
- **Nutrition Info:** Calories: 393; Fat: 17g; Protein:50g; Fiber:0g

133.Kale And Pine Nuts

Servings: 4
Cooking Time: 12 Minutes
Ingredients:
- 10 cups kale; torn
- 1/3 cup pine nuts
- 2 tbsp. lemon zest; grated
- 1 tbsp. lemon juice

- 2 tbsp. olive oil
- Salt and black pepper to taste.

Directions:
1. In a pan that fits the air fryer, combine all the ingredients, toss, introduce the pan in the machine and cook at 380°F for 15 minutes
2. Divide between plates and serve as a side dish.
- **Nutrition Info:** Calories: 121; Fat: 9g; Fiber: 2g; Carbs: 4g; Protein: 5g

134.Herb-roasted Chicken Tenders

Servings: 2
Cooking Time: 10 Minutes
Ingredients:
- 7 ounces chicken tenders
- 1 tablespoon olive oil
- 1/2 teaspoon Herbes de Provence
- 2 tablespoons Dijon mustard
- 1 tablespoon honey
- Salt and pepper

Directions:
1. Start by preheating toaster oven to 450°F.
2. Brush bottom of pan with 1/2 tablespoon olive oil.
3. Season the chicken with herbs, salt, and pepper.
4. Place the chicken in a single flat layer in the pan and drizzle the remaining olive oil over it.
5. Bake for about 10 minutes.
6. While the chicken is baking, mix together the mustard and honey for a tasty condiment.
- **Nutrition Info:** Calories: 297, Sodium: 268 mg, Dietary Fiber: 0.8 g, Total Fat: 15.5 g, Total Carbs: 9.6 g, Protein: 29.8 g.

135.Chives Radishes

Servings: 4
Cooking Time: 12 Minutes
Ingredients:
- 20 radishes; halved
- 2 tbsp. olive oil
- 1 tbsp. garlic; minced
- 1 tsp. chives; chopped.
- Salt and black pepper to taste.

Directions:
1. In your air fryer's pan, combine all the ingredients and toss.
2. Introduce the pan in the machine and cook at 370°F for 15 minutes
3. Divide between plates and serve as a side dish.
- **Nutrition Info:** Calories: 160; Fat: 2g; Fiber: 3g; Carbs: 4g; Protein: 6g

136.Orange Chicken Rice

Servings: 4
Cooking Time: 55 Minutes
Ingredients:
- 3 tablespoons olive oil
- 1 medium onion, chopped
- 1 3/4 cups chicken broth
- 1 cup brown basmati rice
- Zest and juice of 2 oranges
- Salt to taste
- 4 (6-oz.) boneless, skinless chicken thighs
- Black pepper, to taste
- 2 tablespoons fresh mint, chopped
- 2 tablespoons pine nuts, toasted

Directions:
1. Spread the rice in a casserole dish and place the chicken on top.
2. Toss the rest of the Ingredients: in a bowl and liberally pour over the chicken.
3. Press "Power Button" of Air Fry Oven and turn the dial to select the "Bake" mode.
4. Press the Time button and again turn the dial to set the cooking time to 55 minutes.
5. Now push the Temp button and rotate the dial to set the temperature at 350 degrees F.
6. Once preheated, place the casserole dish inside and close its lid.
7. Serve warm.
- **Nutrition Info:** Calories 231 Total Fat 20.1 g Saturated Fat 2.4 g Cholesterol 110 mg Sodium 941 mg Total Carbs 30.1 g Fiber 0.9 g Sugar 1.4 g Protein 14.6 g

137.Sweet & Sour Pork

Servings: 4
Cooking Time: 27 Minutes
Ingredients:
- 2 pounds Pork cut into chunks
- 2 large Eggs
- 1 teaspoon Pure Sesame Oil (optional)
- 1 cup Potato Starch (or cornstarch)
- 1/2 teaspoon Sea Salt
- 1/4 teaspoon Freshly Ground Black Pepper
- 1/16 teaspoon Chinese Five Spice
- 3 Tablespoons Canola Oil
- Oil Mister

Directions:
1. In a mixing bowl, combine salt, potato starch, Chinese Five Spice, and peppers.
2. In another bowl, beat the eggs & add sesame oil.
3. Then dredge the pieces of Pork into the Potato Starch and remove the excess. Then dip each piece into the egg mixture, shake off excess, and then back into the Potato Starch mixture.
4. Place pork pieces into the Instant Pot Duo Crisp Air Fryer Basket after spray the pork with oil.

5. Close the Air Fryer lid and cook at 340°F for approximately 8 to12 minutes (or until pork is cooked), shaking the basket a couple of times for evenly distribution.
   - **Nutrition Info:** Calories 521, Total Fat 21g, Total Carbs 23g, Protein 60g

138.Delightful Turkey Wings

Servings: 4
Cooking Time: 26 Minutes
Ingredients:
- 2 pounds turkey wings
- 4 tablespoons chicken rub
- 3 tablespoons olive oil

Directions:
1. Preheat the Air fryer to 380 degree F and grease an Air fryer basket.
2. Mix the turkey wings, chicken rub, and olive oil in a bowl until well combined.
3. Arrange the turkey wings into the Air fryer basket and cook for about 26 minutes, flipping once in between.
4. Dish out the turkey wings in a platter and serve hot.
   - **Nutrition Info:** Calories: 204, Fat: 15.5g, Carbohydrates: 3g, Sugar: 0g, Protein: 12g, Sodium: 465mg

139.Zucchini Stew

Servings: 4
Cooking Time: 12 Minutes
Ingredients:
- 8 zucchinis, roughly cubed
- ¼ cup tomato sauce
- 1 tbsp. olive oil
- ½ tsp. basil; chopped.
- ¼ tsp. rosemary; dried
- Salt and black pepper to taste.

Directions:
1. Grease a pan that fits your air fryer with the oil, add all the ingredients, toss, introduce the pan in the fryer and cook at 350°F for 12 minutes
2. Divide into bowls and serve.
   - **Nutrition Info:** Calories: 200; Fat: 6g; Fiber: 2g; Carbs: 4g; Protein: 6g

140.Chicken Breasts With Chimichurri

Servings: 1
Cooking Time: 35 Minutes
Ingredients:
- 1 chicken breast, bone-in, skin-on
- Chimichurri
- ½ bunch fresh cilantro
- 1/4 bunch fresh parsley
- ½ shallot, peeled, cut in quarters
- ½ tablespoon paprika ground
- ½ tablespoon chili powder
- ½ tablespoon fennel ground

- ½ teaspoon black pepper, ground
- ½ teaspoon onion powder
- 1 teaspoon salt
- ½ teaspoon garlic powder
- ½ teaspoon cumin ground
- ½ tablespoon canola oil
- Chimichurri
- 2 tablespoons olive oil
- 4 garlic cloves, peeled
- Zest and juice of 1 lemon
- 1 teaspoon kosher salt

Directions:
1. Preheat the Air fryer to 300 degree F and grease an Air fryer basket.
2. Combine all the spices in a suitable bowl and season the chicken with it.
3. Sprinkle with canola oil and arrange the chicken in the Air fryer basket.
4. Cook for about 35 minutes and dish out in a platter.
5. Put all the ingredients in the blender and blend until smooth.
6. Serve the chicken with chimichurri sauce.
   - **Nutrition Info:** Calories: 140, Fats: 7.9g, Carbohydrates: 1.8g, Sugar: 7.1g, Proteins: 7.2g, Sodium: 581mg

141.Parmesan Chicken Meatballs

Servings: 4
Cooking Time: 12 Minutes
Ingredients:
- 1-lb. ground chicken
- 1 large egg, beaten
- ½ cup Parmesan cheese, grated
- ½ cup pork rinds, ground
- 1 teaspoon garlic powder
- 1 teaspoon paprika
- 1 teaspoon kosher salt
- ½ teaspoon pepper
- Crust:
- ½ cup pork rinds, ground

Directions:
1. Toss all the meatball Ingredients: in a bowl and mix well.
2. Make small meatballs out this mixture and roll them in the pork rinds.
3. Place the coated meatballs in the air fryer basket.
4. Press "Power Button" of Air Fry Oven and turn the dial to select the "Bake" mode.
5. Press the Time button and again turn the dial to set the cooking time to 12 minutes.
6. Now push the Temp button and rotate the dial to set the temperature at 400 degrees F.
7. Once preheated, place the air fryer basket inside and close its lid.
8. Serve warm.
   - **Nutrition Info:** Calories 529 Total Fat 17 g Saturated Fat 3 g Cholesterol 65 mg Sodium

391 mg Total Carbs 55 g Fiber 6 g Sugar 8 g Protein 41g

142.Easy Prosciutto Grilled Cheese

Servings: 1
Cooking Time: 5 Minutes
Ingredients:
- 2 slices muenster cheese
- 2 slices white bread
- Four thinly-shaved pieces of prosciutto
- 1 tablespoon sweet and spicy pickles

Directions:
1. Set toaster oven to the Toast setting.
2. Place one slice of cheese on each piece of bread.
3. Put prosciutto on one slice and pickles on the other.
4. Transfer to a baking sheet and toast for 4 minutes or until the cheese is melted.
5. Combine the sides, cut, and serve.
- **Nutrition Info:** Calories: 460, Sodium: 2180 mg, Dietary Fiber: 0 g, Total Fat: 25.2 g, Total Carbs: 11.9 g, Protein: 44.2 g.

143.Air Fryer Fish

Servings: 4
Cooking Time: 17 Minutes
Ingredients:
- 4-6 Whiting Fish fillets cut in half
- Oil to mist
- Fish Seasoning
- ¾ cup very fine cornmeal
- ¼ cup flour
- 2 tsp old bay
- 1 ½ tsp salt
- 1 tsp paprika
- ½ tsp garlic powder
- ½ tsp black pepper

Directions:
1. Put the Ingredients: for fish seasoning in a Ziplock bag and shake it well. Set aside.
2. Rinse and pat dry the fish fillets with paper towels. Make sure that they still are damp.
3. Place the fish fillets in a ziplock bag and shake until they are completely covered with seasoning.
4. Place the fillets on a baking rack to let any excess flour to fall off.
5. Grease the bottom of the Instant Pot Duo Crisp Air Fryer basket tray and place the fillets on the tray. Close the lid, select the Air Fry option and cook filets on 400°F for 10 minutes.
6. Open the Air Fryer lid and spray the fish with oil on the side facing up before flipping it over, ensure that the fish is fully coated. Flip and cook another side of the fish for 7 minutes. Remove the fish and serve.

- **Nutrition Info:** Calories 193, Total Fat 1g, Total Carbs 27g, Protein 19g

144.Ranch Chicken Wings

Servings: 3
Cooking Time: 10 Minutes
Ingredients:
- 1/4 cup almond meal
- 1/4 cup flaxseed meal
- 2 tablespoons butter, melted
- 6 tablespoons parmesan cheese, preferably freshly grated
- 1 tablespoon Ranch seasoning mix
- 2 tablespoons oyster sauce
- 6 chicken wings, bone-in

Directions:
1. Start by preheating your Air Fryer to 370 degrees F.
2. In a resealable bag, place the almond meal, flaxseed meal, butter, parmesan, Ranch seasoning mix, andoyster sauce. Add the chicken wings and shake to coat on all sides.
3. Arrange the chicken wings in the Air Fryer basket. Spritz the chicken wings with a nonstick cooking spray.
4. Cook for 11 minutes. Turn them over and cook an additional 11 minutes. Serve warm with your favorite dipping sauce, if desired. Enjoy!
- **Nutrition Info:** 285 Calories; 22g Fat; 3g Carbs; 12g Protein; 5g Sugars; 6g Fiber

145.Turkey Legs

Servings: 2
Cooking Time: 40 Minutes
Ingredients:
- 2 large turkey legs
- 1 1/2 tsp smoked paprika
- 1 tsp brown sugar
- 1 tsp season salt
- ½ tsp garlic powder
- oil for spraying avocado, canola, etc.

Directions:
1. Mix the smoked paprika, brown sugar, seasoned salt, garlic powder thoroughly.
2. Wash and pat dry the turkey legs.
3. Rub the made seasoning mixture all over the turkey legs making sure to get under the skin also.
4. While preparing for cooking, select the Air Fry option. Press start to begin preheating.
5. Once the preheating temperature is reached, place the turkey legs on the tray in the Instant Pot Duo Crisp Air Fryer basket. Lightly spray them with oil.
6. Air Fry the turkey legs on 400°F for 20 minutes. Then, open the Air Fryer lid and flip the turkey legs and lightly spray with oil.

Close the Instant Pot Duo Crisp Air Fryer lid and cook for 20 more minutes.

7. Remove and Enjoy.
- **Nutrition Info:** Calories 958, Total Fat 46g, Total Carbs 3g, Protein 133g

146. Lobster Tails

Servings: 2
Cooking Time: 8 Minutes
Ingredients:
- 2 6oz lobster tails
- 1 tsp salt
- 1 tsp chopped chives
- 2 Tbsp unsalted butter melted
- 1 Tbsp minced garlic
- 1 tsp lemon juice

Directions:
1. Combine butter, garlic, salt, chives, and lemon juice to prepare butter mixture.
2. Butterfly lobster tails by cutting through shell followed by removing the meat and resting it on top of the shell.
3. Place them on the tray in the Instant Pot Duo Crisp Air Fryer basket and spread butter over the top of lobster meat. Close the Air Fryer lid, select the Air Fry option and cook on 380°F for 4 minutes.
4. Open the Air Fryer lid and spread more butter on top, cook for extra 2-4 minutes until done.
- **Nutrition Info:** Calories 120, Total Fat 12g, Total Carbs 2g, Protein 1g

147. Tomato Avocado Melt

Servings: 2
Cooking Time: 4 Minutes
Ingredients:
- 4 slices of bread
- 1-2 tablespoons mayonnaise
- Cayenne pepper
- 1 small Roma tomato
- 1/2 avocado
- 8 slices of cheese of your choice

Directions:
1. Start by slicing avocado and tomato and set aside.
2. Spread mayonnaise on the bread.
3. Sprinkle cayenne pepper over the mayo to taste.
4. Layer tomato and avocado on top of cayenne pepper.
5. Top with cheese and put on greased baking sheet.
6. Broil on high for 2–4 minutes, until the cheese is melted and bread is toasted.
- **Nutrition Info:** Calories: 635, Sodium: 874 mg, Dietary Fiber: 4.1 g, Total Fat: 50.1 g, Total Carbs: 17.4 g, Protein: 30.5 g.

148. Tomato Frittata

Servings: 2
Cooking Time: 30 Minutes
Ingredients:
- 4 eggs
- ¼ cup onion, chopped
- ½ cup tomatoes, chopped
- ½ cup milk
- 1 cup Gouda cheese, shredded
- Salt, as required

Directions:
1. In a small baking pan, add all the ingredients and mix well.
2. Press "Power Button" of Air Fry Oven and turn the dial to select the "Air Fry" mode.
3. Press the Time button and again turn the dial to set the cooking time to 30 minutes.
4. Now push the Temp button and rotate the dial to set the temperature at 340 degrees F.
5. Press "Start/Pause" button to start.
6. When the unit beeps to show that it is preheated, open the lid.
7. Arrange the baking pan over the "Wire Rack" and insert in the oven.
8. Cut into 2 wedges and serve.
- **Nutrition Info:** Calories: 247 Cal Total Fat: 16.1 g Saturated Fat: 7.5 g Cholesterol: 332 mg Sodium: 417 mg Total Carbs: 7.30 g Fiber: 0.9 g Sugar: 5.2 g Protein: 18.6 g

149. Roasted Grape And Goat Cheese Crostinis

Servings: 10
Cooking Time: 5 Minutes
Ingredients:
- 1 pound seedless red grapes
- 1 teaspoon chopped rosemary
- 4 tablespoons olive oil
- 1 rustic French baguette
- 1 cup sliced shallots
- 2 tablespoons unsalted butter
- 8 ounces goat cheese
- 1 tablespoon honey

Directions:
1. Start by preheating toaster oven to 400°F.
2. Toss grapes, rosemary, and 1 tablespoon of olive oil in a large bowl.
3. Transfer to a roasting pan and roast for 20 minutes.
4. Remove the pan from the oven and set aside to cool.
5. Slice the baguette into 1/2-inch-thick pieces.
6. Brush each slice with olive oil and place on baking sheet.
7. Bake for 8 minutes, then remove from oven and set aside.
8. In a medium skillet add butter and one tablespoon of olive oil.
9. Add shallots and sauté for about 10 minutes.

10. Mix goat cheese and honey in a medium bowl, then add contents of shallot pan and mix thoroughly.
11. Spread shallot mixture onto baguette, top with grapes, and serve.
- **Nutrition Info:** Calories: 238, Sodium: 139 mg, Dietary Fiber: 0.6 g, Total Fat: 16.3 g, Total Carbs: 16.4 g, Protein: 8.4 g.

150. Roasted Beet Salad With Oranges & Beet Greens

Servings: 6
Cooking Time: 1-1/2 Hours
Ingredients:
- 6 medium beets with beet greens attached
- 2 large oranges
- 1 small sweet onion, cut into wedges
- 1/3 cup red wine vinegar
- 1/4 cup extra-virgin olive oil
- 2 garlic cloves, minced
- 1/2 teaspoon grated orange peel

Directions:
1. Start by preheating toaster oven to 400°F.
2. Trim leaves from beets and chop, then set aside.
3. Pierce beets with a fork and place in a roasting pan.
4. Roast beets for 1-1/2 hours.
5. Allow beets to cool, peel, then cut into 8 wedges and put into a bowl.
6. Place beet greens in a sauce pan and cover with just enough water to cover. Heat until water boils, then immediately remove from heat.
7. Drain greens and press to remove liquid from greens, then add to beet bowl.
8. Remove peel and pith from orange and segment, adding each segment to the bowl.
9. Add onion to beet mixture. In a separate bowl mix together vinegar, oil, garlic and orange peel.
10. Combine both bowls and toss, sprinkle with salt and pepper.
11. Let stand for an hour before serving.
- **Nutrition Info:** Calories: 214, Sodium: 183 mg, Dietary Fiber: 6.5 g, Total Fat: 8.9 g, Total Carbs: 32.4 g, Protein: 4.7 g.

151. Duck Rolls

Servings: 3
Cooking Time: 40 Minutes
Ingredients:
- 1 pound duck breast fillet, each cut into 2 pieces
- 3 tablespoons fresh parsley, finely chopped
- 1 small red onion, finely chopped
- 1 garlic clove, crushed
- 1½ teaspoons ground cumin
- 1 teaspoon ground cinnamon

- ½ teaspoon red chili powder
- Salt, to taste
- 2 tablespoons olive oil

Directions:
1. Preheat the Air fryer to 355 degree F and grease an Air fryer basket.
2. Mix the garlic, parsley, onion, spices, and 1 tablespoon of olive oil in a bowl.
3. Make a slit in each duck piece horizontally and coat with onion mixture.
4. Roll each duck piece tightly and transfer into the Air fryer basket.
5. Cook for about 40 minutes and cut into desired size slices to serve.
- **Nutrition Info:** Calories: 239, Fats: 8.2g, Carbohydrates: 3.2g, Sugar: 0.9g, Proteins: 37.5g, Sodium: 46mg

152. Country Comfort Corn Bread

Servings: 12
Cooking Time: 20 Minutes
Ingredients:
- 1 cup yellow cornmeal
- 1-1/2 cups oatmeal
- 1/4 teaspoon salt
- 1/4 cup granulated sugar
- 2 teaspoons baking powder
- 1 cup milk
- 1 large egg
- 1/2 cup applesauce

Directions:
1. Start by blending oatmeal into a fine powder.
2. Preheat toaster oven to 400°F.
3. Mix oatmeal, cornmeal, salt, sugar, and baking powder, and stir to blend.
4. Add milk, egg, and applesauce, and mix well.
5. Pour into a pan and bake for 20 minutes.
- **Nutrition Info:** Calories: 113, Sodium: 71 mg, Dietary Fiber: 1.9 g, Total Fat: 1.9 g, Total Carbs: 21.5 g, Protein: 3.4 g.

153. Okra And Green Beans Stew

Servings: 4
Cooking Time: 12 Minutes
Ingredients:
- 1 lb. green beans; halved
- 4 garlic cloves; minced
- 1 cup okra
- 3 tbsp. tomato sauce
- 1 tbsp. thyme; chopped.
- Salt and black pepper to taste.

Directions:
1. In a pan that fits your air fryer, mix all the ingredients, toss, introduce the pan in the air fryer and cook at 370°F for 15 minutes
2. Divide the stew into bowls and serve.
- **Nutrition Info:** Calories: 183; Fat: 5g; Fiber: 2g; Carbs: 4g; Protein: 8g

154. Oregano Chicken Breast

Servings: 6
Cooking Time: 25 Minutes
Ingredients:
- 2 lbs. chicken breasts, minced
- 1 tablespoon avocado oil
- 1 teaspoon smoked paprika
- 1 teaspoon garlic powder
- 1 teaspoon oregano
- 1/2 teaspoon salt
- Black pepper, to taste

Directions:
1. Toss all the meatball Ingredients: in a bowl and mix well.
2. Make small meatballs out this mixture and place them in the air fryer basket.
3. Press "Power Button" of Air Fry Oven and turn the dial to select the "Air Fry" mode.
4. Press the Time button and again turn the dial to set the cooking time to 25 minutes.
5. Now push the Temp button and rotate the dial to set the temperature at 375 degrees F.
6. Once preheated, place the air fryer basket inside and close its lid.
7. Serve warm.
- **Nutrition Info:** Calories 352 Total Fat 14 g Saturated Fat 2 g Cholesterol 65 mg Sodium 220 mg Total Carbs 15.8 g Fiber 0.2 g Sugar 1 g Protein 26 g

155. Turkey-stuffed Peppers

Servings: 6
Cooking Time: 35 Minutes
Ingredients:
- 1 pound lean ground turkey
- 1 tablespoon olive oil
- 2 cloves garlic, minced
- 1/3 onion, minced
- 1 tablespoon cilantro (optional)
- 1 teaspoon garlic powder
- 1 teaspoon cumin powder
- 1/2 teaspoon salt
- Pepper to taste
- 3 large red bell peppers
- 1 cup chicken broth
- 1/4 cup tomato sauce
- 1-1/2 cups cooked brown rice
- 1/4 cup shredded cheddar
- 6 green onions

Directions:
1. Start by preheating toaster oven to 400°F.
2. Heat a skillet on medium heat.
3. Add olive oil to the skillet, then mix in onion and garlic.
4. Sauté for about 5 minutes, or until the onion starts to look opaque.
5. Add the turkey to the skillet and season with cumin, garlic powder, salt, and pepper.
6. Brown the meat until thoroughly cooked, then mix in chicken broth and tomato sauce.
7. Reduce heat and simmer for about 5 minutes, stirring occasionally.
8. Add the brown rice and continue stirring until it is evenly spread through the mix.
9. Cut the bell peppers lengthwise down the middle and remove all of the seeds.
10. Grease a pan or line it with parchment paper and lay all peppers in the pan with the outside facing down.
11. Spoon the meat mixture evenly into each pepper and use the back of the spoon to level.
12. Bake for 30 minutes.
13. Remove pan from oven and sprinkle cheddar over each pepper, then put it back in for another 3 minutes, or until the cheese is melted.
14. While the cheese melts, dice the green onions. Remove pan from oven and sprinkle onions over each pepper and serve.
- **Nutrition Info:** Calories: 394, Sodium: 493 mg, Dietary Fiber: 4.1 g, Total Fat: 12.9 g, Total Carbs: 44.4 g, Protein: 27.7 g.

156. Spicy Green Crusted Chicken

Servings: 6
Cooking Time: 40 Minutes
Ingredients:
- 6 eggs, beaten
- 6 teaspoons parsley
- 4 teaspoons thyme
- 1 pound chicken pieces
- 6 teaspoons oregano
- Salt and freshly ground black pepper, to taste
- 4 teaspoons paprika

Directions:
1. Preheat the Air fryer to 360 degree F and grease an Air fryer basket.
2. Whisk eggs in a bowl and mix all the ingredients in another bowl except chicken pieces.
3. Dip the chicken in eggs and then coat generously with the dry mixture.
4. Arrange half of the chicken pieces in the Air fryer basket and cook for about 20 minutes.
5. Repeat with the remaining mixture and dish out to serve hot.
- **Nutrition Info:** Calories: 218, Fat: 10.4g, Carbohydrates: 2.6g, Sugar: 0.6g, Protein: 27.9g, Sodium: 128mg

157. Chicken & Rice Casserole

Servings: 6
Cooking Time: 40 Minutes
Ingredients:
- 2 lbs. bone-in chicken thighs

- Salt and black pepper
- 1 teaspoon olive oil
- 5 cloves garlic, chopped
- 2 large onions, chopped
- 2 large red bell peppers, chopped
- 1 tablespoon sweet Hungarian paprika
- 1 teaspoon hot Hungarian paprika
- 2 tablespoons tomato paste
- 2 cups chicken broth
- 3 cups brown rice, thawed
- 2 tablespoons parsley, chopped
- 6 tablespoons sour cream

Directions:
1. Mix broth, tomato paste, and all the spices in a bowl.
2. Add chicken and mix well to coat.
3. Spread the rice in a casserole dish and add chicken along with its marinade.
4. Top the casserole with the rest of the Ingredients:.
5. Press "Power Button" of Air Fry Oven and turn the dial to select the "Bake" mode.
6. Press the Time button and again turn the dial to set the cooking time to 40 minutes.
7. Now push the Temp button and rotate the dial to set the temperature at 350 degrees F.
8. Once preheated, place the baking pan inside and close its lid.
9. Serve warm.
- **Nutrition Info:** Calories 440 Total Fat 7.9 g Saturated Fat 1.8 g Cholesterol 5 mg Sodium 581 mg Total Carbs 21.8 g Sugar 7.1 g Fiber 2.6 g Protein 37.2 g

158.Roasted Delicata Squash With Kale

Servings: 2
Cooking Time: 10 Minutes
Ingredients:
- 1 medium delicata squash
- 1 bunch kale
- 1 clove garlic
- 2 tablespoons olive oil
- Salt and pepper

Directions:
1. Start by preheating toaster oven to 425°F.
2. Clean squash and cut off each end. Cut in half and remove the seeds. Quarter the halves.
3. Toss the squash in 1 tablespoon of olive oil.
4. Place the squash on a greased baking sheet and roast for 25 minutes, turning halfway through.
5. Rinse kale and remove stems. Chop garlic.
6. Heat the leftover oil in a medium skillet and add kale and salt to taste.
7. Sauté the kale until it darkens, then mix in the garlic.
8. Cook for another minute then remove from heat and add 2 tablespoons of water.

9. Remove squash from oven and lay it on top of the garlic kale.
10. Top with salt and pepper to taste and serve.
- **Nutrition Info:** Calories: 159, Sodium: 28 mg, Dietary Fiber: 1.8 g, Total Fat: 14.2 g, Total Carbs: 8.2 g, Protein: 2.6 g.

159.Coriander Potatoes

Servings: 4
Cooking Time: 25 Minutes
Ingredients:
- 1 pound gold potatoes, peeled and cut into wedges
- Salt and black pepper to the taste
- 1 tablespoon tomato sauce
- 2 tablespoons coriander, chopped
- ½ teaspoon garlic powder
- 1 teaspoon chili powder
- 1 tablespoon olive oil

Directions:
1. In a bowl, combine the potatoes with the tomato sauce and the other Ingredients:, toss, and transfer to the air fryer's basket.
2. Cook at 370 degrees F for 25 minutes, divide between plates and serve as a side dish.
- **Nutrition Info:** Calories 210, fat 5, fiber 7, carbs 12, protein 5

160.Herb-roasted Turkey Breast

Servings: 8
Cooking Time: 60 Minutes
Ingredients:
- 3 lb turkey breast
- Rub Ingredients:
- 2 tbsp olive oil
- 2 tbsp lemon juice
- 1 tbsp minced Garlic
- 2 tsp ground mustard
- 2 tsp kosher salt
- 1 tsp pepper
- 1 tsp dried rosemary
- 1 tsp dried thyme
- 1 tsp ground sage

Directions:
1. Take a small bowl and thoroughly combine the Rub Ingredients: in it. Rub this on the outside of the turkey breast and under any loose skin.
2. Place the coated turkey breast keeping skin side up on a cooking tray.
3. Place the drip pan at the bottom of the cooking chamber of the Instant Pot Duo Crisp Air Fryer. Select Air Fry option, post this, adjust the temperature to 360°F and the time to one hour, then touch start.
4. When preheated, add the food to the cooking tray in the lowest position. Close the lid for cooking.

5. When the Air Fry program is complete, check to make sure that the thickest portion of the meat reads at least 160°F, remove the turkey and let it rest for 10 minutes before slicing and serving.
- **Nutrition Info:** Calories 214, Total Fat 10g, Total Carbs 2g, Protein 29g

161.Roasted Fennel, Ditalini, And Shrimp

Servings: 4
Cooking Time: 30 Minutes
Ingredients:
- 1 pound extra large, thawed, tail-on shrimp
- 1 teaspoon fennel seeds
- 1 teaspoon salt
- 1 fennel bulb, halved and sliced crosswise
- 4 garlic cloves, chopped
- 2 tablespoons olive oil
- 1/2 teaspoon freshly ground black pepper
- Grated zest of 1 lemon
- 1/2 pound whole wheat ditalini

Directions:
1. Start by preheating toaster oven to 450°F.
2. Toast the seeds in a medium pan over medium heat for about 5 minutes, then toss with shrimp.
3. Add water and 1/2 teaspoon salt to the pan and bring the mixture to a boil.
4. Reduce heat and simmer for 30 minutes.
5. Combine fennel, garlic, oil, pepper, and remaining salt in a roasting pan.
6. Roast for 20 minutes, then add shrimp mixture and roast for another 5 minutes or until shrimp are cooked.
7. While the fennel is roasting, cook pasta per the directions on the package, drain, and set aside.
8. Remove the shrimp mixture and mix in pasta, roast for another 5 minutes.
- **Nutrition Info:** Calories: 420, Sodium: 890 mg, Dietary Fiber: 4.2 g, Total Fat: 10.2 g, Total Carbs: 49.5 g, Protein: 33.9 g.

162.Chicken And Celery Stew

Servings: 6
Cooking Time: 12 Minutes
Ingredients:
- 1 lb. chicken breasts, skinless; boneless and cubed
- 4 celery stalks; chopped.
- ½ cup coconut cream
- 2 red bell peppers; chopped.
- 2 tsp. garlic; minced
- 1 tbsp. butter, soft
- Salt and black pepper to taste.

Directions:
1. Grease a baking dish that fits your air fryer with the butter, add all the ingredients in the pan and toss them.

2. Introduce the dish in the fryer, cook at 360°F for 30 minutes, divide into bowls and serve
- **Nutrition Info:** Calories: 246; Fat: 12g; Fiber: 2g; Carbs: 6g; Protein: 12g

163.Lemon Pepper Turkey

Servings: 6
Cooking Time: 45 Minutes
Ingredients:
- 3 lbs. turkey breast
- 2 tablespoons oil
- 1 tablespoon Worcestershire sauce
- 1 teaspoon lemon pepper
- 1/2 teaspoon salt

Directions:
1. Whisk everything in a bowl and coat the turkey liberally.
2. Place the turkey in the Air fryer basket.
3. Press "Power Button" of Air Fry Oven and turn the dial to select the "Air Fry" mode.
4. Press the Time button and again turn the dial to set the cooking time to 45 minutes.
5. Now push the Temp button and rotate the dial to set the temperature at 375 degrees F.
6. Once preheated, place the air fryer basket inside and close its lid.
7. Serve warm.
- **Nutrition Info:** Calories 391 Total Fat 2.8 g Saturated Fat 0.6 g Cholesterol 330 mg Sodium 62 mg Total Carbs 36.5 g Fiber 9.2 g Sugar 4.5 g Protein 6.6

164.Creamy Green Beans And Tomatoes

Servings: 4
Cooking Time: 20 Minutes
Ingredients:
- 1 pound green beans, trimmed and halved
- ½ pound cherry tomatoes, halved
- 2 tablespoons olive oil
- 1 teaspoon oregano, dried
- 1 teaspoon basil, dried
- Salt and black pepper to the taste
- 1 cup heavy cream
- ½ tablespoon cilantro, chopped

Directions:
1. In your air fryer's pan, combine the green beans with the tomatoes and the other Ingredients:, toss and cook at 360 degrees F for 20 minutes.
2. Divide the mix between plates and serve.
- **Nutrition Info:** Calories 174, fat 5, fiber 7, carbs 11, protein 4

165.Crispy Breaded Pork Chop

Servings: 6
Cooking Time: 12 Minutes
Ingredients:
- olive oil spray

- 6 3/4-inch thick center-cut boneless pork chops, fat trimmed (5 oz each)
- kosher salt
- 1 large egg, beaten
- 1/2 cup panko crumbs, check labels for GF
- 1/3 cup crushed cornflakes crumbs
- 2 tbsp grated parmesan cheese
- 1 1/4 tsp sweet paprika
- 1/2 tsp garlic powder
- 1/2 tsp onion powder
- 1/4 tsp chili powder
- 1/8 tsp black pepper

Directions:
1. Preheat the Instant Pot Duo Crisp Air Fryer for 12 minutes at 400°F.
2. On both sides, season pork chops with half teaspoon kosher salt.
3. Then combine cornflake crumbs, panko, parmesan cheese, 3/4 tsp kosher salt, garlic powder, paprika, onion powder, chili powder, and black pepper in a large bowl.
4. Place the egg beat in another bowl. Dip the pork in the egg & then crumb mixture.
5. When the air fryer is ready, place 3 of the chops into the Instant Pot Duo Crisp Air Fryer Basket and spritz the top with oil.
6. Close the Air Fryer lid and cook for 12 minutes turning halfway, spritzing both sides with oil.
7. Set aside and repeat with the remaining.
- **Nutrition Info:** Calories 281, Total Fat 13g, Total Carbs 8g, Protein 33g

166.Pork Stew

Servings: 4
Cooking Time: 12 Minutes
Ingredients:
- 2 lb. pork stew meat; cubed
- 1 eggplant; cubed
- ½ cup beef stock
- 2 zucchinis; cubed
- ½ tsp. smoked paprika
- Salt and black pepper to taste.
- A handful cilantro; chopped.

Directions:
1. In a pan that fits your air fryer, mix all the ingredients, toss, introduce in your air fryer and cook at 370°F for 30 minutes
2. Divide into bowls and serve right away.
- **Nutrition Info:** Calories: 245; Fat: 12g; Fiber: 2g; Carbs: 5g; Protein: 14g

167.Garlic Chicken Potatoes

Servings: 4
Cooking Time: 30 Minutes
Ingredients:
- 2 lbs. red potatoes, quartered
- 3 tablespoons olive oil
- 1/2 teaspoon cumin seeds

- Salt and black pepper, to taste
- 4 garlic cloves, chopped
- 2 tablespoons brown sugar
- 1 lemon (1/2 juiced and 1/2 cut into wedges)
- Pinch of red pepper flakes
- 4 skinless, boneless chicken breasts
- 2 tablespoons cilantro, chopped

Directions:
1. Place the chicken, lemon, garlic, and potatoes in a baking pan.
2. Toss the spices, herbs, oil, and sugar in a bowl.
3. Add this mixture to the chicken and veggies then toss well to coat.
4. Press "Power Button" of Air Fry Oven and turn the dial to select the "Bake" mode.
5. Press the Time button and again turn the dial to set the cooking time to 30 minutes.
6. Now push the Temp button and rotate the dial to set the temperature at 400 degrees F.
7. Once preheated, place the baking pan inside and close its lid.
8. Serve warm.
- **Nutrition Info:** Calories 545 Total Fat 36.4 g Saturated Fat 10.1 g Cholesterol 200 mg Sodium 272 mg Total Carbs 40.7 g Fiber 0.2 g Sugar 0.1 g Protein 42.5 g

168.Basic Roasted Tofu

Servings: 4
Cooking Time: 45 Minutes
Ingredients:
- 1 or more (16-ounce) containers extra-firm tofu
- 1 tablespoon sesame oil
- 1 tablespoon soy sauce
- 1 tablespoon rice vinegar
- 1 tablespoon water

Directions:
1. Start by drying the tofu: first pat dry with paper towels, then lay on another set of paper towels or a dish towel.
2. Put a plate on top of the tofu then put something heavy on the plate (like a large can of vegetables). Leave it there for at least 20 minutes.
3. While tofu is being pressed, whip up marinade by combining oil, soy sauce, vinegar, and water in a bowl and set aside.
4. Cut the tofu into squares or sticks. Place the tofu in the marinade for at least 30 minutes.
5. Preheat toaster oven to 350°F. Line a pan with parchment paper and add as many pieces of tofu as you can, giving each piece adequate space.
6. Bake 20–45 minutes; tofu is done when the outside edges look golden brown. Time will vary depending on tofu size and shape.

- **Nutrition Info:** Calories: 114, Sodium: 239 mg, Dietary Fiber: 1.1 g, Total Fat: 8.1 g, Total Carbs: 2.2 g, Protein: 9.5 g.

169.Persimmon Toast With Sour Cream & Cinnamon

Servings: 1
Cooking Time: 5 Minutes
Ingredients:
- 1 slice of wheat bread
- 1/2 persimmon
- Sour cream to taste
- Sugar to taste
- Cinnamon to taste

Directions:
1. Spread a thin layer of sour cream across the bread.
2. Slice the persimmon into 1/4 inch pieces and lay them across the bread.
3. Sprinkle cinnamon and sugar over persimmon.
4. Toast in toaster oven until bread and persimmon begin to brown.
- **Nutrition Info:** Calories: 89, Sodium: 133 mg, Dietary Fiber: 2.0 g, Total Fat: 1.1 g, Total Carbs: 16.5 g, Protein: 3.8 g.

170.Okra Casserole

Servings: 4
Cooking Time: 12 Minutes
Ingredients:
- 2 red bell peppers; cubed
- 2 tomatoes; chopped.
- 3 garlic cloves; minced
- 3 cups okra
- ½ cup cheddar; shredded
- ¼ cup tomato puree
- 1 tbsp. cilantro; chopped.
- 1 tsp. olive oil
- 2 tsp. coriander, ground
- Salt and black pepper to taste.

Directions:
1. Grease a heat proof dish that fits your air fryer with the oil, add all the ingredients except the cilantro and the cheese and toss them really gently
2. Sprinkle the cheese and the cilantro on top, introduce the dish in the fryer and cook at 390°F for 20 minutes.
3. Divide between plates and serve for lunch.
- **Nutrition Info:** Calories: 221; Fat: 7g; Fiber: 2g; Carbs: 4g; Protein: 9g

171.Bbq Chicken Breasts

Servings: 4
Cooking Time: 15 Minutes
Ingredients:
- 4 boneless skinless chicken breast about 6 oz each
- 1-2 Tbsp bbq seasoning

Directions:
1. Cover both sides of chicken breast with the BBQ seasoning. Cover and marinate the in the refrigerator for 45 minutes.
2. Choose the Air Fry option and set the temperature to 400°F. Push start and let it preheat for 5 minutes.
3. Upon preheating, place the chicken breast in the Instant Pot Duo Crisp Air Fryer basket, making sure they do not overlap. Spray with oil.
4. Cook for 13-14 minutes
5. flipping halfway.
6. Remove chicken when the chicken reaches an internal temperature of 160°F. Place on a plate and allow to rest for 5 minutes before slicing.
- **Nutrition Info:** Calories 131, Total Fat 3g, Total Carbs 2g, Protein 24g

172.Crisp Chicken Casserole

Servings: 4
Cooking Time: 15 Minutes
Ingredients:
- 3 cup chicken, shredded
- 12 oz bag egg noodles
- 1/2 large onion
- 1/2 cup chopped carrots
- 1/4 cup frozen peas
- 1/4 cup frozen broccoli pieces
- 2 stalks celery chopped
- 5 cup chicken broth
- 1 tsp garlic powder
- salt and pepper to taste
- 1 cup cheddar cheese, shredded
- 1 package French's onions
- 1/4 cup sour cream
- 1 can cream of chicken and mushroom soup

Directions:
1. Place the chicken, vegetables, garlic powder, salt and pepper, and broth and stir. Then place it into the Instant Pot Duo Crisp Air Fryer Basket.
2. Press or lightly stir the egg noodles into the mix until damp/wet.
3. Select the option Air Fryer and cook for 4 minutes.
4. Stir in the sour cream, can of soup, cheese, and 1/3 of the French's onions.
5. Top with the remaining French's onions and close the Air Fryer lid and cook for about 10 more minutes.
- **Nutrition Info:** Calories 301, Total Fat 17g, Total Carbs 17g, Protein 20g

173.Saucy Chicken With Leeks

Servings: 6
Cooking Time: 10 Minutes

Ingredients:
- 2 leeks, sliced
- 2 large-sized tomatoes, chopped
- 3 cloves garlic, minced
- ½ teaspoon dried oregano
- 6 chicken legs, boneless and skinless
- ½ teaspoon smoked cayenne pepper
- 2 tablespoons olive oil
- A freshly ground nutmeg

Directions:
1. In a mixing dish, thoroughly combine all ingredients, minus the leeks. Place in the refrigerator and let it marinate overnight.
2. Lay the leeks onto the bottom of an Air Fryer cooking basket. Top with the chicken legs.
3. Roast chicken legs at 375 degrees F for 18 minutes, turning halfway through. Serve with hoisin sauce.
- **Nutrition Info:** 390 Calories; 16g Fat; 2g Carbs; 59g Protein; 8g Sugars; 4g Fiber

174.Air Fried Steak Sandwich

Servings: 4
Cooking Time: 16 Minutes
Ingredients:
- Large hoagie bun, sliced in half
- 6 ounces of sirloin or flank steak, sliced into bite-sized pieces
- ½ tablespoon of mustard powder
- ½ tablespoon of soy sauce
- 1 tablespoon of fresh bleu cheese, crumbled
- 8 medium-sized cherry tomatoes, sliced in half
- 1 cup of fresh arugula, rinsed and patted dry

Directions:
1. Preparing the ingredients. In a small mixing bowl, combine the soy sauce and onion powder; stir with a fork until thoroughly combined.
2. Lay the raw steak strips in the soy-mustard mixture, and fully immerse each piece to marinate.
3. Set the instant crisp air fryer to 320 degrees for 10 minutes.
4. Arrange the soy-mustard marinated steak pieces on a piece of tin foil, flat and not overlapping, and set the tin foil on one side of the instant crisp air fryer basket. The foil should not take up more than half of the surface.
5. Lay the hoagie-bun halves, crusty-side up and soft-side down, on the other half of the air-fryer.
6. Air frying. Close air fryer lid.
7. After 10 minutes, the instant crisp air fryer will shut off; the hoagie buns should be

starting to crisp and the steak will have begun to cook.
8. Carefully, flip the hoagie buns so they are now crusty-side down and soft-side up; crumble a layer of the bleu cheese on each hoagie half.
9. With a long spoon, gently stir the marinated steak in the foil to ensure even coverage.
10. Set the instant crisp air fryer to 360 degrees for 6 minutes.
11. After 6 minutes, when the fryer shuts off, the bleu cheese will be perfectly melted over the toasted bread, and the steak will be juicy on the inside and crispy on the outside.
12. Remove the cheesy hoagie halves first, using tongs, and set on a serving plate; then cover one side with the steak, and top with the cherry-tomato halves and the arugula. Close with the other cheesy hoagie-half, slice into two pieces, and enjoy.
- **Nutrition Info:** Calories 284 Total fat 7.9 g Saturated fat 1.4 g Cholesterol 36 mg Sodium 704 mg Total carbs 46 g Fiber 3.6 g Sugar 5.5 g Protein 17.9 g

175.Dijon And Swiss Croque Monsieur

Servings: 2
Cooking Time: 13 Minutes
Ingredients:
- 4 slices white bread
- 2 tablespoons unsalted butter
- 1 tablespoon all-purpose flour
- 1/2 cup whole milk
- 3/4 cups shredded Swiss cheese
- 1/4 teaspoon freshly ground black pepper
- 1/8 teaspoon salt
- 1 tablespoon Dijon mustard
- 4 slices ham

Directions:
1. Start by cutting crusts off bread and placing them on a pan lined with parchment paper.
2. Melt 1 tablespoon of butter in a sauce pan, then dab the top sides of each piece of bread with butter.
3. Toast bread inoven for 3-5 minutes until each piece is golden brown.
4. Melt the second tablespoon of butter in the sauce pan and add the flour, mix together until they form a paste.
5. Add the milk and continue to mix until the sauce begins to thicken.
6. Remove from heat and mix in 1 tablespoon of Swiss cheese, salt, and pepper; continue stirring until cheese is melted.
7. Flip the bread over in the pan so the untoasted side is facing up.
8. Set two slices aside and spread Dijon on the other two slices.
9. Add ham and sprinkle 1/4 cup Swiss over each piece.

10. Broil for about 3 minutes.
11. Top the sandwiches off with the other slices of bread, soft-side down.
12. Top with sauce and sprinkle with remaining Swiss. Toast for another 5 minutes or until the cheese is golden brown.
13. Serve immediately.
- **Nutrition Info:** Calories: 452, Sodium: 1273 mg, Dietary Fiber: 1.6 g, Total Fat: 30.5 g, Total Carbs: 19.8 g, Protein: 24.4 g.

176.Sweet Potato And Parsnip Spiralized Latkes

Servings: 12
Cooking Time: 20 Minutes
Ingredients:
- 1 medium sweet potato
- 1 large parsnip
- 4 cups water
- 1 egg + 1 egg white
- 2 scallions
- 1/2 teaspoon garlic powder
- 1/2 teaspoon sea salt
- 1/2 teaspoon ground pepper

Directions:
1. Start by spiralizing the sweet potato and parsnip and chopping the scallions, reserving only the green parts.
2. Preheat toaster oven to 425°F.
3. Bring 4 cups of water to a boil. Place all of your noodles in a colander and pour the boiling water over the top, draining well.
4. Let the noodles cool, then grab handfuls and place them in a paper towel; squeeze to remove as much liquid as possible.
5. In a large bowl, beat egg and egg white together. Add noodles, scallions, garlic powder, salt, and pepper, mix well.
6. Prepare a baking sheet; scoop out 1/4 cup of mixture at a time and place on sheet.
7. Slightly press down each scoop with your hands, then bake for 20 minutes, flipping halfway through.
- **Nutrition Info:** Calories: 24, Sodium: 91 mg, Dietary Fiber: 1.0 g, Total Fat: 0.4 g, Total Carbs: 4.3 g, Protein: 0.9 g.

177.Coriander Artichokes(3)

Servings: 4
Cooking Time: 12 Minutes
Ingredients:
- 12 oz. artichoke hearts
- 1 tbsp. lemon juice
- 1 tsp. coriander, ground
- ½ tsp. cumin seeds
- ½ tsp. olive oil
- Salt and black pepper to taste.

Directions:

1. In a pan that fits your air fryer, mix all the ingredients, toss, introduce the pan in the fryer and cook at 370°F for 15 minutes
2. Divide the mix between plates and serve as a side dish.
- **Nutrition Info:** Calories: 200; Fat: 7g; Fiber: 2g; Carbs: 5g; Protein: 8g

178.Eggplant And Leeks Stew

Servings: 4
Cooking Time: 12 Minutes
Ingredients:
- 2 big eggplants, roughly cubed
- ½ bunch cilantro; chopped.
- 1 cup veggie stock
- 2 garlic cloves; minced
- 3 leeks; sliced
- 2 tbsp. olive oil
- 1 tbsp. hot sauce
- 1 tbsp. sweet paprika
- 1 tbsp. tomato puree
- Salt and black pepper to taste.

Directions:
1. In a pan that fits the air fryer, mix all the ingredients, toss, introduce in the fryer and cook at 380°F for 20 minutes
2. Divide the stew into bowls and serve for lunch.
- **Nutrition Info:** Calories: 183; Fat: 4g; Fiber: 2g; Carbs: 4g; Protein: 12g

179.Turkey Meatballs With Manchego Cheese

Servings: 4
Cooking Time: 10 Minutes
Ingredients:
- 1 pound ground turkey
- 1/2 pound ground pork
- 1 egg, well beaten
- 1 teaspoon dried basil
- 1 teaspoon dried rosemary
- 1/4 cup Manchego cheese, grated
- 2 tablespoons yellow onions, finely chopped
- 1 teaspoon fresh garlic, finely chopped
- Sea salt and ground black pepper, to taste

Directions:
1. In a mixing bowl, combine all the ingredients until everything is well incorporated.
2. Shape the mixture into 1-inch balls.
3. Cook the meatballs in the preheated Air Fryer at 380 degrees for 7 minutes. Shake halfway through the cooking time. Work in batches.
4. Serve with your favorite pasta.
- **Nutrition Info:** 386 Calories; 24g Fat; 9g Carbs; 41g Protein; 3g Sugars; 2g Fiber

180.Butter Fish With Sake And Miso

Servings: 4
Cooking Time: 11 Minutes
Ingredients:

- 4 (7-ounce) pieces of butter fish
- 1/3 cup sake
- 1/3 cup mirin
- 2/3 cup sugar
- 1 cup white miso

Directions:

1. Start by combining sake, mirin, and sugar in a sauce pan and bring to a boil.
2. Allow to boil for 5 minutes, then reduce heat and simmer for another 10 minutes.
3. Remove from heat completely and mix in miso.
4. Marinate the fish in the mixture for as long as possible, up to 3 days if possible.
5. Preheat toaster oven to 450°F and bake fish for 8 minutes.
6. Switch your setting to Broil and broil another 2-3 minutes, until the sauce is caramelized.
- **Nutrition Info:** Calories: 529, Sodium: 2892 mg, Dietary Fiber: 3.7 g, Total Fat: 5.8 g, Total Carbs: 61.9 g, Protein: 53.4 g.

181.Chicken Breast With Rosemary

Servings: 4
Cooking Time: 60 Minutes
Ingredients:

- 4 bone-in chicken breast halves
- 3 tablespoons softened butter
- 1/2 teaspoon salt
- 1/4 teaspoon pepper
- 1 tablespoon rosemary
- 1 tablespoon extra-virgin olive oil

Directions:

1. Start by preheating toaster oven to 400°F.
2. Mix butter, salt, pepper, and rosemary in a bowl.
3. Coat chicken with the butter mixture and place in a shallow pan.
4. Drizzle oil over chicken and roast for 25 minutes.
5. Flip chicken and roast for another 20 minutes.
6. Flip chicken one more time and roast for a final 15 minutes.
- **Nutrition Info:** Calories: 392, Sodium: 551 mg, Dietary Fiber: 0 g, Total Fat: 18.4 g, Total Carbs: 0.6 g, Protein: 55.4 g.

182.Seven-layer Tostadas

Servings: 6
Cooking Time: 5 Minutes
Ingredients:

- 1 (16-ounce) can refried pinto beans
- 1-1/2 cups guacamole
- 1 cup light sour cream
- 1/2 teaspoon taco seasoning
- 1 cup shredded Mexican cheese blend
- 1 cup chopped tomatoes
- 1/2 cup thinly sliced green onions
- 1/2 cup sliced black olives
- 6-8 whole wheat flour tortillas small enough to fit in your oven
- Olive oil

Directions:

1. Start by placing baking sheet into toaster oven while preheating it to 450°F. Remove pan and drizzle with olive oil.
2. Place tortillas on pan and cook in oven until they are crisp, turn at least once, this should take about 5 minutes or less.
3. In a medium bowl, mash refried beans to break apart any chunks, then microwave for 2 1/2 minutes.
4. Stir taco seasoning into the sour cream. Chop vegetables and halve olives.
5. Top tortillas with ingredients in this order: refried beans, guacamole, sour cream, shredded cheese, tomatoes, onions, and olives.
- **Nutrition Info:** Calories: 657, Sodium: 581 mg, Dietary Fiber: 16.8 g, Total Fat: 31.7 g, Total Carbs: 71.3 g, Protein: 28.9 g.

183.Onion Omelet

Servings: 2
Cooking Time: 15 Minutes
Ingredients:

- 4 eggs
- ¼ teaspoon low-sodium soy sauce
- Ground black pepper, as required
- 1 teaspoon butter
- 1 medium yellow onion, sliced
- ¼ cup Cheddar cheese, grated

Directions:

1. In a skillet, melt the butter over medium heat and cook the onion and cook for about 8-10 minutes.
2. Remove from the heat and set aside to cool slightly.
3. Meanwhile, in a bowl, add the eggs, soy sauce and black pepper and beat well.
4. Add the cooked onion and gently, stir to combine.
5. Place the zucchini mixture into a small baking pan.
6. Press "Power Button" of Air Fry Oven and turn the dial to select the "Air Fry" mode.
7. Press the Time button and again turn the dial to set the cooking time to 5 minutes.
8. Now push the Temp button and rotate the dial to set the temperature at 355 degrees F.
9. Press "Start/Pause" button to start.

10. When the unit beeps to show that it is preheated, open the lid.
11. Arrange pan over the "Wire Rack" and insert in the oven.
12. Cut the omelet into 2 portions and serve hot.
- **Nutrition Info:** Calories: 222 Cal Total Fat: 15.4 g Saturated Fat: 6.9 g Cholesterol: 347 mg Sodium: 264 mg Total Carbs: 6.1 g Fiber: 1.2 g Sugar: 3.1 g Protein: 15.3 g

184.Rosemary Lemon Chicken

Servings: 8
Cooking Time: 45 Minutes
Ingredients:
- 4-lb. chicken, cut into pieces
- Salt and black pepper, to taste
- Flour for dredging 3 tablespoons olive oil
- 1 large onion, sliced
- Peel of ½ lemon
- 2 large garlic cloves, minced
- 1 1/2 teaspoons rosemary leaves
- 1 tablespoon honey
- 1/4 cup lemon juice
- 1 cup chicken broth

Directions:
1. Dredges the chicken through the flour then place in the baking pan.
2. Whisk broth with the rest of the Ingredients: in a bowl.
3. Pour this mixture over the dredged chicken in the pan.
4. Press "Power Button" of Air Fry Oven and turn the dial to select the "Bake" mode.
5. Press the Time button and again turn the dial to set the cooking time to 45 minutes.
6. Now push the Temp button and rotate the dial to set the temperature at 400 degrees F.
7. Once preheated, place the baking pan inside and close its lid.
8. Baste the chicken with its sauce every 15 minutes.
9. Serve warm.
- **Nutrition Info:** Calories 405 Total Fat 22.7 g Saturated Fat 6.1 g Cholesterol 4 mg Sodium 227 mg Total Carbs 26.1 g Fiber 1.4 g Sugar 0.9 g Protein 45.2 g

185.Portobello Pesto Burgers

Servings: 4
Cooking Time: 26 Minutes
Ingredients:
- 4 portobello mushrooms
- 1/4 cup sundried tomato pesto
- 4 whole-grain hamburger buns
- 1 large ripe tomato

- 1 log fresh goat cheese
- 8 large fresh basil leaves

Directions:
1. Start by preheating toaster oven to 425°F.
2. Place mushrooms on a pan, round sides facing up.
3. Bake for 14 minutes.
4. Pull out tray, flip the mushrooms and spread 1 tablespoon of pesto on each piece.
5. Return to oven and bake for another 10 minutes.
6. Remove the mushrooms and toast the buns for 2 minutes.
7. Remove the buns and build the burger by placing tomatoes, mushroom, 2 slices of cheese, and a sprinkle of basil, then topping with the top bun.
- **Nutrition Info:** Calories: 297, Sodium: 346 mg, Dietary Fiber: 1.8 g, Total Fat: 18.1 g, Total Carbs: 19.7 g, Protein: 14.4 g.

186.Easy Italian Meatballs

Servings: 4
Cooking Time: 13 Minutes
Ingredients:
- 2-lb. lean ground turkey
- ¼ cup onion, minced
- 2 cloves garlic, minced
- 2 tablespoons parsley, chopped
- 2 eggs
- 1½ cup parmesan cheese, grated
- ½ teaspoon red pepper flakes
- ½ teaspoon Italian seasoning Salt and black pepper to taste

Directions:
1. Toss all the meatball Ingredients: in a bowl and mix well.
2. Make small meatballs out this mixture and place them in the air fryer basket.
3. Press "Power Button" of Air Fry Oven and turn the dial to select the "Air Fry" mode.
4. Press the Time button and again turn the dial to set the cooking time to 13 minutes.
5. Now push the Temp button and rotate the dial to set the temperature at 350 degrees F.
6. Once preheated, place the air fryer basket inside and close its lid.
7. Flip the meatballs when cooked halfway through.
8. Serve warm.
- **Nutrition Info:** Calories 472 Total Fat 25.8 g Saturated Fat .4 g Cholesterol 268 mg Sodium 503 mg Total Carbs 1.7 g Fiber 0.3 g Sugar 0.6 g Protein 59.6 g

DINNER RECIPES

187. Christmas Filet Mignon Steak

Servings: 6
Cooking Time: 20 Minutes
Ingredients:
- 1/3 stick butter, at room temperature
- 1/2 cup heavy cream
- 1/2 medium-sized garlic bulb, peeled and pressed
- 6 filet mignon steaks
- 2 teaspoons mixed peppercorns, freshly cracked
- 1 ½ tablespoons apple cider
- A dash of hot sauce
- 1 ½ teaspoons sea salt flakes

Directions:
1. Season the mignon steaks with the cracked peppercorns and salt flakes. Roast the mignon steaks in the preheated Air Fryer for 24 minutes at 385 degrees F, turning once. Check for doneness and set aside, keeping it warm.
2. In a small nonstick saucepan that is placed over a moderate flame, mash the garlic to a smooth paste. Whisk in the rest of the above ingredients. Whisk constantly until it has a uniform consistency.
3. To finish, lay the filet mignon steaks on serving plates; spoon a little sauce onto each filet mignon.
- **Nutrition Info:** 452 Calories; 32g Fat; 8g Carbs; 26g Protein; 6g Sugars; 1g Fiber

188. Roasted Butternut Squash With Brussels Sprouts & Sweet Potato Noodles

Servings: 2
Cooking Time: 15 Minutes
Ingredients:
- Squash:
- 3 cups chopped butternut squash
- 2 teaspoons extra light olive oil
- 1/8 teaspoon sea salt
- Veggies:
- 5-6 Brussels sprouts
- 5 fresh shiitake mushrooms
- 2 cloves garlic
- 1/2 teaspoon black sesame seeds
- 1/2 teaspoon white sesame seeds
- A few sprinkles ground pepper
- A small pinch red pepper flakes
- 1 tablespoon extra light olive oil
- 1 teaspoon sesame oil
- 1 teaspoon onion powder
- 1 teaspoon garlic powder
- 1/4 teaspoon sea salt
- Noodles:
- 1 bundle sweet potato vermicelli
- 2-3 teaspoons low-sodium soy sauce

Directions:
1. Start by soaking potato vermicelli in water for at least 2 hours.
2. Preheat toaster oven to 375°F.
3. Place squash on a baking sheet with edges, then drizzle with olive oil and sprinkle with salt and pepper. Mix together well on pan.
4. Bake the squash for 30 minutes, mixing and flipping half way through.
5. Remove the stems from the mushrooms and chop the Brussels sprouts.
6. Chop garlic and mix the veggies.
7. Drizzle sesame and olive oil over the mixture, then add garlic powder, onion powder, sesame seeds, red pepper flakes, salt, and pepper.
8. Bake veggie mix for 15 minutes.
9. While the veggies bake, put noodles in a small sauce pan and add just enough water to cover.
10. Bring water to a rolling boil and boil noodles for about 8 minutes.
11. Drain noodles and combine with squash and veggies in a large bowl.
12. Drizzle with soy sauce, sprinkle with sesame seeds, and serve.
- **Nutrition Info:** Calories: 409, Sodium: 1124 mg, Dietary Fiber: 12.2 g, Total Fat: 15.6 g, Total Carbs: 69.3 g, Protein: 8.8 g.

189. Irish Whisky Steak

Servings: 6
Cooking Time: 20 Minutes
Ingredients:
- 2 pounds sirloin steaks
- 1 ½ tablespoons tamari sauce
- 1/3 teaspoon cayenne pepper
- 1/3 teaspoon ground ginger
- 2 garlic cloves, thinly sliced
- 2 tablespoons Irish whiskey
- 2 tablespoons olive oil
- Fine sea salt, to taste

Directions:
1. Firstly, add all the ingredients, minus the olive oil and the steak, to a resealable plastic bag.
2. Throw in the steak and let it marinate for a couple of hours. After that, drizzle the sirloin steaks with 2 tablespoons olive oil.
3. Roast for approximately 22 minutes at 395 degrees F, turning it halfway through the time.
- **Nutrition Info:** 260 Calories; 17g Fat; 8g Carbs; 35g Protein; 2g Sugars; 1g Fiber

190.Chinese-style Spicy And Herby Beef

Servings: 4
Cooking Time: 20 Minutes
Ingredients:
- 1 pound flank steak, cut into small pieces
- 1 teaspoon fresh sage leaves, minced
- 1/3 cup olive oil
- 3 teaspoons sesame oil
- 3 tablespoons Shaoxing wine
- 2 tablespoons tamari
- 1 teaspoon hot sauce
- 1/8 teaspoon xanthum gum
- 1 teaspoon seasoned salt
- 3 cloves garlic,minced
- 1 teaspoon fresh rosemary leaves, finely minced
- 1/2 teaspoon freshly cracked black pepper

Directions:
1. Warm the oil in a sauté pan over a moderate heat. Now, sauté the garlic until just tender and fragrant.
2. Now, add the remaining ingredients. Toss to coat well.
3. Then, roast for about 18 minutes at 345 degrees F. Check doneness and serve warm.
- **Nutrition Info:** 354 Calories; 24g Fat; 8g Carbs; 21g Protein; 3g Sugars; 3g Fiber

191.Grandma's Meatballs With Spicy Sauce

Servings: 4
Cooking Time: 20 Minutes
Ingredients:
- 4 tablespoons pork rinds
- 1/3 cup green onion
- 1 pound beef sausage meat
- 3 garlic cloves, minced
- 1/3 teaspoon ground black pepper
- Sea salt, to taste
- For the sauce:
- 2 tablespoons Worcestershire sauce
- 1/3 yellow onion, minced
- Dash of Tabasco sauce
- 1/3 cup tomato paste
- 1 teaspoon cumin powder
- 1/2 tablespoon balsamic vinegar

Directions:
1. Knead all of the above ingredients until everything is well incorporated.
2. Roll into balls and cook in the preheated Air Fryer at 365 degrees for 13 minutes.
3. In the meantime, in a saucepan, cook the ingredients for the sauce until thoroughly warmed. Serve your meatballs with the tomato sauce and enjoy!
- **Nutrition Info:** 360 Calories; 23g Fat; 6g Carbs; 23g Protein; 4g Sugars; 2g Fiber

192.Pesto & White Wine Salmon

Servings: 4
Cooking Time: 10 Minutes
Ingredients:
- 1-1/4 pounds salmon filet
- 2 tablespoons white wine
- 2 tablespoons pesto
- 1 lemon

Directions:
1. Cut the salmon into 4 pieces and place on a greased baking sheet.
2. Slice the lemon into quarters and squeeze 1 quarter over each piece of salmon.
3. Drizzle wine over salmon and set aside to marinate while preheating the toaster oven on broil.
4. Spread pesto over each piece of salmon.
5. Broil for at least 10 minutes, or until the fish is cooked to desired doneness and the pesto is browned.
- **Nutrition Info:** Calories: 236, Sodium: 111 mg, Dietary Fiber: 0.9 g, Total Fat: 12.1 g, Total Carbs: 3.3 g, Protein: 28.6 g.

193.Scallops With Capers Sauce

Servings: 2
Cooking Time: 6 Minutes
Ingredients:
- 10: 1-ouncesea scallops, cleaned and patted very dry
- 2 tablespoons fresh parsley, finely chopped
- 2 teaspoons capers, finely chopped
- Salt and ground black pepper, as required
- ¼ cup extra-virgin olive oil
- 1 teaspoon fresh lemon zest, finely grated
- ½ teaspoon garlic, finely chopped

Directions:
1. Preheat the Air fryer to 390 degree F and grease an Air fryer basket.
2. Season the scallops evenly with salt and black pepper.
3. Arrange the scallops in the Air fryer basket and cook for about 6 minutes.
4. Mix parsley, capers, olive oil, lemon zest and garlic in a bowl.
5. Dish out the scallops in a platter and top with capers sauce.
- **Nutrition Info:** Calories: 344, Fat: 26.3g, Carbohydrates: 4.2g, Sugar: 0.1g, Protein: 24g, Sodium: 393mg

194.Hasselback Potatoes

Servings: 4
Cooking Time: 30 Minutes
Ingredients:
- 4 potatoes
- 2 tablespoons Parmesan cheese, shredded
- 1 tablespoon fresh chives, chopped
- 2 tablespoons olive oil

Directions:
1. Preheat the Air fryer to 355 ºF and grease an Air fryer basket.
2. Cut slits along each potato about ¼-inch apart with a sharp knife, making sure slices should stay connected at the bottom.
3. Coat the potatoes with olive oil and arrange into the Air fryer basket.
4. Cook for about 30 minutes and dish out in a platter.
5. Top with chives and Parmesan cheese to serve.
- **Nutrition Info:** Calories: 218, Fat: 7.9g, Carbohydrates: 33.6g, Sugar: 2.5g, Protein: 4.6g, Sodium: 55mg

195.Crumbly Oat Meatloaf

Servings: 8
Cooking Time: 60 Minutes
Ingredients:
- 2 lbs. ground beef
- 1 cup of salsa
- 3/4 cup Quaker Oats
- 1/2 cup chopped onion
- 1 large egg, beaten
- 1 tablespoon Worcestershire sauce
- Salt and black pepper to taste

Directions:
1. Thoroughly mix ground beef with salsa, oats, onion, egg, and all the ingredients in a bowl.
2. Grease a meatloaf pan with oil or butter and spread the minced beef in the pan.
3. Press "Power Button" of Air Fry Oven and turn the dial to select the "Bake" mode.
4. Press the Time button and again turn the dial to set the cooking time to 60 minutes.
5. Now push the Temp button and rotate the dial to set the temperature at 350 degrees F.
6. Once preheated, place the beef baking pan in the oven and close its lid.
7. Slice and serve.
- **Nutrition Info:** Calories: 412 Cal Total Fat: 24.8 g Saturated Fat: 12.4 g Cholesterol: 3 mg Sodium: 132 mg Total Carbs: 43.8 g Fiber: 3.9 g Sugar: 2.5 g Protein: 18.9 g

196.Salsa Stuffed Eggplants

Servings: 2
Cooking Time: 25 Minutes
Ingredients:
- 1 large eggplant
- 8 cherry tomatoes, quartered
- ½ tablespoon fresh parsley
- 2 teaspoons olive oil, divided
- 2 teaspoons fresh lemon juice, divided
- 2 tablespoons tomato salsa
- Salt and black pepper, as required

Directions:

1. Preheat the Air fryer to 390 degree F and grease an Air fryer basket.
2. Arrange the eggplant into the Air fryer basket and cook for about 15 minutes.
3. Cut the eggplant in half lengthwise and drizzle evenly with one teaspoon of oil.
4. Set the Air fryer to 355 degree F and arrange the eggplant into the Air fryer basket, cut-side up.
5. Cook for another 10 minutes and dish out in a bowl.
6. Scoop out the flesh from the eggplant and transfer into a bowl.
7. Stir in the tomatoes, salsa, parsley, salt, black pepper, remaining oil, and lemon juice.
8. Squeeze lemon juice on the eggplant halves and stuff with the salsa mixture to serve.
- **Nutrition Info:** Calories: 192, Fat: 6.1g, Carbohydrates: 33.8g, Sugar: 20.4g, Protein: 6.9g, Sodium: 204mg

197.Green Beans And Mushroom Casserole

Servings: 6
Cooking Time: 12 Minutes
Ingredients:
- 24 ounces fresh green beans, trimmed
- 2 cups fresh button mushrooms, sliced
- 1/3 cup French fried onions
- 3 tablespoons olive oil
- 2 tablespoons fresh lemon juice
- 1 teaspoon ground sage
- 1 teaspoon garlic powder
- 1 teaspoon onion powder
- Salt and black pepper, to taste

Directions:
1. Preheat the Air fryer to 400 ºF and grease an Air fryer basket.
2. Mix the green beans, mushrooms, oil, lemon juice, sage, and spices in a bowl and toss to coat well.
3. Arrange the green beans mixture into the Air fryer basket and cook for about 12 minutes.
4. Dish out in a serving dish and top with fried onions to serve.
- **Nutrition Info:** Calories: 65, Fat: 1.6g, Carbohydrates: 11g, Sugar: 2.4g, Protein: 3g, Sodium: 52mg

198.Baby Portabellas With Romano Cheese

Servings: 4
Cooking Time: 20 Minutes
Ingredients:
- 1 pound baby portabellas
- 1/2 cup almond meal
- 2 eggs
- 2 tablespoons milk

- 1 cup Romano cheese, grated
- Sea salt and ground black pepper
- 1/2 teaspoon shallot powder
- 1 teaspoon garlic powder
- 1/2 teaspoon cumin powder
- 1/2 teaspoon cayenne pepper

Directions:
1. Pat the mushrooms dry with a paper towel.
2. To begin, set up your breading station. Place the almond meal in a shallow dish. In a separate dish, whisk the eggs with milk.
3. Finally, place grated Romano cheese and seasonings in the third dish.
4. Start by dredging the baby portabellas in the almond meal mixture; then, dip them into the egg wash. Press the baby portabellas into Romano cheese, coating evenly.
5. Spritz the Air Fryer basket with cooking oil. Add the baby portabellas and cook at 400 degrees F for 6 minutes, flipping them halfway through the cooking time.
- **Nutrition Info:** 230 Calories; 13g Fat; 2g Carbs; 11g Protein; 8g Sugars; 6g Fiber

199.Sesame Seeds Bok Choy

Servings: 4
Cooking Time: 6 Minutes
Ingredients:
- 4 bunches baby bok choy, bottoms removed and leaves separated
- 1 teaspoon sesame seeds
- Olive oil cooking spray
- 1 teaspoon garlic powder

Directions:
1. Preheat the Air fryer to 325 ºF and grease an Air fryer basket.
2. Arrange the bok choy leaves into the Air fryer basket and spray with the cooking spray.
3. Sprinkle with garlic powder and cook for about 6 minutes, shaking twice in between.
4. Dish out in the bok choy onto serving plates and serve garnished with sesame seeds.
- **Nutrition Info:** Calories: 26, Fat: 0.7g, Carbohydrates: 4g, Sugar: 1.9g, Protein: 2.5g, Sodium: 98mg

200.Creamy Lemon Turkey

Servings: 4
Cooking Time: 20 Minutes
Ingredients:
- 1/3 cup sour cream
- 2 cloves garlic, finely minced 1/3 tsp. lemon zest
- 2 small-sized turkey breasts, skinless and cubed 1/3 cup thickened cream
- 2 tablespoons lemon juice
- 1 tsp. fresh marjoram, chopped

- Salt and freshly cracked mixed peppercorns, to taste 1/2 cup scallion, chopped
- 1/2 can tomatoes, diced
- 1½ tablespoons canola oil

Directions:
1. Firstly, pat dry the turkey breast. Mix the remaining items; marinate the turkey for 2 hours.
2. Set the air fryer to cook at 355 ºF. Brush the turkey with a nonstick spray; cook for 23 minutes, turning once. Serve with naan and enjoy!
- **Nutrition Info:** 260 Calories; 15.3g Fat; 8.9g Carbs; 28.6g Protein; 1.9g Sugars

201.Almond Pork Bites

Servings: 10
Cooking Time: 40 Minutes
Ingredients:
- 16 oz sausage meat
- 1 whole egg, beaten
- 3 ½ oz onion, chopped
- 2 tbsp dried sage
- 2 tbsp almonds, chopped
- ½ tsp pepper
- 3 ½ oz apple, sliced
- ½ tsp salt

Directions:
1. Preheat your air fryer to 350 f. In a bowl, mix onion, almonds, sliced apples, egg, pepper and salt. Add the almond mixture and sausage in a ziploc bag. Mix to coat well and set aside for 15 minutes.
2. Use the mixture to form cutlets. Add cutlets to your fryer's basket and cook for 25 minutes. Serve with heavy cream and enjoy!
- **Nutrition Info:** Calories: 491.7 Cal Total Fat: 25.9 g Saturated Fat: 4.4 g Cholesterol: 42 mg Sodium: 364.3 mg Total Carbs: 40.4 g Fiber: 3.3 g Sugar: 0.7 g Protein: 21.8 g

202.Almond Asparagus

Servings: 3
Cooking Time: 6 Minutes
Ingredients:
- 1 pound asparagus
- 1/3 cup almonds, sliced
- 2 tablespoons olive oil
- 2 tablespoons balsamic vinegar
- Salt and black pepper, to taste

Directions:
1. Preheat the Air fryer to 400 ºF and grease an Air fryer basket.
2. Mix asparagus, oil, vinegar, salt, and black pepper in a bowl and toss to coat well.
3. Arrange asparagus into the Air fryer basket and sprinkle with the almond slices.
4. Cook for about 6 minutes and dish out to serve hot.

- **Nutrition Info:** Calories: 173, Fat: 14.8g, Carbohydrates: 8.2g, Sugar: 3.3g, Protein: 5.6g, Sodium: 54mg

203.Steak With Cascabel-garlic Sauce

Servings: 4
Cooking Time: 20 Minutes
Ingredients:
- 2 teaspoons brown mustard
- 2 tablespoons mayonnaise
- 1 ½ pounds beef flank steak, trimmed and cubed
- 2 teaspoons minced cascabel
- ½ cup scallions, finely chopped
- 1/3 cup Crème fraîche
- 2 teaspoons cumin seeds
- 3 cloves garlic, pressed
- Pink peppercorns to taste, freshly cracked
- 1 teaspoon fine table salt
- 1/3 teaspoon black pepper, preferably freshly ground

Directions:
1. Firstly, fry the cumin seeds just about 1 minute or until they pop.
2. After that, season your beef flank steak with fine table salt, black pepper and the fried cumin seeds; arrange the seasoned beef cubes on the bottom of your baking dish that fits in the air fryer.
3. Throw in the minced cascabel, garlic, and scallions; air-fry approximately 8 minutes at 390 degrees F.
4. Once the beef cubes start to tender, add your favorite mayo, Crème fraîche, freshly cracked pink peppercorns and mustard; air-fry 7 minutes longer. Serve over hot wild rice.
- **Nutrition Info:** 329 Calories; 16g Fat; 8g Carbs; 37g Protein; 9g Sugars; 6g Fiber

204.Salmon Steak Grilled With Cilantro Garlic Sauce

Servings: 2
Cooking Time: 15 Minutes
Ingredients:
- 2 salmon steaks
- Salt and pepper to taste
- 2 tablespoons vegetable oil
- 2 cloves of garlic, minced
- 1 cup cilantro leaves
- ½ cup Greek yogurt
- 1 teaspoon honey

Directions:
1. Place the instant pot air fryer lid on and preheat the instant pot at 390 degrees F.
2. Place the grill pan accessory in the instant pot.
3. Season the salmon steaks with salt and pepper. Brush with oil.
4. Place on the grill pan, close the air fryer lid and grill for 15 minutes and make sure to flip halfway through the cooking time.
5. In a food processor, mix the garlic, cilantro leaves, yogurt, and honey. Season with salt and pepper to taste. Pulse until smooth.
6. Serve the salmon steaks with the cilantro sauce.
- **Nutrition Info:** Calories: 485; Carbs: 6.3g; Protein: 47.6g; Fat: 29.9g

205.Sautéed Green Beans

Servings: 2
Cooking Time: 10 Minutes
Ingredients:
- 8 ounces fresh green beans, trimmed and cut in half
- 1 teaspoon sesame oil
- 1 tablespoon soy sauce

Directions:
1. Preheat the Air fryer to 390 ºF and grease an Air fryer basket.
2. Mix green beans, soy sauce, and sesame oil in a bowl and toss to coat well.
3. Arrange green beans into the Air fryer basket and cook for about 10 minutes, tossing once in between.
4. Dish out onto serving plates and serve hot.
- **Nutrition Info:** Calories: 59, Fats: 2.4g, Carbohydrates: 59g, Sugar: 1.7g, Proteins: 2.6g, Sodium: 458mg

206.Fennel & Tomato Chicken Paillard

Servings: 1
Cooking Time: 12 Minutes
Ingredients:
- 1/4 cup olive oil
- 1 boneless skinless chicken breast
- Salt and pepper
- 1 garlic clove, thinly sliced
- 1 small diced Roma tomato
- 1/2 fennel bulb, shaved
- 1/4 cup sliced mushrooms
- 2 tablespoons sliced black olives
- 1-1/2 teaspoons capers
- 2 sprigs fresh thyme
- 1 tablespoon chopped fresh parsley

Directions:
1. Start by pounding the chicken until it is about 1/2-inch thick.
2. Preheat the toaster oven to 400°F and brush the bottom of a baking pan with olive oil.
3. Sprinkle salt and pepper on both sides of the chicken and place it in the baking pan.
4. In a bowl, mix together all other ingredients, including the remaining olive oil.
5. Spoon mixture over chicken and bake for 12 minutes.

- **Nutrition Info:** Calories: 797, Sodium: 471 mg, Dietary Fiber: 6.0 g, Total Fat: 63.7 g, Total Carbs: 16.4 g, Protein: 45.8 g.

207.Shrimps, Zucchini, And Tomatoes On The Grill

Servings: 2
Cooking Time: 15 Minutes
Ingredients:
- 10 jumbo shrimps, peeled and deveined
- Salt and pepper to taste
- 1 clove of garlic, minced
- 1 medium zucchini, sliced
- 1-pint cherry tomatoes
- ¼ cup feta cheese

Directions:
1. Place the instant pot air fryer lid on and preheat the instant pot at 390 degrees F.
2. Place the grill pan accessory in the instant pot.
3. In a mixing bowl, season the shrimps with salt and pepper. Stir in the garlic, zucchini, and tomatoes.
4. Place on the grill pan, close the air fryer lid and cook for 15 minutes.
5. Once cooked, transfer to a bowl and sprinkle with feta cheese.
- **Nutrition Info:** Calories: 257; Carbs:4.2 g; Protein: 48.9g; Fat: 5.3g

208.Amazing Bacon And Potato Platter

Servings: 4
Cooking Time: 40 Minutes
Ingredients:
- 4 potatoes, halved
- 6 garlic cloves, squashed
- 4 streaky cut rashers bacon
- 2 sprigs rosemary
- 1 tbsp olive oil

Directions:
1. Preheat your air fryer to 392 f. In a mixing bowl, mix garlic, bacon, potatoes and rosemary; toss in oil. Place the mixture in your air fryer's cooking basket and roast for 25-30 minutes. Serve and enjoy!
- **Nutrition Info:** Calories: 336 Cal Total Fat: 18.5 g Saturated Fat: 0 g Cholesterol: 82 mg Sodium: 876 mg Total Carbs: 69.9 g Fiber: 0 g Sugar: 0 g Protein: 0 g

209.Artichoke Spinach Casserole

Servings: 4
Cooking Time: 20 Minutes
Ingredients:
- ⅓cup full-fat mayonnaise
- oz. full-fat cream cheese; softened.
- ¼ cup diced yellow onion
- ⅓cup full-fat sour cream.
- ¼ cup chopped pickled jalapeños.

- 2 cups fresh spinach; chopped
- 2 cups cauliflower florets; chopped
- 1 cup artichoke hearts; chopped
- 1 tbsp. salted butter; melted.

Directions:
1. Take a large bowl, mix butter, onion, cream cheese, mayonnaise and sour cream. Fold in jalapeños, spinach, cauliflower and artichokes.
2. Pour the mixture into a 4-cup round baking dish. Cover with foil and place into the air fryer basket
3. Adjust the temperature to 370 Degrees F and set the timer for 15 minutes. In the last 2 minutes of cooking, remove the foil to brown the top. Serve warm.
- **Nutrition Info:** Calories: 423; Protein: 7g; Fiber: 3g; Fat: 33g; Carbs: 11g

210.Beef, Olives And Tomatoes

Servings: 4
Cooking Time: 35 Minutes
Ingredients:
- 2pounds beef stew meat, cubed
- 1cup black olives, pitted and halved
- 1cup cherry tomatoes, halved
- 1tablespoon smoked paprika
- 3tablespoons olive oil
- 1teaspoon coriander, ground
- Salt and black pepper to the taste

Directions:
1. In the air fryer's pan, mix the beef with the olives and the other ingredients, toss and cook at 390 degrees F for 35 minutes.
2. Divide between plates and serve.
- **Nutrition Info:** Calories 291, Fat 12, Fiber 9, Carbs 20, Protein 26

211.Grilled Chicken Tikka Masala

Servings: 4
Cooking Time: 20 Minutes
Ingredients:
- 1 tsp. Tikka Masala 1 tsp. fine sea salt
- 2 heaping tsps. whole grain mustard
- 2 tsps. coriander, ground 2 tablespoon olive oil
- 2 large-sized chicken breasts, skinless and halved lengthwise
- 2 tsp.s onion powder
- 1½ tablespoons cider vinegar Basmati rice, steamed
- 1/3 tsp. red pepper flakes, crushed

Directions:
1. Preheat the air fryer to 335 °For 4 minutes.
2. Toss your chicken together with the other ingredients, minus basmati rice. Let it stand at least 3 hours.

3. Cook for 25 minutes in your air fryer; check for doneness because the time depending on the size of the piece of chicken.
4. Serve immediately over warm basmati rice. Enjoy!
- **Nutrition Info:** 319 Calories; 20.1g Fat; 1.9g Carbs; 30.5g Protein; 0.1g Sugars

212.Chat Masala Grilled Snapper

Servings: 5
Cooking Time: 25 Minutes
Ingredients:
- 2 ½ pounds whole fish
- Salt to taste
- 1/3 cup chat masala
- 3 tablespoons fresh lime juice
- 5 tablespoons olive oil

Directions:
1. Place the instant pot air fryer lid on and preheat the instant pot at 390 degrees F.
2. Place the grill pan accessory in the instant pot.
3. Season the fish with salt, chat masala and lime juice.
4. Brush with oil
5. Place the fish on a foil basket and place it inside the grill.
6. Close the air fryer lid and cook for 25 minutes.
- **Nutrition Info:** Calories:308; Carbs: 0.7g; Protein: 35.2g; Fat: 17.4g

213.Pollock With Kalamata Olives And Capers

Servings: 3
Cooking Time: 20 Minutes
Ingredients:
- 2 tablespoons olive oil
- 1 red onion, sliced
- 2 cloves garlic, chopped
- 1 Florina pepper, deveined and minced
- 3 pollock fillets,skinless
- 2 ripe tomatoes, diced
- 12 Kalamata olives, pitted and chopped
- 2 tablespoons capers
- 1 teaspoon oregano
- 1 teaspoon rosemary
- Sea salt, to taste
- 1/2 cup white wine

Directions:
1. Start by preheating your Air Fryer to 360 degrees F. Heat the oil in a baking pan. Once hot, sauté the onion, garlic, and pepper for 2 to 3 minutes or until fragrant.
2. Add the fish fillets to the baking pan. Top with the tomatoes, olives, and capers. Sprinkle with the oregano, rosemary, and salt. Pour in white wine and transfer to the cooking basket.

3. Turn the temperature to 395 degrees F and bake for 10 minutes. Taste for seasoning and serve on individual plates, garnished with some extra Mediterranean herbs if desired. Enjoy!
- **Nutrition Info:** 480 Calories; 37g Fat; 9g Carbs; 49g Protein; 5g Sugars; 2g Fiber

214.Easy Air Fryed Roasted Asparagus

Servings: 4
Cooking Time: 10 Minutes
Ingredients:
- 1 bunch fresh asparagus
- 1 ½ tsp herbs de provence
- Fresh lemon wedge (optional)
- 1 tablespoon olive oil or cooking spray
- Salt and pepper to taste

Directions:
1. Wash asparagus and trim off hard ends
2. Drizzle asparagus with olive oil and add seasonings
3. Place asparagus in air fryer and cook on 360F for 6 to 10 minutes
4. Drizzle squeezed lemon over roasted asparagus.
- **Nutrition Info:** Calories 46 protein 2g fat 3g net carbs 1g

215.Filet Mignon With Chili Peanut Sauce

Servings: 4
Cooking Time: 20 Minutes
Ingredients:
- 2 pounds filet mignon, sliced into bite-sized strips
- 1 tablespoon oyster sauce
- 2 tablespoons sesame oil
- 2 tablespoons tamari sauce
- 1 tablespoon ginger-garlic paste
- 1 tablespoon mustard
- 1 teaspoon chili powder
- 1/4 cup peanut butter
- 2 tablespoons lime juice
- 1 teaspoon red pepper flakes
- 2 tablespoons water

Directions:
1. Place the beef strips, oyster sauce, sesame oil, tamari sauce, ginger-garlic paste, mustard, and chili powder in a large ceramic dish.
2. Cover and allow it to marinate for 2 hours in your refrigerator.
3. Cook in the preheated Air Fryer at 400 degrees F for 18 minutes, shaking the basket occasionally.
4. Mix the peanut butter with lime juice, red pepper flakes, and water. Spoon the sauce onto the air fried beef strips and serve warm.

- **Nutrition Info:** 420 Calories; 21g Fat; 5g Carbs; 50g Protein; 7g Sugars; 1g Fiber

216.Party Stuffed Pork Chops

Servings: 4
Cooking Time: 40 Minutes
Ingredients:
- 8 pork chops
- ¼ tsp pepper
- 4 cups stuffing mix
- ½ tsp salt
- 2 tbsp olive oil
- 4 garlic cloves, minced
- 2 tbsp sage leaves

Directions:
1. Preheat your air fryer to 350 f. cut a hole in pork chops and fill chops with stuffing mix. In a bowl, mix sage leaves, garlic cloves, oil, salt and pepper. Cover chops with marinade and let marinate for 10 minutes. Place the chops in your air fryer's cooking basket and cook for 25 minutes. Serve and enjoy!
- **Nutrition Info:** Calories: 364 Cal Total Fat: 13 g Saturated Fat: 4 g Cholesterol: 119 mg Sodium: 349 mg Total Carbs: 19 g Fiber: 3 g Sugar: 6 g Protein: 40 g

217.Keto Lamb Kleftiko

Servings: 6
Cooking Time: 30 Minutes
Ingredients:
- 2 oz. garlic clove, peeled
- 1 tablespoon dried oregano
- ½ lemon
- ¼ tablespoon ground cinnamon
- 3 tablespoon butter, frozen
- 18 oz. leg of lamb
- 1 cup heavy cream
- 1 teaspoon bay leaf
- 1 teaspoon dried mint
- 1 tablespoon olive oil

Directions:
1. Crush the garlic cloves and combine them with the dried oregano, and ground cinnamon. Mix it.
2. Then chop the lemon.
3. Sprinkle the leg of lamb with the crushed garlic mixture.
4. Then rub it with the chopped lemon.
5. Combine the heavy cream, bay leaf, and dried mint together.
6. Whisk the mixture well.
7. After this, add the olive oil and whisk it one more time more.
8. Then pour the cream mixture on the leg of lamb and stir it carefully.
9. Leave the leg of lamb for 10 minutes to marinate.
10. Preheat the air fryer to 380 F.
11. Chop the butter and sprinkle the marinated lamb.
12. Then place the leg of lamb in the air fryer basket tray and sprinkle it with the remaining cream mixture.
13. Then sprinkle the meat with the chopped butter.
14. Cook the meat for 30 minutes.
15. When the time is over – remove the meat from the air fryer and sprinkle it gently with the remaining cream mixture.
16. Serve it!
- **Nutrition Info:** calories 318, fat 21.9, fiber 0.9, carbs 4.9, protein 25.1

218.Lemon Duck Legs

Servings: 6
Cooking Time: 25 Minutes
Ingredients:
- 1 lemon
- 2-pound duck legs
- 1 teaspoon ground coriander
- 1 teaspoon ground nutmeg
- 1 teaspoon kosher salt
- ½ teaspoon dried rosemary
- 1 tablespoon olive oil
- 1 teaspoon stevia extract
- ¼ teaspoon sage

Directions:
1. Squeeze the juice from the lemon and grate the zest.
2. Combine the lemon juice and lemon zest together in the big mixing bowl.
3. Add the ground coriander, ground nutmeg, kosher salt, dried rosemary, and sage.
4. Sprinkle the liquid with the olive oil and stevia extract.
5. Whisk it carefully and put the duck legs there.
6. Stir the duck legs and leave them for 15 minutes to marinate.
7. Meanwhile, preheat the air fryer to 380 F.
8. Put the marinated duck legs in the air fryer and cook them for 25 minutes.
9. Turn the duck legs into another side after 15 minutes of cooking.
10. When the duck legs are cooked – let them cool little.
11. Serve and enjoy!
- **Nutrition Info:** calories 296, fat 11.5, fiber 0.5, carbs 1.6, protein 44.2

219.Red Hot Chili Fish Curry

Servings: 4
Cooking Time: 20 Minutes
Ingredients:
- 2 tablespoons sunflower oil
- 1 pound fish, chopped
- 2 red chilies, chopped

- 1 tablespoon coriander powder
- 1 teaspoon red curry paste
- 1 cup coconut milk
- Salt and white pepper, to taste
- 1/2 teaspoon fenugreek seeds
- 1 shallot, minced
- 1 garlic clove, minced
- 1 ripe tomato, pureed

Directions:
1. Preheat your Air Fryer to 380 degrees F; brush the cooking basket with 1 tablespoon of sunflower oil.
2. Cook your fish for 10 minutes on both sides. Transfer to the baking pan that is previously greased with the remaining tablespoon of sunflower oil.
3. Add the remaining ingredients and reduce the heat to 350 degrees F. Continue to cook an additional 10 to 12 minutes or until everything is heated through. Enjoy!
- **Nutrition Info:** 298 Calories; 18g Fat; 4g Carbs; 23g Protein; 7g Sugars; 7g Fiber

220.Air Fryer Roasted Broccoli

Servings: 4
Cooking Time: 10 Minutes
Ingredients:
- 1 tsp. herbes de provence seasoning (optional)
- 4 cups fresh broccoli
- 1 tablespoon olive oil
- Salt and pepper to taste

Directions:
1. Drizzle or spray broccoli with olive and sprinkle seasoning throughout
2. Spray air fryer basket with cooking oil, place broccoli and cook for 5-8 minutes on 360F
3. Open air fryer and examine broccoli after 5 minutes because different fryer brands cook at different rates.
- **Nutrition Info:** Calories 61 Fat 4g protein 3g net carbs 4g

221.Morning Ham And Cheese Sandwich

Servings: 4
Cooking Time: 15 Minutes
Ingredients:
- 8 slices whole wheat bread
- 4 slices lean pork ham
- 4 slices cheese
- 8 slices tomato

Directions:
1. Preheat your air fryer to 360 f. Lay four slices of bread on a flat surface. Spread the slices with cheese, tomato, turkey and ham. Cover with the remaining slices to form sandwiches. Add the sandwiches to the air

fryer cooking basket and cook for 10 minutes.
- **Nutrition Info:** Calories: 361 Cal Total Fat: 16.7 g Saturated Fat: 0 g Cholesterol: 0 mg Sodium: 1320 mg Total Carbs: 32.5 g Fiber: 2.3 g Sugar: 5.13 g Protein: 19.3 g

222.Lemon Garlic Shrimps

Servings: 2
Cooking Time: 8 Minutes
Ingredients:
- ¾ pound medium shrimp, peeled and deveined
- 1½ tablespoons fresh lemon juice
- 1 tablespoon olive oil
- 1 teaspoon lemon pepper
- ¼ teaspoon paprika
- ¼ teaspoon garlic powder

Directions:
1. Preheat the Air fryer to 400 degree F and grease an Air fryer basket.
2. Mix lemon juice, olive oil, lemon pepper, paprika and garlic powder in a large bowl.
3. Stir in the shrimp and toss until well combined.
4. Arrange shrimp into the Air fryer basket in a single layer and cook for about 8 minutes.
5. Dish out the shrimp in serving plates and serve warm.
- **Nutrition Info:** Calories: 260, Fat: 12.4g, Carbohydrates: 0.3g, Sugar: 0.1g, Protein: 35.6g, Sodium: 619mg

223.Salmon Casserole

Servings: 8
Cooking Time: 12 Minutes
Ingredients:
- 7 oz Cheddar cheese, shredded
- ½ cup cream
- 1-pound salmon fillet
- 1 tablespoon dried dill
- 1 teaspoon dried parsley
- 1 teaspoon salt
- 1 teaspoon ground coriander
- ½ teaspoon ground black pepper
- 2 green pepper, chopped
- 4 oz chive stems, diced
- 7 oz bok choy, chopped
- 1 tablespoon olive oil

Directions:
1. Sprinkle the salmon fillet with the dried dill, dried parsley, ground coriander, and ground black pepper.
2. Massage the salmon fillet gently and leave it for 5 minutes to make the fish soaks the spices.
3. Meanwhile, sprinkle the air fryer casserole tray with the olive oil inside.

4. After this, cut the salmon fillet into the cubes.
5. Separate the salmon cubes into 2 parts.
6. Then place the first part of the salmon cubes in the casserole tray.
7. Sprinkle the fish with the chopped bok choy, diced chives, and chopped green pepper.
8. After this, place the second part of the salmon cubes over the vegetables.
9. Then sprinkle the casserole with the shredded cheese and heavy cream.
10. Preheat the air fryer to 380 F.
11. Cook the salmon casserole for 12 minutes.
12. When the dish is cooked – it will have acrunchy light brown crust.
13. Serve it and enjoy!
- **Nutrition Info:** calories 216, fat 14.4, fiber 1.1, carbs 4.3, protein 18.2

224.Spicy Paprika Steak

Servings: 2
Cooking Time: 20 Minutes
Ingredients:
- 1/2 Ancho chili pepper, soaked in hot water before using
- 1 tablespoon brandy
- 2 teaspoons smoked paprika
- 1 1/2 tablespoons olive oil
- 2 beef steaks
- Kosher salt, to taste
- 1 teaspoon ground allspice
- 3 cloves garlic, sliced

Directions:
1. Sprinkle the beef steaks with salt, paprika, and allspice. Add the steak to a baking dish that fits your fryer. Scatter the sliced garlic over the top.
2. Now, drizzle it with brandy and olive oil; spread minced Ancho chili pepper over the top.
3. Bake at 385 degrees F for 14 minutes, turning halfway through. Serve warm.
- **Nutrition Info:** 450 Calories; 26g Fat; 4g Carbs; 58g Protein; 3g Sugars; 3g Fiber

225.Cinnamon Pork Rinds

Servings: 2
Cooking Time: 20 Minutes
Ingredients:
- 2 oz. pork rinds
- ¼ cup powdered erythritol
- 2 tbsp. unsalted butter; melted.
- ½ tsp. ground cinnamon.

Directions:
1. Take a large bowl, toss pork rinds and butter. Sprinkle with cinnamon and erythritol, then toss to evenly coat.
2. Place pork rinds into the air fryer basket. Adjust the temperature to 400 Degrees F

and set the timer for 5 minutes. Serve immediately.
- **Nutrition Info:** Calories: 264; Protein: 13g; Fiber: 4g; Fat: 28g; Carbs: 15g

226.Marinated Cajun Beef

Servings: 2
Cooking Time: 20 Minutes
Ingredients:
- 1/3 cup beef broth
- 2 tablespoons Cajun seasoning, crushed
- 1/2 teaspoon garlic powder
- 3/4 pound beef tenderloins
- ½ tablespoon pear cider vinegar
- 1/3 teaspoon cayenne pepper
- 1 ½ tablespoon olive oil
- 1/2 teaspoon freshly ground black pepper
- 1 teaspoon salt

Directions:
1. Firstly, coat the beef tenderloins with salt, cayenne pepper, and black pepper.
2. Mix the remaining items in a medium-sized bowl; let the meat marinate for 40 minutes in this mixture.
3. Roast the beef for about 22 minutes at 385 degrees F, turning it halfway through the cooking time.
- **Nutrition Info:** 483 Calories; 23g Fat; 5g Carbs; 53g Protein; 6g Sugars; 4g Fiber

227.Cheese Breaded Pork

Servings: 6
Cooking Time: 15 Minutes
Ingredients:
- 6 pork chops
- 6 tbsp seasoned breadcrumbs
- 2 tbsp parmesan cheese, grated
- 1 tbsp melted butter
- ½ cup mozzarella cheese, shredded
- 1 tbsp marinara sauce

Directions:
1. Preheat your air fryer to 390 f. Grease the cooking basket with cooking spray. In a small bowl, mix breadcrumbs and parmesan cheese. In another microwave proof bowl, add butter and melt in the microwave.
2. Brush the pork with butter and dredge into the breadcrumbs. Add pork to the cooking basket and cook for 6 minutes. Turnover and top with marinara sauce and shredded mozzarella; cook for 3 more minutes
- **Nutrition Info:** Calories: 431 Cal Total Fat: 0 g Saturated Fat: 0 g Cholesterol: 0 mg Sodium: 0 mg Total Carbs: 0 g Fiber: 0 g Sugar: 0 g Protein: 0 g

228.Veggie Stuffed Bell Peppers

Servings: 6

Cooking Time: 25 Minutes

Ingredients:

- 6 large bell peppers, tops and seeds removed
- 1 carrot, peeled and finely chopped
- 1 potato, peeled and finely chopped
- ½ cup fresh peas, shelled
- 1/3 cup cheddar cheese, grated
- 2 garlic cloves, minced
- Salt and black pepper, to taste

Directions:

1. Preheat the Air fryer to 350 ºF and grease an Air fryer basket.
2. Mix vegetables, garlic, salt and black pepper in a bowl.
3. Stuff the vegetable mixture in each bell pepper and arrange in the Air fryer pan.
4. Cook for about 20 minutes and top with cheddar cheese.
5. Cook for about 5 more minutes and dish out to serve warm.
- **Nutrition Info:** Calories: 101, Fat: 2.5g, Carbohydrates: 17.1g, Sugar: 7.4g, Protein: 4.1g, Sodium: 51mg

229.Cheddar Pork Meatballs

Servings: 4 To 6
Cooking Time: 25 Minutes

Ingredients:

- 1 lb ground pork
- 1 large onion, chopped
- ½ tsp maple syrup
- 2 tsp mustard
- ½ cup chopped basil leaves
- Salt and black pepper to taste
- 2 tbsp. grated cheddar cheese

Directions:

1. In a mixing bowl, add the ground pork, onion, maple syrup, mustard, basil leaves, salt, pepper, and cheddar cheese; mix well. Use your hands to form bite-size balls. Place in the fryer basket and cook at 400 f for 10 minutes.
2. Slide out the fryer basket and shake it to toss the meatballs. Cook further for 5 minutes. Remove them onto a wire rack and serve with zoodles and marinara sauce.
- **Nutrition Info:** Calories: 300 Cal Total Fat: 24 g Saturated Fat: 9 g Cholesterol: 70 mg Sodium: 860 mg Total Carbs: 3 g Fiber: 0 g Sugar: 0 g Protein: 16 g

230.Dinner Avocado Chicken Sliders

Servings: 4
Cooking Time: 20 Minutes

Ingredients:

- ½ pounds ground chicken meat 4 burger buns
- 1/2 cup Romaine lettuce, loosely packed

- ½ tsp. dried parsley flakes 1/3 tsp. mustard seeds
- 1 tsp. onion powder
- 1 ripe fresh avocado, mashed 1 tsp. garlic powder
- 1 ½ tablespoon extra-virgin olive oil
- 1 cloves garlic, minced Nonstick cooking spray
- Salt and cracked black pepper (peppercorns, to taste)

Directions:

1. Firstly, spritz an air fryer cooking basket with a nonstick cooking spray.
2. Mix ground chicken meat, mustard seeds, garlic powder, onion powder, parsley, salt, and black pepper until everything is thoroughly combined. Make sure not to overwork the meat to avoid tough chicken burgers.
3. Shape the meat mixture into patties and roll them in breadcrumbs; transfer your burgers to the prepared cooking basket. Brush the patties with the cooking spray.
4. Air-fry at 355 F for 9 minutes, working in batches. Slice burger buns into halves. In the meantime, combine olive oil with mashed avocado and pressed garlic.
5. To finish, lay Romaine lettuce and avocado spread on bun bottoms; now, add burgers and bun tops.
- **Nutrition Info:** 321 Calories; 18.7g Fat; 15.8g Carbs; 1.2g Sugars

231.Beef With Apples And Plums

Servings: 4
Cooking Time: 30 Minutes

Ingredients:

- 2pounds beef stew meat, cubed
- 1cup apples, cored and cubed
- 1cup plums, pitted and halved
- 2tablespoons butter, melted
- Salt and black pepper to the taste
- ½ cup red wine
- 1tablespoon chives, chopped

Directions:

1. In the air fryer's pan, mix the beef with the apples and the other ingredients, toss, put the pan in the machine and cook at 390 degrees F for 30 minutes.
2. Divide the mix between plates and serve right away.
- **Nutrition Info:** Calories 290, Fat 12, Fiber 5, Carbs 19, Protein 28

232.Garlic Lamb Shank

Servings: 5
Cooking Time: 24 Minutes

Ingredients:

- 17 oz. lamb shanks

- 2 tablespoon garlic, peeled
- 1 teaspoon kosher salt
- 1 tablespoon dried parsley
- 4 oz chive stems, chopped
- ½ cup chicken stock
- 1 teaspoon butter
- 1 teaspoon dried rosemary
- 1 teaspoon nutmeg
- ½ teaspoon ground black pepper

Directions:
1. Chop the garlic roughly.
2. Make the cuts in the lamb shank and fill the cuts with the chopped garlic.
3. Then sprinkle the lamb shank with the kosher salt, dried parsley, dried rosemary, nutmeg, and ground black pepper.
4. Stir the spices on the lamb shank gently.
5. Then put the butter and chicken stock in the air fryer basket tray.
6. Preheat the air fryer to 380 F.
7. Put the chives in the air fryer basket tray.
8. Add the lamb shank and cook the meat for 24 minutes.
9. When the lamb shank is cooked – transfer it to the serving plate and sprinkle with the remaining liquid from the cooked meat.
10. Enjoy!
- **Nutrition Info:** calories 205, fat 8.2, fiber 0.8, carbs 3.8, protein 27.2

233.Herbed Eggplant

Servings: 2
Cooking Time: 15 Minutes
Ingredients:
- 1 large eggplant, cubed
- ½ teaspoon dried marjoram, crushed
- ½ teaspoon dried oregano, crushed
- ½ teaspoon dried thyme, crushed
- ½ teaspoon garlic powder
- Salt and black pepper, to taste
- Olive oil cooking spray

Directions:
1. Preheat the Air fryer to 390 degree F and grease an Air fryer basket.
2. Mix herbs, garlic powder, salt, and black pepper in a bowl.
3. Spray the eggplant cubes with cooking spray and rub with the herb mixture.
4. Arrange the eggplant cubes in the Air fryer basket and cook for about 15 minutes, flipping twice in between.
5. Dish out onto serving plates and serve hot.
- **Nutrition Info:** Calories: 62, Fat: 0.5g, Carbohydrates: 14.5g, Sugar: 7.1g, Protein: 2.4g, Sodium: 83mg

234.Broccoli With Olives

Servings: 4
Cooking Time: 19 Minutes

Ingredients:
- 2 pounds broccoli, stemmed and cut into 1-inch florets
- 1/3 cup Kalamata olives, halved and pitted
- ¼ cup Parmesan cheese, grated
- 2 tablespoons olive oil
- Salt and ground black pepper, as required
- 2 teaspoons fresh lemon zest, grated

Directions:
1. Preheat the Air fryer to 400 ºF and grease an Air fryer basket.
2. Boil the broccoli for about 4 minutes and drain well.
3. Mix broccoli, oil, salt, and black pepper in a bowl and toss to coat well.
4. Arrange broccoli into the Air fryer basket and cook for about 15 minutes.
5. Stir in the olives, lemon zest and cheese and dish out to serve.
- **Nutrition Info:** Calories: 169, Fat: 10.2g, Carbohydrates: 16g, Sugar: 3.9g, Protein: 8.5g, Sodium: 254mg

235.Beef Roast

Servings: 4
Cooking Time:x
Ingredients:
- 2 lbs. beef roast
- 1 tbsp. smoked paprika
- 3 tbsp. garlic; minced
- 3 tbsp. olive oil
- Salt and black pepper to taste

Directions:
1. In a bowl, combine all the ingredients and coat the roast well.
2. Place the roast in your air fryer and cook at 390°F for 55 minutes. Slice the roast, divide it between plates and serve with a side salad

236.Broccoli And Avocado Tacos

Servings: 3
Cooking Time: 5 Minutes
Ingredients:
- 6-10 authentic Mexican corn tortillas
- 1 large ripe avocado
- 1 large head broccoli
- 6-8 white mushrooms, sliced
- 1/2 bunch cilantro
- 1/2 teaspoon garlic powder
- Sea salt and pepper
- Olive oil

Directions:
1. Start by preheating toaster oven to 400°F.
2. Slice avocado into thin slices and chop the broccoli into bite-sized florets.
3. Arrange the broccoli and mushrooms on a baking sheet; drizzle oil and sprinkle salt, pepper, and garlic powder over the veggies.

4. Bake for 20 minutes. Warm the tortillas, then fill with mushrooms and broccoli, and top with avocado.
5. Sprinkle cilantro over tacos and serve.
- **Nutrition Info:** Calories: 313, Sodium: 99 mg, Dietary Fiber: 12.6 g, Total Fat: 15.3 g, Total Carbs: 40.5 g, Protein: 10.4 g.

237.Tasty Grilled Red Mullet

Servings: 8
Cooking Time: 15 Minutes
Ingredients:
- 8 whole red mullets, gutted and scales removed
- Salt and pepper to taste
- Juice from 1 lemon
- 1 tablespoon olive oil

Directions:
1. Place the instant pot air fryer lid on and preheat the instant pot at 390 degrees F.
2. Place the grill pan accessory in the instant pot.
3. Season the red mullet with salt, pepper, and lemon juice.
4. Place red mullets on the grill pan and brush with olive oil.
5. Close the air fryer lid and grill for 15 minutes.
- **Nutrition Info:** Calories: 152; Carbs: 0.9g; Protein: 23.1g; Fat: 6.2g

238.Corned Beef With Carrots

Servings: 3
Cooking Time: 35 Minutes
Ingredients:
- 1 tbsp beef spice
- 1 whole onion, chopped
- 4 carrots, chopped
- 12 oz bottle beer
- 1½ cups chicken broth
- 4 pounds corned beef

Directions:
1. Preheat your air fryer to 380 f. Cover beef with beer and set aside for 20 minutes. Place carrots, onion and beef in a pot and heat over high heat. Add in broth and bring to a boil. Drain boiled meat and veggies; set aside.
2. Top with beef spice. Place the meat and veggies in your air fryer's cooking basket and cook for 30 minutes.
- **Nutrition Info:** Calories: 464 Cal Total Fat: 17 g Saturated Fat: 6.8 g Cholesterol: 91.7 mg Sodium: 1904.2 mg Total Carbs: 48.9 g Fiber: 7.2 g Sugar: 5.8 g Protein: 30.6 g

239.Air Fryer Veggie Quesdillas

Servings: 4
Cooking Time: 40 Minutes

Ingredients:
- 4 sprouted whole-grain flour tortillas (6-in.)
- 1 cup sliced red bell pepper
- 4 ounces reduced-fat Cheddar cheese, shredded
- 1 cup sliced zucchini
- 1 cup canned black beans, drained and rinsed (no salt)
- Cooking spray
- 2 ounces plain 2% reduced-fat Greek yogurt
- 1 teaspoon lime zest
- 1 Tbsp. fresh juice (from 1 lime)
- ¼ tsp. ground cumin
- 2 tablespoons chopped fresh cilantro
- 1/2 cup drained refrigerated pico de gallo

Directions:
1. Place tortillas on work surface, sprinkle 2 tablespoons shredded cheese over half of each tortilla and top with cheese on each tortilla with 1/4 cup each red pepper slices, zucchini slices, and black beans. Sprinkle evenly with remaining 1/2 cup cheese.
2. Fold tortillas over to form half-moon shaped quesadillas, lightly coat with cooking spray, and secure with toothpicks.
3. Lightly spray air fryer basket with cooking spray. Place 2 quesadillas in the basket, and cook at 400°F for 10 minutes until tortillas are golden brown and slightly crispy, cheese is melted, and vegetables are slightly softened. Turn quesadillas over halfway through cooking.
4. Repeat with remaining quesadillas.
5. Meanwhile, stir yogurt, lime juice, lime zest and cumin in a small bowl.
6. Cut each quesadilla into wedges and sprinkle with cilantro.
7. Serve with 1 tablespoon cumin cream and 2 tablespoons pico de gallo each.
- **Nutrition Info:** Calories 291 Fat 8g Saturated fat 4g Unsaturated fat 3g Protein 17g Carbohydrate 36g Fiber 8g Sugars 3g Sodium 518mg Calcium 30% DV Potassium 6% DV

240.Venetian Liver

Servings: 6
Cooking Time: 15-30;
Ingredients:
- 500g veal liver
- 2 white onions
- 100g of water
- 2 tbsp vinegar
- Salt and pepper to taste

Directions:
1. Chop the onion and put it inside the pan with the water. Set the air fryer to 1800C and cook for 20 minutes.

2. Add the liver cut into small pieces and vinegar, close the lid, and cook for an additional 10 minutes.
3. Add salt and pepper.
- **Nutrition Info:** Calories 131, Fat 14.19 g, Carbohydrates 16.40 g, Sugars 5.15 g, Protein 25.39 g, Cholesterol 350.41 mg

241.Garlic Parmesan Shrimp

Servings: 2
Cooking Time: 10 Minutes
Ingredients:
- 1 pound shrimp, deveined and peeled
- ½ cup parmesan cheese, grated
- ¼ cup cilantro, diced
- 1 tablespoon olive oil
- 1 teaspoon salt
- 1 teaspoon fresh cracked pepper
- 1 tablespoon lemon juice
- 6 garlic cloves, diced

Directions:
1. Preheat the Air fryer to 350 degree F and grease an Air fryer basket.
2. Drizzle shrimp with olive oil and lemon juice and season with garlic, salt and cracked pepper.
3. Cover the bowl with plastic wrap and refrigerate for about 3 hours.
4. Stir in the parmesan cheese and cilantro to the bowl and transfer to the Air fryer basket.
5. Cook for about 10 minutes and serve immediately.
- **Nutrition Info:** Calories: 602, Fat: 23.9g, Carbohydrates: 46.5g, Sugar: 2.9g, Protein: 11.3g, Sodium: 886mg

242.Oven-fried Herbed Chicken

Servings: 2
Cooking Time: 15 Minutes
Ingredients:
- 1/2 cup buttermilk
- 2 cloves garlic, minced
- 1-1/2 teaspoons salt
- 1 tablespoon oil
- 1/2 pound boneless, skinless chicken breasts
- 1 cup rolled oats
- 1/2 teaspoon red pepper flakes
- 1/2 cup grated parmesan cheese
- 1/4 cup fresh basil leaves or rosemary needles
- Olive oil spray

Directions:
1. Mix together buttermilk, oil, 1/2 teaspoon salt, and garlic in a shallow bowl.
2. Roll chicken in buttermilk and refrigerate in bowl overnight.
3. Preheat your toaster oven to 425°F.
4. Mix together the oats, red pepper, salt, parmesan, and basil, and mix roughly to break up oats.
5. Place the mixture on a plate.
6. Remove the chicken from the buttermilk mixture and let any excess drip off.
7. Roll the chicken in the oat mixture and transfer to a baking sheet lightly coated with olive oil spray.
8. Spray the chicken with oil spray and bake for 15 minutes.
- **Nutrition Info:** Calories: 651, Sodium: 713 mg, Dietary Fiber: 4.4 g, Total Fat: 31.2 g, Total Carbs: 34.1 g, Protein: 59.5 g.

243.Crispy Scallops

Servings: 4
Cooking Time: 6 Minutes
Ingredients:
- 18 sea scallops, cleaned and patted very dry
- 1/8 cup all-purpose flour
- 1 tablespoon 2% milk
- ½ egg
- ¼ cup cornflakes, crushed
- ½ teaspoon paprika
- Salt and black pepper, as required

Directions:
1. Preheat the Air fryer to 400 degree F and grease an Air fryer basket.
2. Mix flour, paprika, salt, and black pepper in a bowl.
3. Whisk egg with milk in another bowl and place the cornflakes in a third bowl.
4. Coat each scallop with the flour mixture, dip into the egg mixture and finally, dredge in the cornflakes.
5. Arrange scallops in the Air fryer basket and cook for about 6 minutes.
6. Dish out the scallops in a platter and serve hot.
- **Nutrition Info:** Calories: 150, Fat: 1.7g, Carbohydrates: 8g, Sugar: 0.4g, Protein: 24g, Sodium: 278mg

244.Zingy Dilled Salmon

Servings: 2
Cooking Time: 20 Minutes
Ingredients:
- 2 salmon steaks
- Coarse sea salt, to taste
- 1/4 teaspoon freshly ground black pepper, or more to taste
- 1 tablespoon sesame oil
- Zest of 1 lemon
- 1 tablespoon fresh lemon juice
- 1 teaspoon garlic, minced
- 1/2 teaspoon smoked cayenne pepper
- 1/2 teaspoon dried dill

Directions:

1. Preheat your Air Fryer to 380 degrees F. Pat dry the salmon steaks with a kitchen towel.
2. In a ceramic dish, combine the remaining ingredients until everything is well whisked.
3. Add the salmon steaks to the ceramic dish and let them sit in the refrigerator for 1 hour. Now, place the salmon steaks in the cooking basket. Reserve the marinade.
4. Cook for 12 minutes, flipping halfway through the cooking time.
5. Meanwhile, cook the marinade in a small sauté pan over a moderate flame. Cook until the sauce has thickened.
6. Pour the sauce over the steaks and serve.
- **Nutrition Info:** 476 Calories; 18g Fat; 2g Carbs; 47g Protein; 8g Sugars; 4g Fiber

245.Portuguese Bacalao Tapas

Servings: 4
Cooking Time: 26 Minutes
Ingredients:
- 1-pound codfish fillet, chopped
- 2 Yukon Gold potatoes, peeled and diced
- 2 tablespoon butter
- 1 yellow onion, thinly sliced
- 1 clove garlic, chopped, divided
- 1/4 cup chopped fresh parsley, divided
- 1/4 cup olive oil
- 3/4 teaspoon red pepper flakes
- freshly ground black pepper to taste
- 2 hard-cooked eggs, chopped
- 5 pitted green olives
- 5 pitted black olives

Directions:
1. Place the instant pot air fryer lid on, lightly grease baking pan of the instant pot with cooking spray. Add butter and place the baking pan in the instant pot.
2. Close the air fryer lid and melt butter at 360 ºF. Stir in onions and cook for 6 minutes until caramelized.
3. Stir in black pepper, red pepper flakes, half of the parsley, garlic, olive oil, diced potatoes, and chopped fish. For 10 minutes, cook on 360 ºF. Halfway through cooking time, stir well to mix.
4. Cook for 10 minutes at 390 ºF until tops are lightly browned.
5. Garnish with remaining parsley, eggs, black and green olives.
6. Serve and enjoy with chips.
- **Nutrition Info:** Calories: 691; Carbs: 25.2g; Protein: 77.1g; Fat: 31.3g

246.Homemade Beef Stroganoff

Servings: 3
Cooking Time: 20 Minutes
Ingredients:
- 1 pound thin steak

- 4 tbsp butter
- 1 whole onion, chopped
- 1 cup sour cream
- 8 oz mushrooms, sliced
- 4 cups beef broth
- 16 oz egg noodles, cooked

Directions:
1. Preheat your Air Fryer to 400 F. Using a microwave proof bowl, melt butter in a microwave oven. In a mixing bowl, mix the melted butter, sliced mushrooms, cream, onion, and beef broth.
2. Pour the mixture over steak and set aside for 10 minutes. Place the marinated beef in your fryer's cooking basket, and cook for 10 minutes. Serve with cooked egg noodles and enjoy!
- **Nutrition Info:** 456 Calories; 37g Fat; 1g Carbs; 21g Protein; 5g Sugars; 6g Fiber

247.Creole Beef Meatloaf

Servings: 6
Cooking Time: 15 Minutes
Ingredients:
- 1 lb. ground beef
- 1/2 tablespoon butter
- 1 red bell pepper diced
- 1/3 cup red onion diced
- 1/3 cup cilantro diced
- 1/3 cup zucchini diced
- 1 tablespoon creole seasoning
- 1/2 teaspoon turmeric
- 1/2 teaspoon cumin
- 1/2 teaspoon coriander
- 2 garlic cloves minced
- Salt and black pepper to taste

Directions:
1. Mix the beef minced with all the meatball ingredients in a bowl.
2. Make small meatballs out of this mixture and place them in the Air fryer basket.
3. Press "Power Button" of Air Fry Oven and turn the dial to select the "Air Fry" mode.
4. Press the Time button and again turn the dial to set the cooking time to 15 minutes.
5. Now push the Temp button and rotate the dial to set the temperature at 370 degrees F.
6. Once preheated, place the Air fryer basket in the oven and close its lid.
7. Slice and serve warm.
- **Nutrition Info:** Calories: 331 Cal Total Fat: 2.5 g Saturated Fat: 0.5 g Cholesterol: 35 mg Sodium: 595 mg Total Carbs: 69 g Fiber: 12.2 g Sugar: 12.5 g Protein: 26.7 g

248.Baked Veggie Egg Rolls

Servings: 2
Cooking Time: 20 Minutes
Ingredients:

- 1/2 tablespoon olive or vegetable oil
- 2 cups thinly-sliced chard
- 1/4 cup grated carrot
- 1/2 cup chopped pea pods
- 3 shiitake mushrooms
- 2 scallions
- 2 medium cloves garlic
- 1/2 tablespoon fresh ginger
- 1/2 tablespoon soy sauce
- 6 egg roll wrappers
- Olive oil spray for cookie sheet and egg rolls

Directions:
1. Start by mincing mushrooms, garlic, and ginger and slicing scallions.
2. Heat oil on medium heat in a medium skillet and char peas, carrots, scallions, and mushrooms.
3. Cook 3 minutes, then add ginger. Stir in soy sauce and remove from heat.
4. Preheat toaster oven to 400°F and spray cookie sheet. Spoon even portions of vegetable mix over each egg roll wrapper, and wrap them up.
5. Place egg rolls on cookie sheet and spray with olive oil. Bake for 20 minutes until egg roll shells are browned.
- **Nutrition Info:** Calories: 421, Sodium: 1166 mg, Dietary Fiber: 8.2 g, Total Fat: 7.7 g, Total Carbs: 76.9 g, Protein: 13.7 g.

MEAT RECIPES

249.Greek Chicken Paillard

Servings: 8
Cooking Time: 25 Minutes
Ingredients:
- 4 chicken breasts, skinless and boneless
- 1/2 cup olives, diced
- 1 small onion, sliced
- 1 fennel bulb, sliced
- 28 oz can tomatoes, diced
- 1/4 cup fresh basil, chopped
- 1/4 cup fresh parsley, chopped
- 1/4 cup pine nuts
- 2 tbsp olive oil
- Pepper
- Salt

Directions:
1. Fit the oven with the rack in position
2. Season chicken with pepper and salt and place in baking dish. Drizzle with oil.
3. In a bowl, mix together olives, tomatoes, pine nuts, onion, fennel, pepper, and salt.
4. Pour olive mixture over chicken.
5. Set to bake at 450 F for 30 minutes. After 5 minutes place the baking dish in the preheated oven.
6. Garnish with basil and parsley and serve.
- **Nutrition Info:** Calories 242 Fat 12.8 g Carbohydrates 9.3 g Sugar 3.9 g Protein 23.2 g Cholesterol 65 mg

250.Goat Cheese Meatballs

Servings: 8
Cooking Time: 12 Minutes
Ingredients:
- 1 lb ground beef
- 1 lb ground pork
- 2 eggs, lightly beaten
- 1/4 cup fresh parsley, chopped
- 1 tbsp garlic, minced
- 1 onion, chopped
- 1 tbsp Worcestershire sauce
- 1/2 cup goat cheese, crumbled
- 1/2 cup breadcrumbs
- Pepper
- Salt

Directions:
1. Fit the oven with the rack in position 2.
2. Line the air fryer basket with parchment paper.
3. Add all ingredients into a large bowl and mix until well combined.
4. Make small balls from meat mixture and place in the air fryer basket then place an air fryer basket in the baking pan.
5. Place a baking pan on the oven rack. Set to air fry at 400 F for 12 minutes.

6. Serve and enjoy.
- **Nutrition Info:** Calories 253 Fat 8.1 g Carbohydrates 7.2 g Sugar 1.6 g Protein 35.6 g Cholesterol 136 mg

251.Provençal Chicken With Peppers

Servings:2
Cooking Time: 20 Minutes
Ingredients:
- 2 chicken tenders
- Salt and black pepper to taste
- ½ tsp herbs de Provence
- 1 tbsp butter, softened
- 2 mini red peppers, sliced
- 1 onion, sliced

Directions:
1. Preheat on AirFry function to 390 F. Lay a foil on a flat surface. Place the chicken, red peppers, and onion on the foil, sprinkle with herbs de Provence and brush with butter. Season with salt and black pepper. Wrap the foil around the breasts.
2. Place the wrapped chicken in the basket and press Start; cook for 12 minutes. Remove and carefully unwrap. Serve with the sauce extract and veggies.

252.Meatloaf(1)

Servings: 4
Cooking Time: 20 Minutes
Ingredients:
- 1 lb ground pork
- 1 egg, lightly beaten
- 1 tbsp thyme, chopped
- 1/4 tsp garlic powder
- 4 tbsp breadcrumbs
- 1 onion, chopped
- 1/2 tsp Italian seasoning
- Pepper
- Salt

Directions:
1. Fit the oven with the rack in position
2. Add all ingredients into the mixing bowl and mix until well combined.
3. Pour meat mixture into the greased loaf pan.
4. Set to bake at 375 F for 25 minutes. After 5 minutes place the loaf pan in the preheated oven.
5. Serve and enjoy.
- **Nutrition Info:** Calories 220 Fat 5.7 g Carbohydrates 8.2 g Sugar 1.8 g Protein 32.4 g Cholesterol 124 mg

253.Baked Italian Lemon Chicken

Servings: 4
Cooking Time: 25 Minutes
Ingredients:

- 1 1/4 lbs chicken breasts, skinless and boneless
- 3 tbsp butter, melted
- 1 tsp Italian seasoning
- 1 tbsp olive oil
- 1 tbsp fresh parsley, chopped
- 2 tbsp fresh lemon juice
- 1/4 cup water
- Pepper
- Salt

Directions:
1. Fit the oven with the rack in position
2. Season chicken with Italian seasoning, pepper, and salt.
3. Heat oil in a pan over medium-high heat.
4. Add chicken to the pan and cook for 3-5 minutes on each side.
5. Transfer chicken to a baking dish.
6. In a small bowl, mix together butter, lemon juice, and water.
7. Pour butter mixture over chicken.
8. Set to bake at 400 F for 30 minutes. After 5 minutes place the baking dish in the preheated oven.
9. Garnish with parsley and serve.
- **Nutrition Info:** Calories 382 Fat 23.1 g Carbohydrates 0.4 g Sugar 0.3 g Protein 41.2 g Cholesterol 150 mg

254.Crispy Cajun Chicken Breast

Servings: 2
Cooking Time: 25 Minutes
Ingredients:
- 2 chicken breasts
- 3/4 cup breadcrumbs
- 1 tsp garlic powder
- 1 tsp paprika
- 1 tsp Cajun seasoning
- 2 tbsp mayonnaise
- 1/2 tsp pepper
- 1/2 tsp salt

Directions:
1. Fit the oven with the rack in position
2. In a shallow dish, mix breadcrumbs, Cajun seasoning, paprika, garlic powder, pepper, and salt.
3. Brush chicken with mayonnaise and coat with breadcrumbs.
4. Place coated chicken breasts into the baking pan.
5. Set to bake at 425 F for 30 minutes. After 5 minutes place the baking pan in the preheated oven.
6. Serve and enjoy.
- **Nutrition Info:** Calories 504 Fat 18.1 g Carbohydrates 34.6 g Sugar 3.9 g Protein 48.3 g Cholesterol 134 mg

255.Tandoori Chicken

Servings:x
Cooking Time:x
Ingredients:
- 4 tsp. fennel
- 2 tbsp. ginger-garlic paste
- 1 small onion
- 6-7 flakes garlic (optional)
- Salt to taste
- 1 lb. chicken (Cut the chicken into cubes of one inch each. Make sure that
- they have been deboned well)
- 1 big capsicum (Cut this capsicum into big cubes)
- 1 onion (Cut it into quarters. Now separate the layers carefully.)
- 5 tbsp. gram flour
- A pinch of salt to taste
- For sauce:
- 2 cup fresh green coriander
- ½ cup mint leaves
- 3 tbsp. lemon juice

Directions:
1. You will first need to make the sauce. Add the ingredients to a blender and make a thick paste. Slit the pieces of chicken and stuff half the paste into the cavity obtained. Take the remaining paste and add it to the gram flour and salt.
2. Toss the pieces of chicken in this mixture and set aside. Apply a little bit of the mixture on the capsicum and onion. Place these on a stick along with the chicken pieces.
3. Pre heat the oven at 290 Fahrenheit for around 5 minutes. Open the basket. Arrange the satay sticks properly. Close the basket.
4. Keep the sticks with the chicken at 180 degrees for around half an hour while the sticks with the vegetables are to be kept at the same temperature for only 7 minutes. Turn the sticks in between so that one side does not get burnt and also to provide a uniform cook.

256.Mustard Chicken Breasts

Servings:4
Cooking Time: 20 Minutes
Ingredients:
- ¼ cup flour
- 1 lb chicken breasts, sliced
- 1 tbsp Worcestershire sauce
- ¼ cup onions, chopped
- 1 ½ cups brown sugar
- ¼ cup yellow mustard
- ¾ cup water
- ½ cup ketchup

Directions:

1. Preheat on AirFry function to 360 F. In a bowl, mix sugar, water, ketchup, onions, mustard, Worcestershire sauce, salt, and pepper. Stir until the sugar dissolves.
2. Flour the chicken slices and then dip it in the mustard mixture. Let marinate for 10 minutes. Place the chicken in a greased baking dish and press Start. Cook for 15 minutes. Serve immediately.

257.Spicy Pork Chops With Carrots And Mushrooms

Servings:4
Cooking Time: 15 Minutes
Ingredients:
- 2 carrots, cut into sticks
- 1 cup mushrooms, sliced
- 2 garlic cloves, minced
- 2 tablespoons olive oil
- 1 pound (454 g) boneless pork chops
- 1 teaspoon dried oregano
- 1 teaspoon dried thyme
- 1 teaspoon cayenne pepper
- Salt and ground black pepper, to taste
- Cooking spray

Directions:
1. In a mixing bowl, toss together the carrots, mushrooms, garlic, olive oil and salt until well combined.
2. Add the pork chops to a different bowl and season with oregano, thyme, cayenne pepper, salt and black pepper.
3. Lower the vegetable mixture in the greased basket. Place the seasoned pork chops on top.
4. Put the air fryer basket on the baking pan and slide into Rack Position 2, select Air Fry, set temperature to 360ºF (182ºC) and set time to 15 minutes.
5. After 7 minutes, remove from the oven. Flip the pork and stir the vegetables. Return to the oven and continue cooking.
6. When cooking is complete, the pork chops should be browned and the vegetables should be tender.
7. Transfer the pork chops to the serving dishes and let cool for 5 minutes. Serve warm with vegetable on the side.

258.Juicy Pork Ribs Ole

Servings: 4
Cooking Time: 25 Minutes
Ingredients:
- 1 rack of pork ribs
- 1/2 cup low-fat milk
- 1 tablespoon envelope taco seasoning mix
- 1 can tomato sauce
- 1/2 teaspoon ground black pepper
- 1 teaspoon seasoned salt

- 1 tablespoon cornstarch
- 1 teaspoon canola oil

Directions:
1. Preparing the Ingredients. Place all ingredients in a mixing dish; let them marinate for 1 hour.
2. Air Frying. Cook the marinated ribs approximately 25 minutes at 390 degrees F
3. Work with batches. Enjoy .

259.Basil Cheese Chicken

Servings: 4
Cooking Time: 20 Minutes
Ingredients:
- 4 chicken breasts, cubed
- 1 tbsp garlic powder
- 1 cup mayonnaise
- ½ tsp pepper
- ½ cup soft cheese
- ½ tbsp salt
- Chopped basil for garnish

Directions:
1. In a bowl, mix cheese, mayonnaise, garlic powder, and salt to form a marinade. Cover your chicken with the marinade. Place the marinated chicken in the basket and fit in the baking tray; cook for 15 minutes at 380 F on Air Fry function. Serve garnished with chopped fresh basil.

260.Worcestershire Ribeye Steaks

Servings:2 To 4
Cooking Time: 10 To 12 Minutes
Ingredients:
- 2 (8-ounce / 227-g) boneless ribeye steaks
- 4 teaspoons Worcestershire sauce
- ½ teaspoon garlic powder
- Salt and ground black pepper, to taste
- 4 teaspoons olive oil

Directions:
1. Brush the steaks with Worcestershire sauce on both sides. Sprinkle with garlic powder and coarsely ground black pepper. Drizzle the steaks with olive oil. Allow steaks to marinate for 30 minutes.
2. Transfer the steaks into the basket.
3. Put the air fryer basket on the baking pan and slide into Rack Position 2, select Roast, set the temperature to 400ºF (205ºC) and set time to 4 minutes.
4. After 2 minutes, remove from the oven. Flip the steaks. Return to the oven and continue cooking.
5. When cooking is complete, the steaks should be well browned.
6. Remove the steaks from the basket and let sit for 5 minutes. Salt and serve.

261.Perfect Beef Hash Brown Bake

Servings: 4
Cooking Time: 40 Minutes
Ingredients:
- 1 lb ground beef
- 2 cups cheddar cheese, shredded
- 1 cup milk
- 10 oz can cream of mushroom soup
- 30 oz frozen shredded hash browns
- 1 tsp garlic powder
- 1 tbsp onion, minced
- Pepper
- Salt

Directions:
1. Fit the oven with the rack in position
2. In a pan, brown ground beef with garlic powder, onion, pepper, and salt. Drain.
3. In a bowl, mix meat, shredded cheese, milk, soup, and hash browns.
4. Pour meat mixture into the greased 9*13-inch baking dish.
5. Set to bake at 350 F for 45 minutes. After 5 minutes place the baking dish in the preheated oven.
6. Serve and enjoy.
- **Nutrition Info:** Calories 514 Fat 28.3 g Carbohydrates 11.4 g Sugar 4.8 g Protein 51.6 g Cholesterol 168 mg

262.Pheasant Chili

Servings:x
Cooking Time:x
Ingredients:
- 1 lb. cubed pheasant
- 2 ½ tsp. ginger-garlic paste
- 1 tsp. red chili sauce
- ¼ tsp. salt
- ¼ tsp. red chili powder/black pepper
- A few drops of edible orange food coloring
- For sauce:
- 2 tbsp. olive oil
- 1 ½ tsp. ginger garlic paste
- ½ tbsp. red chili sauce
- 2 tbsp. tomato ketchup
- 2 tsp. soya sauce
- 1-2 tbsp. honey
- ¼ tsp. Ajinomoto
- 1-2 tsp. red chili flakes

Directions:
1. Mix all the ingredients for the marinade and put the pheasant cubes inside and let it rest overnight. Mix the breadcrumbs, oregano and red chili flakes well and place the marinated Oregano Fingers on this mixture.
2. Cover it with plastic wrap and leave it till right before you serve to cook. Pre heat the oven at 160 degrees Fahrenheit for 5 minutes. Place the Oregano Fingers in the

fry basket and close it. Let them cook at the same temperature for another 15 minutes or so. Toss the Oregano Fingers well so that they are cooked uniformly.

263.Copycat Taco Bell Crunch Wraps

Servings: 6
Cooking Time: 2 Minutes
Ingredients:
- 6 wheat tostadas
- 2 C. sour cream
- 2 C. Mexican blend cheese
- 2 C. shredded lettuce
- 12 ounces low-sodium nacho cheese
- 3 Roma tomatoes
- 6 12-inch wheat tortillas
- 1 1/3 C. water
- 2 packets low-sodium taco seasoning
- 2 pounds of lean ground beef

Directions:
1. Preparing the Ingredients. Ensure your air fryer oven is preheated to 400 degrees.
2. Make beef according to taco seasoning packets.
3. Place 2/3 C. prepared beef, 4 tbsp. cheese, 1 tostada, 1/3 C. sour cream, 1/3 C. lettuce, 1/6th of tomatoes and 1/3 C. cheese on each tortilla.
4. Fold up tortillas edges and repeat with remaining ingredients.
5. Lay the folded sides of tortillas down into the air fryer oven and spray with olive oil.
6. Air Frying. Set temperature to 400°F, and set time to 2 minutes. Cook 2 minutes till browned.
- **Nutrition Info:** CALORIES: 311; FAT: 9G; PROTEIN:22G; SUGAR:2

264.Juicy Baked Chicken Wings

Servings: 4
Cooking Time: 40 Minutes
Ingredients:
- 2 lbs chicken wings
- 1 tbsp garlic, minced
- 2 tbsp mayonnaise
- 2 tbsp ketchup
- Pepper
- Salt

Directions:
1. Fit the oven with the rack in position
2. Add chicken wings and remaining ingredients into the bowl and mix well. Let marinate chicken wings for 3 hours.
3. Place marinated chicken wings into the baking dish.
4. Set to bake at 400 F for 45 minutes. After 5 minutes place the baking dish in the preheated oven.
5. Serve and enjoy.

- **Nutrition Info:** Calories 470 Fat 19.3 g Carbohydrates 4.4 g Sugar 2.2 g Protein 65.9 g Cholesterol 204 mg

265.Sherry Grilled Chicken

Servings: 2
Cooking Time: 25 Minutes
Ingredients:
- 2 chicken breasts, cubed
- 2 garlic clove, minced
- ½ cup ketchup
- ½ tbsp ginger, minced
- ½ cup soy sauce
- 2 tbsp sherry
- ½ cup pineapple juice
- 2 tbsp apple cider vinegar
- ½ cup brown sugar

Directions:
1. In a bowl, mix ketchup, pineapple juice, sugar, cider vinegar, and ginger. Heat the mixture in a frying pan over low heat. Cover chicken with the soy sauce and sherry; pour the hot sauce on top. Set aside for 15 minutes to marinate.
2. Preheat your oven on Broil function to 360 F. Remove the chicken from the marinade, pat dry, and place it in the greased basket. Fit in a baking tray and cook for 15 minutes.

266.Baked Pork Ribs

Servings: 8
Cooking Time: 30 Minutes
Ingredients:
- 2 lbs pork ribs, boneless
- 1 tbsp onion powder
- 1 1/2 tbsp garlic powder
- Pepper
- Salt

Directions:
1. Fit the oven with the rack in position
2. Place pork ribs in baking pan and season with onion powder, garlic powder, pepper, and salt.
3. Set to bake at 350 F for 35 minutes. After 5 minutes place the baking pan in the preheated oven.
4. Serve and enjoy.
- **Nutrition Info:** Calories 318 Fat 20.1 g Carbohydrates 1.9 g Sugar 0.7 g Protein 30.4 g Cholesterol 117 mg

267.One-pot Farfalle Pasta

Servings:x
Cooking Time:x
Ingredients:
- olive oil
- 5 slices bacon, chopped 1 (25-oz) jar marinara sauce with basil
- 2 cups water
- Salt and freshly ground black pepper, to taste
- 2 cups dried farfalle pasta
- 3 cups baby spinach
- 1½ cups fresh Mozzarella cheese, sliced
- Fresh basil leaves
- Grated Parmesan cheese

Directions:
1. Preheat the oven to 375°F.
2. In oven over medium heat, heat the olive oil until hot.
3. Add the bacon crumbles and cook for5 minutes.
4. Add the marinara sauce and water. Bring to a boil. Season with salt and pepper.
5. Add the pasta and spinach, and mix.
6. Tuck a few slices of fresh mozzarella into the mix, and place the rest
7. on top. Cover and bake for 20 minutes, or until the pasta is tender.
8. Sprinkle fresh basil and Parmesan cheese on top, and serve.

268.Corn Flour Lamb Fries With Red Chili

Servings:x
Cooking Time:x
Ingredients:
- 2 tsp. salt
- 1 tsp. pepper powder
- 1 lb. boneless lamb cut into Oregano Fingers
- 2 cup dry breadcrumbs
- 2 tsp. oregano
- 2 tsp. red chili flakes
- 1 ½ tbsp. ginger-garlic paste
- 4 tbsp. lemon juice
- 1 tsp. red chili powder
- 6 tbsp. corn flour
- 4 eggs

Directions:
1. Mix all the ingredients for the marinade and put the lamb Oregano Fingers inside and let it rest overnight.
2. Mix the breadcrumbs, oregano and red chili flakes well and place the
3. marinated Oregano Fingers on this mixture. Cover it with plastic wrap and leave it till right before you serve to cook.
4. Pre heat the oven at 160 degrees Fahrenheit for 5 minutes. Place the Oregano Fingers in the fry basket and close it. Let them cook at the same temperature for another 15 minutes or so. Toss the Oregano Fingers well so that they are cooked uniformly.

269.Crispy Pork Tenderloin

Servings:6
Cooking Time: 10 Minutes
Ingredients:

- 2 large egg whites
- 1½ tablespoons Dijon mustard
- 2 cups crushed pretzel crumbs
- 1½ pounds (680 g) pork tenderloin, cut into ¼-pound (113-g) sections
- Cooking spray

Directions:
1. Spritz the air fryer basket with cooking spray.
2. Whisk the egg whites with Dijon mustard in a bowl until bubbly. Pour the pretzel crumbs in a separate bowl.
3. Dredge the pork tenderloin in the egg white mixture and press to coat. Shake the excess off and roll the tenderloin over the pretzel crumbs.
4. Arrange the well-coated pork tenderloin in the pan and spritz with cooking spray.
5. Put the air fryer basket on the baking pan and slide into Rack Position 2, select Air Fry, set temperature to 350ºF (180ºC) and set time to 10 minutes.
6. After 5 minutes, remove from the oven. Flip the pork. Return to the oven and continue cooking.
7. When cooking is complete, the pork should be golden brown and crispy.
8. Serve immediately.

270.Pork Burger Cutlets With Fresh Coriander Leaves

Servings:x
Cooking Time:x
Ingredients:
- ½ lb. pork (Make sure that you mince the pork fine)
- ½ cup breadcrumbs
- ½ cup of boiled peas
- ¼ tsp. cumin powder
- A pinch of salt to taste
- ¼ tsp. ginger finely chopped
- 1 green chili finely chopped
- 1 tsp. lemon juice
- 1 tbsp. fresh coriander leaves. Chop them finely
- ¼ tsp. red chili powder
- ¼ tsp. dried mango powder

Directions:
1. Take a container and into it pour all the masalas, onions, green chilies, peas, coriander leaves, lemon juice, and ginger and 1-2 tbsp. breadcrumbs. Add the minced pork as well. Mix all the ingredients well.
2. Mold the mixture into round Cutlets. Press them gently. Now roll them out carefully. Pre heat the oven at 250 Fahrenheit for 5 minutes.
3. Open the basket of the Fryer and arrange the Cutlets in the basket. Close it carefully.

Keep the fryer at 150 degrees for around 10 or 12 minutes. In between the cooking process, turn the Cutlets over to get a uniform cook. Serve hot with mint sauce.

271.Tender Baby Back Ribs

Servings: 4
Cooking Time: 45 Minutes
Ingredients:
- 1 rack baby back ribs, separated in 2-3 rib sections
- 1 tsp salt
- 1 tsp pepper
- 2 cloves garlic, crushed
- 1 bay leaf
- 3 tbsp. white wine
- 2 tbsp. olive oil
- 1 tsp lemon juice
- ¼ tsp paprika
- 1 tsp soy sauce
- 2 thyme stems
- Nonstick cooking spray

Directions:
1. In a large bowl, combine all ingredients, except ribs, and mix well.
2. Add ribs and turn to coat all sides. Let marinate at room temperature 30 minutes.
3. Lightly spray fryer basket with cooking spray. Place baking pan in position 1 of the oven.
4. Add ribs to basket, in a single layer, and place on baking pan. Set oven to air fry on 360°F for 45 minutes. Baste ribs with marinade and turn a few times while cooking. Serve immediately.
- **Nutrition Info:** Calories 772, Total Fat 52g, Saturated Fat 10g, Total Carbs 2g, Net Carbs 2g, Protein 74g, Sugar 0g, Fiber 0g, Sodium 864mg, Potassium 1255mg, Phosphorus 749mg

272.Sweet-and-sour Chicken Nuggets

Servings:4
Cooking Time: 15 Minutes
Ingredients:
- 1 cup cornstarch
- Chicken seasoning or rub, to taste
- Salt and ground black pepper, to taste
- 2 eggs
- 2 (4-ounce/ 113-g) boneless, skinless chicken breasts, cut into 1-inch pieces
- 1½ cups sweet-and-sour sauce
- Cooking spray

Directions:
1. Spritz the air fryer basket with cooking spray.
2. Combine the cornstarch, chicken seasoning, salt, and pepper in a large bowl. Stir to mix well. Whisk the eggs in a separate bowl.

3. Dredge the chicken pieces in the bowl of cornstarch mixture first, then in the bowl of whisked eggs, and then in the cornstarch mixture again.
4. Arrange the well-coated chicken pieces in the basket. Spritz with cooking spray.
5. Put the air fryer basket on the baking pan and slide into Rack Position 2, select Air Fry, set temperature to 360ºF (182ºC) and set time to 15 minutes.
6. Flip the chicken halfway through.
7. When cooking is complete, the chicken should be golden brown and crispy.
8. Transfer the chicken pieces on a large serving plate, then baste with sweet-and-sour sauce before serving.

273.Fried Chicken Tenderloins

Servings: 4
Cooking Time: 15 Minutes
Ingredients:
- 8 chicken tenderloins
- 2 tbsp butter, softened
- 2 oz breadcrumbs
- 1 large egg, whisked

Directions:
1. Preheat on Air Fry function to 380 F. Combine butter and breadcrumbs in a bowl. Keep mixing and stirring until the mixture gets crumbly. Dip the chicken in the egg, then in the crumb mix. Place in the greased basket and fit in the baking tray; cook for 10 minutes, flipping once until crispy. Set on Broil function for crispier taste. Serve.

274.Bacon Ranch Chicken

Servings: 6
Cooking Time: 45 Minutes
Ingredients:
- 2 lbs chicken breasts
- 1 packet dry ranch dressing mix
- 2 cups cheddar cheese, shredded
- 1 tsp garlic powder
- 4 oz cream cheese
- 1 cup sour cream
- 12 oz broccoli, steam
- 1 lb bacon, cooked & chopped

Directions:
1. Fit the oven with the rack in position
2. Place chicken breasts and broccoli into the greased baking pan.
3. Mix together sour cream, cream cheese, garlic powder, bacon, and ranch dressing mix and pour over chicken and broccoli.
4. Sprinkle cheddar cheese on top of chicken and broccoli mixture.
5. Set to bake at 350 F for 50 minutes. After 5 minutes place the baking pan in the preheated oven.

6. Serve and enjoy.
- **Nutrition Info:** Calories 844 Fat 60.8 g Carbohydrates 11.8 g Sugar 1.5 g Protein 65.6 g Cholesterol 212 mg

275.Venison Tandoor

Servings:x
Cooking Time:x
Ingredients:
- 2 cups sliced venison
- 1 big capsicum (Cut this capsicum into big cubes)
- 1 onion (Cut it into quarters. Now separate the layers carefully.)
- 5 tbsp. gram flour
- A pinch of salt to taste
- For the filling:
- 2 cup fresh green coriander
- ½ cup mint leaves
- 4 tsp. fennel
- 2 tbsp. ginger-garlic paste
- 1 small onion
- 6-7 flakes garlic (optional)
- Salt to taste
- 3 tbsp. lemon juice

Directions:
1. You will first need to make the sauce. Add the ingredients to a blender and make a thick paste. Slit the pieces of venison and stuff half the paste into the cavity obtained. Take the remaining paste and add it to the gram flour and salt.
2. Toss the pieces of venison in this mixture and set aside. Apply a little bit of the mixture on the capsicum and onion. Place these on a stick along with the venison pieces. Pre heat the oven at 290 Fahrenheit for around 5 minutes.
3. Open the basket. Arrange the satay sticks properly. Close the basket. Keep the sticks with the venison at 180 degrees for around half an hour while the sticks with the vegetables are to be kept at the same temperature for only 7 minutes. Turn the sticks in between so that one side does not get burnt and also to provide a uniform cook.

276.Pork Sausages Bites With Almonds & Apples

Servings:6
Cooking Time: 25 Minutes
Ingredients:
- 16 oz sausage meat
- 1 whole egg, beaten
- 3 ½ oz onion, chopped
- 2 tbsp dried sage
- 2 tbsp almonds, chopped
- ½ tsp pepper

- 3 ½ oz apple, sliced
- ½ tsp salt

Directions:
1. Preheat oven to 350 F on AirFry function. In a bowl, mix onion, almonds, apples, egg, pepper, and salt. Add in the sausages and mix well with your hands. Form bite-size shapes from the mixture and add them to the frying basket. Cook for 20 minutes until golden. Serve warm.

277.Rosemary Pork Chops

Servings: 4
Cooking Time: 30 Minutes
Ingredients:
- 4 pork chops, boneless
- 1 tsp dried rosemary, crushed
- 4 garlic cloves, minced
- 1 tbsp fresh rosemary, chopped
- 1/4 tsp pepper
- 1/4 tsp salt

Directions:
1. Fit the oven with the rack in position
2. Season pork chops with pepper and salt and set aside.
3. In a small bowl, mix together garlic and rosemary and rub over pork chops.
4. Place pork chops in a baking pan.
5. Set to bake at 425 F for 35 minutes. After 5 minutes place the baking pan in the preheated oven.
6. Serve and enjoy.
- **Nutrition Info:** Calories 265 Fat 20.1 g Carbohydrates 1.8 g Sugar 0 g Protein 18.2 g Cholesterol 69 mg

278.Drumsticks With Barbecue-honey Sauce

Servings:5
Cooking Time: 18 Minutes
Ingredients:
- 1 tablespoon olive oil
- 10 chicken drumsticks
- Chicken seasoning or rub, to taste
- Salt and ground black pepper, to taste
- 1 cup barbecue sauce
- ¼ cup honey

Directions:
1. Grease the basket with olive oil.
2. Rub the chicken drumsticks with chicken seasoning or rub, salt and ground black pepper on a clean work surface.
3. Arrange the chicken drumsticks in the basket.
4. Put the air fryer basket on the baking pan and slide into Rack Position 2, select Air Fry, set temperature to 390ºF (199ºC) and set time to 18 minutes.
5. Flip the drumsticks halfway through.

6. When cooking is complete, the drumsticks should be lightly browned.
7. Meanwhile, combine the barbecue sauce and honey in a small bowl. Stir to mix well.
8. Remove the drumsticks from the oven and baste with the sauce mixture to serve.

279.Cheesy Baked Burger Patties

Servings: 6
Cooking Time: 15 Minutes
Ingredients:
- 2 lbs ground beef
- 1 tsp onion powder
- 1 tsp garlic powder
- 1/2 cup mozzarella cheese, shredded
- 1/2 cup cheddar cheese, shredded
- Pepper
- Salt

Directions:
1. Fit the oven with the rack in position
2. Add all ingredients into the large bowl and mix until well combined.
3. Make patties from the meat mixture and place it into the baking pan.
4. Set to bake at 400 F for 20 minutes. After 5 minutes place the baking pan in the preheated oven.
5. Serve and enjoy.
- **Nutrition Info:** Calories 329 Fat 13 g Carbohydrates 0.9 g Sugar 0.3 g Protein 49 g Cholesterol 146 mg

280.Korean Flavor Glazed Chicken Wings

Servings:4
Cooking Time: 25 Minutes
Ingredients:
- Wings:
- 2 pounds (907 g) chicken wings
- 1 teaspoon salt
- 1 teaspoon ground black pepper
- Sauce:
- 2 tablespoons gochujang
- 1 tablespoon mayonnaise
- 1 tablespoon minced ginger
- 1 tablespoon minced garlic
- 1 teaspoon agave nectar
- 2 packets Splenda
- 1 tablespoon sesame oil
- For Garnish:
- 2 teaspoons sesame seeds
- ¼ cup chopped green onions

Directions:
1. Line the baking pan with aluminum foil, then arrange the rack on the pan.
2. On a clean work surface, rub the chicken wings with salt and ground black pepper, then arrange the seasoned wings on the rack.

3. Put the air fryer basket on the baking pan and slide into Rack Position 2, select Air Fry, set temperature to 400ºF (205ºC) and set time to 20 minutes.
4. Flip the wings halfway through.
5. When cooking is complete, the wings should be well browned.
6. Meanwhile, combine the ingredients for the sauce in a small bowl. Stir to mix well. Reserve half of the sauce in a separate bowl until ready to serve.
7. Remove the air fried chicken wings from the oven and toss with remaining half of the sauce to coat well.
8. Place the wings back to the oven. Put the air fryer basket on the baking pan and slide into Rack Position 2, select Air Fry, and set time to 5 minutes.
9. When cooking is complete, the internal temperature of the wings should reach at least 165ºF (74ºC).
10. Remove the wings from the oven and place on a large plate. Sprinkle with sesame seeds and green onions. Serve with reserved sauce.

281.Mexican Chicken Burgers

Servings: 6
Cooking Time: 10 Minutes
Ingredients:
- 1 jalapeno pepper
- 1 tsp. cayenne pepper
- 1 tbsp. mustard powder
- 1 tbsp. oregano
- 1 tbsp. thyme
- 3 tbsp. smoked paprika
- 1 beaten egg
- 1 small head of cauliflower
- 4 chicken breasts

Directions:
1. Preparing the Ingredients. Ensure your air fryer oven is preheated to 350 degrees.
2. Add seasonings to a blender. Slice cauliflower into florets and add to blender.
3. Pulse till mixture resembles that of breadcrumbs.
4. Take out ¾ of cauliflower mixture and add to a bowl. Set to the side. In another bowl, beat your egg and set to the side.
5. Remove skin and bones from chicken breasts and add to blender with remaining cauliflower mixture. Season with pepper and salt.
6. Take out mixture and form into burger shapes. Roll each patty in cauliflower crumbs, then the egg, and back into crumbs again.
7. Air Frying. Place coated patties into the air fryer oven. Set temperature to 350°F, and set time to 10 minutes.

8. Flip over at 10-minute mark. They are done when crispy!
- **Nutrition Info:** CALORIES: 234; FAT: 18G; PROTEIN:24G; SUGAR:1G

282.Bo Luc Lac

Servings:4
Cooking Time: 4 Minutes
Ingredients:
- For the Meat:
- 2 teaspoons soy sauce
- 4 garlic cloves, minced
- 1 teaspoon kosher salt
- 2 teaspoons sugar
- ¼ teaspoon ground black pepper
- 1 teaspoon toasted sesame oil
- 1½ pounds (680 g) top sirloin steak, cut into 1-inch cubes
- Cooking spray
- For the Salad:
- 1 head Bibb lettuce, leaves separated and torn into large pieces
- ¼ cup fresh mint leaves
- ½ cup halved grape tomatoes
- ½ red onion, halved and thinly sliced
- 2 tablespoons apple cider vinegar
- 1 garlic clove, minced
- 2 teaspoons sugar
- ¼ teaspoon kosher salt
- ¼ teaspoon ground black pepper
- 2 tablespoons vegetable oil
- For Serving:
- Lime wedges, for garnish
- Coarse salt and freshly cracked black pepper, to taste

Directions:
1. Combine the ingredients for the meat, except for the steak, in a large bowl. Stir to mix well.
2. Dunk the steak cubes in the bowl and press to coat. Wrap the bowl in plastic and marinate under room temperature for at least 30 minutes.
3. Spritz the air fryer basket with cooking spray.
4. Discard the marinade and transfer the steak cubes in the prepared basket.
5. Put the air fryer basket on the baking pan and slide into Rack Position 2, select Air Fry, set temperature to 450ºF (235ºC) and set time to 4 minutes.
6. Flip the steak cubes halfway through.
7. When cooking is complete, the steak cubes should be lightly browned but still have a little pink.
8. Meanwhile, combine the ingredients for the salad in a separate large bowl. Toss to mix well.

9. Pour the salad in a large serving bowl and top with the steak cubes. Squeeze the lime wedges over and sprinkle with salt and black pepper before serving.

283.Honey & Garlic Chicken Thighs

Servings: 4
Cooking Time: 30 Minutes
Ingredients:
- 4 thighs, skin-on
- 3 tbsp honey
- 2 tbsp Dijon mustard
- ½ tbsp garlic powder
- Salt and black pepper to taste

Directions:
1. In a bowl, mix honey, mustard, garlic, salt, and black pepper. Coat the thighs in the mixture and arrange them on the greased basket. Fit in the baking tray and cook for 16 minutes at 400 F on Air Fry function, turning once halfway through. Serve warm.

284.Savory Honey & Garlic Chicken

Servings: 2
Cooking Time: 20 Minutes + Marinating Time
Ingredients:
- 2 chicken drumsticks, skin removed
- 2 tbsp olive oil
- 2 tbsp honey
- ½ tbsp garlic, minced

Directions:
1. Add garlic, olive oil, and honey to a sealable zip bag. Add chicken and toss to coat; set aside for 30 minutes. Add the coated chicken to the basket and fit in the baking sheet; cook for 15 minutes at 400 F on Air Fry function, flipping once. Serve and enjoy!

285.Quail Fried Baked Pastry

Servings:x
Cooking Time:x
Ingredients:
- 2 tbsp. unsalted butter
- 1 ½ cup all-purpose flour
- 1 tsp. coarsely crushed coriander
- 1 dry red chili broken into pieces
- A small amount of salt (to taste)
- ½ tsp. dried mango powder
- ½ tsp. red chili power.
- A pinch of salt to taste
- Add as much water as required to make the dough stiff and firm
- 1 lb. quail
- ¼ cup boiled peas
- 1 tsp. powdered ginger
- 1 or 2 green chilies that are finely chopped or mashed
- ½ tsp. cumin
- 1-2 tbsp. coriander.

Directions:
1. You will first need to make the outer covering. In a large bowl, add the flour, butter and enough water to knead it into dough that is stiff. Transfer this to a container and leave it to rest for five minutes. Place a pan on medium flame and add the oil. Roast the mustard seeds and once roasted, add the coriander seeds and the chopped dry red chilies. Add all the dry ingredients for the filling and mix the ingredients well. Add a little water and continue to stir the ingredients.
2. Make small balls out of the dough and roll them out. Cut the rolled-out dough into halves and apply a little water on the edges to help you fold the halves into a cone. Add the filling to the cone and close up the samosa.
3. Pre-heat the oven for around 5 to 6 minutes at 300 Fahrenheit. Place all the samosas in the fry basket and close the basket properly. Keep the oven at 200 degrees for another 20 to 25 minutes. Around the halfway point, open the basket and turn the samosas over for uniform cooking. After this, fry at 250 degrees for around 10 minutes in order to give them the desired golden-brown color. Serve hot. Recommended sides are tamarind or mint sauce.

286.Carne Asada

Servings:4
Cooking Time: 15 Minutes
Ingredients:
- 3 chipotle peppers in adobo, chopped
- $1/3$ cup chopped fresh oregano
- $1/3$ cup chopped fresh parsley
- 4 cloves garlic, minced
- Juice of 2 limes
- 1 teaspoon ground cumin seeds
- $1/3$ cup olive oil
- 1 to 1½ pounds (454 g to 680 g) flank steak
- Salt, to taste

Directions:
1. Combine the chipotle, oregano, parsley, garlic, lime juice, cumin, and olive oil in a large bowl. Stir to mix well.
2. Dunk the flank steak in the mixture and press to coat well. Wrap the bowl in plastic and marinate under room temperature for at least 30 minutes.
3. Discard the marinade and place the steak in the basket. Sprinkle with salt.
4. Put the air fryer basket on the baking pan and slide into Rack Position 2, select Air Fry, set temperature to 390ºF (199ºC) and set time to 15 minutes.

5. Flip the steak halfway through the cooking time.
6. When cooking is complete, the steak should be medium-rare or reach your desired doneness.
7. Remove the steak from the oven and slice to serve.

287. Seafood Grandma's Easy To Cook Wontons

Servings:x
Cooking Time:x
Ingredients:
- 1 ½ cup all-purpose flour
- ½ tsp. salt
- 5 tbsp. water
- For filling:
- 2 cups minced seafood (prawns, shrimp, oysters, scallops)
- 2 tbsp. oil
- 2 tsp. ginger-garlic paste
- 2 tsp. soya sauce
- 2 tsp. vinegar

Directions:
1. Squeeze the dough and cover it with plastic wrap and set aside. Next, cook the ingredients for the filling and try to ensure that the seafood is covered well with the sauce. Roll the dough and place the filling in the center. Now, wrap the dough to cover the filling and pinch the edges together. Pre heat the oven at 200° F for 5 minutes.
2. Place the wontons in the fry basket and close it. Let them cook at the same temperature for another 20 minutes. Recommended sides are chili sauce or ketchup.

288. Copycat Chicken Sandwich

Servings: 4
Cooking Time: 15 Minutes
Ingredients:
- 2 chicken breasts, boneless & skinless
- 1 cup buttermilk
- 1 tbsp. + 2 tsp paprika, divided
- 1 tbsp. + 1 ½ tsp garlic powder, divided
- 2 tsp salt, divided
- 2 tsp pepper, divided
- 4 brioche buns
- 1 cup flour
- ½ cup corn starch
- 1 tbsp. onion powder
- 1 tbsp. cayenne pepper
- ½ cup mayonnaise
- 1 tsp hot sauce
- Sliced pickles

Directions:
1. Place chicken between two sheets of plastic wrap and pound to ½-inch thick. Cut crosswise to get 4 cutlets.
2. In a large bowl, whisk together buttermilk and one teaspoon each paprika, garlic powder, salt, and pepper. Add chicken, cover, and refrigerate overnight.
3. Place the buns on the baking pan and place in position 2 of the oven. Set to toast for about 2-5 minutes depending how toasted you want them. Set aside.
4. In a medium shallow dish, combine flour, cornstarch, onion powder, cayenne pepper, and remaining paprika, garlic powder, salt, and pepper.
5. Whisk in 2-3 tablespoons of the buttermilk batter chicken was marinating in until smooth.
6. Lightly spray fryer basket with cooking spray.
7. Dredge chicken in the flour mixture forming a thick coating of the batter. Place in fryer basket.
8. Place basket in the oven. Set oven to air fryer on 375°F for 10 minutes. Cook until crispy and golden brown, turning chicken over halfway through cooking time.
9. In a small bowl, whisk together mayonnaise, hot sauce, 1 teaspoon paprika, and ½ teaspoon garlic powder.
10. To serve, spread top of buns with mayonnaise mixture. Place chicken on bottom buns and top with pickles then top bun.
- **Nutrition Info:** Calories 689, Total Fat 27g, Saturated Fat 5g, Total Carbs 71g, Net Carbs 67g, Protein 38g, Sugar 7g, Fiber 4g, Sodium 1734mg, Potassium 779mg, Phosphorus 435mg

289. Honey Glazed Chicken Breasts

Servings:4
Cooking Time: 10 Minutes
Ingredients:
- 4 (4-ounce / 113-g) boneless, skinless chicken breasts
- Chicken seasoning or rub, to taste
- Salt and ground black pepper, to taste
- ¼ cup honey
- 2 tablespoons soy sauce
- 2 teaspoons grated fresh ginger
- 2 garlic cloves, minced
- Cooking spray

Directions:
1. Spritz the air fryer basket with cooking spray.
2. Rub the chicken breasts with chicken seasoning, salt, and black pepper on a clean work surface.

3. Arrange the chicken breasts in the basket and spritz with cooking spray.
4. Put the air fryer basket on the baking pan and slide into Rack Position 2, select Air Fry, set temperature to 400ºF (205ºC) and set time to 10 minutes.
5. Flip the chicken breasts halfway through.
6. When cooking is complete, the internal temperature of the thickest part of the chicken should reach at least 165ºF (74ºC).
7. Meanwhile, combine the honey, soy sauce, ginger, and garlic in a saucepan and heat over medium-high heat for 3 minutes or until thickened. Stir constantly.
8. Remove the chicken from the oven and serve with the honey glaze.

290.Garlic Lemony Chicken Breast

Servings:2
Cooking Time: 20 Minutes
Ingredients:
- 1 chicken breast
- 2 lemon, juiced and rind reserved
- 1 tbsp chicken seasoning
- 1 tbsp garlic puree
- A handful of peppercorns
- Salt and black pepper to taste

Directions:
1. Place a silver foil sheet on a flat surface. Add all seasonings alongside the lemon rind. Lay the chicken breast onto a chopping board and trim any fat and little bones; season.
2. Rub the chicken seasoning on both sides. Place on the foil sheet and seal tightly; flatten with a rolling pin. Place the breast in the basket and cook for 15 minutes at 350 F on AirFry function.

291.Hot Chicken Wings

Servings: 2
Cooking Time: 20 Minutes + Chilling Time
Ingredients:
- 8 chicken wings
- 1 tbsp water
- 2 tbsp potato starch
- 2 tbsp hot curry paste
- ½ tbsp baking powder

Directions:
1. Combine hot curry paste and water in a small bowl. Add in the wings toss to coat. Cover the bowl with plastic wrap and refrigerate for 30 minutes.
2. Preheat on Air Fry function to 370 degrees. In a bowl, mix the baking powder with potato starch. Remove the wings from the fridge and dip them in the starch mixture.
3. Place on a lined baking dish and cook in your for 7 minutes. Flip over and cook for 5 minutes.

292.Quail Marinade Cutlet

Servings:x
Cooking Time:x
Ingredients:
- ½ cup mint leaves
- 4 tsp. fennel
- 2 tbsp. ginger-garlic paste
- 1 small onion
- 6-7 flakes garlic (optional)
- Salt to taste
- 2 cups sliced quail
- 1 big capsicum (Cut this capsicum into big cubes)
- 1 onion (Cut it into quarters. Now separate the layers carefully.)
- 5 tbsp. gram flour
- A pinch of salt to taste
- For the filling:
- 2 cup fresh green coriander
- 3 tbsp. lemon juice

Directions:
1. You will first need to make the sauce. Add the ingredients to a blender and make a thick paste. Slit the pieces of quail and stuff half the paste into the cavity obtained.
2. Take the remaining paste and add it to the gram flour and salt. Toss the pieces of quail in this mixture and set aside.
3. Apply a little bit of the mixture on the capsicum and onion. Place these on a stick along with the quail pieces.
4. Pre heat the oven at 290 Fahrenheit for around 5 minutes. Open the basket. Arrange the satay sticks properly. Close the basket. Keep the sticks with the quail at 180 degrees for around half an hour while the sticks with the vegetables are to be kept at the same temperature for only 7 minutes.
5. Turn the sticks in between so that one side does not get burnt and also to provide a uniform cook.

293.Ham And Eggs

Servings:x
Cooking Time:x
Ingredients:
- Bread slices (brown or white)
- 1 egg white for every 2 slices
- 1 tsp sugar for every 2 slices
- ½ lb. sliced ham

Directions:
1. Put two slices together and cut them along the diagonal. In a bowl, whisk the egg whites and add some sugar.
2. Dip the bread triangles into this mixture. Cook the chicken now. Pre heat the oven at 180° C for 4 minutes. Place the coated bread triangles in the fry basket and close it. Let

them cook at the same temperature for another 20 minutes at least.

3. Halfway through the process, turn the triangles over so that you get a uniform cook. Top with ham and serve.

294.Mango Marinated Chicken Breasts

Servings: 2
Cooking Time: 20 Minutes + Marinating Time
Ingredients:
- 2 chicken breasts, cubed
- 1 large mango, cubed
- 1 red pepper, chopped
- 2 tbsp balsamic vinegar
- 5 tbsp olive oil
- 2 garlic cloves, minced
- 1 tbsp fresh parsley, chopped
- Salt to taste

Directions:
1. In a bowl, mix mango, garlic, red pepper, olive oil, salt, and balsamic vinegar. Add the mixture to a blender and pulse until smooth. Transfer to a bowl and add in the chicken cubes. Toss to coat and place in the fridge for 30 minutes.
2. Preheat on Air Fry function to 360 F. Remove the chicken from the fridge and place cubes in the greased basket. Fit in the baking tray and cook in the air fryer oven for 12 minutes, shaking once. Garnish with parsley and serve.

295.Minced Venison Grandma's Easy To Cook Wontons With Garlic Paste

Servings:x
Cooking Time:x
Ingredients:
- 1 ½ cup all-purpose flour
- ½ tsp. salt
- 2 tsp. soya sauce
- 5 tbsp. water
- 2 cups minced venison
- 2 tbsp. oil
- 2 tsp. ginger-garlic paste
- 2 tsp. vinegar

Directions:
1. Squeeze the dough and cover it with plastic wrap and set aside. Next, cook the ingredients for the filling and try to ensure that the venison is covered well with the sauce. Roll the dough and place the filling in the center.
2. Now, wrap the dough to cover the filling and pinch the edges together. Pre heat the oven at 200° F for 5 minutes.
3. Place the wontons in the fry basket and close it. Let them cook at the same temperature for another 20 minutes.

Recommended sides are chili sauce or ketchup.

296.Pork Spicy Lemon Kebab

Servings:x
Cooking Time:x
Ingredients:
- 1 lb. boneless pork cubed
- 3 onions chopped
- 5 green chilies-roughly chopped
- 1 ½ tbsp. ginger paste
- 4 tbsp. fresh mint chopped
- 3 tbsp. chopped capsicum
- 3 eggs
- 2 ½ tbsp. white sesame seeds
- 1 ½ tsp. garlic paste
- 1 ½ tsp. salt
- 3 tsp. lemon juice
- 2 tsp. garam masala
- 4 tbsp. chopped coriander
- 3 tbsp. cream
- 2 tbsp. coriander powder

Directions:
1. Mix the dry ingredients in a bowl. Make the mixture into a smooth paste and coat the pork cubes with the mixture. Beat the eggs in a bowl and add a little salt to them. Dip the cubes in the egg mixture and coat them with sesame seeds and leave them in the refrigerator for an hour. Pre heat the oven at 290 Fahrenheit for around 5 minutes.
2. Place the kebabs in the basket and let them cook for another 25 minutes at the same temperature. Turn the kebabs over in between the cooking process to get a uniform cook. Serve the kebabs with mint sauce.

297.Balsamic Chicken With Mozzarella Cheese

Servings:4
Cooking Time: 25 Minutes
Ingredients:
- 4 chicken breasts, cubed
- 4 fresh basil leaves
- ¼ cup balsamic vinegar
- 2 tomatoes, chopped
- 1 tbsp butter, melted
- 4 mozzarella cheese, grated

Directions:
1. In a bowl, mix butter and balsamic vinegar. Add in the chicken and toss to coat. Transfer to a baking tray and press Start. Cook for 20 minutes at 400 F on AirFry function. Top with mozzarella cheese and Bake until the cheese melts. Top with basil and tomatoes and serve.

298.Meatballs(5)

Servings: 6
Cooking Time: 20 Minutes
Ingredients:
- 2 lbs ground beef
- 1 egg, lightly beaten
- 1 tsp cinnamon
- 2 tsp cumin
- 2 tsp coriander
- 1 tsp garlic, minced
- 1 tbsp fresh basil, chopped
- 1/4 cup fresh parsley, minced
- 1 tsp smoked paprika
- 1 tsp oregano
- 1 onion, grated
- 1/4 tsp pepper
- 1/2 tsp salt

Directions:
1. Fit the oven with the rack in position
2. Add all ingredients into the large mixing bowl and mix until well combined.
3. Make small balls from the meat mixture and place it into the parchment-lined baking pan.
4. Set to bake at 400 F for 25 minutes. After 5 minutes place the baking pan in the preheated oven.
5. Serve and enjoy.
- **Nutrition Info:** Calories 306 Fat 10.4 g Carbohydrates 3.1 g Sugar 0.9 g Protein 47.3 g Cholesterol 162 mg

299.Simple Pork Meatballs With Red Chili

Servings:4
Cooking Time: 15 Minutes
Ingredients:
- 1 pound (454 g) ground pork
- 2 cloves garlic, finely minced
- 1 cup scallions, finely chopped
- 1½ tablespoons Worcestershire sauce
- ½ teaspoon freshly grated ginger root
- 1 teaspoon turmeric powder
- 1 tablespoon oyster sauce
- 1 small sliced red chili, for garnish
- Cooking spray

Directions:
1. Spritz the air fryer basket with cooking spray.
2. Combine all the ingredients, except for the red chili in a large bowl. Toss to mix well.
3. Shape the mixture into equally sized balls, then arrange them in the basket and spritz with cooking spray.
4. Put the air fryer basket on the baking pan and slide into Rack Position 2, select Air Fry, set temperature to 350ºF (180ºC) and set time to 15 minutes.

5. After 7 minutes, remove from the oven. Flip the balls. Return to the oven and continue cooking.
6. When cooking is complete, the balls should be lightly browned.
7. Serve the pork meatballs with red chili on top.

300.Cripsy Crusted Pork Chops

Servings: 4
Cooking Time: 40 Minutes
Ingredients:
- 4 pork chops, boneless
- 1 cup parmesan cheese
- 1 tbsp olive oil
- 1 tsp garlic powder
- 1 cup breadcrumbs
- 1/2 tsp Italian seasoning
- Pepper
- Salt

Directions:
1. Fit the oven with the rack in position
2. In a shallow dish, mix breadcrumbs, parmesan cheese, Italian seasoning, garlic powder, pepper, and salt.
3. Brush pork chops with oil and coat with breadcrumb mixture.
4. Place coated pork chops in a baking pan.
5. Set to bake at 350 F for 45 minutes. After 5 minutes place the baking pan in the preheated oven.
6. Serve and enjoy.
- **Nutrition Info:** Calories 469 Fat 29.8 g Carbohydrates 20.8 g Sugar 1.9 g Protein 28.9 g Cholesterol 85 mg

301.Pesto & Spinach Beef Rolls

Servings:4
Cooking Time: 30 Minutes
Ingredients:
- 2 lb beef steak, thinly sliced
- Salt and black pepper to taste
- 3 tbsp pesto
- ½ cup mozzarella cheese; shredded
- 1 cup spinach, chopped
- 1 bell pepper, deseeded and sliced

Directions:
1. Preheat oven to 400 F on Bake function. Place the beef slices between 2 baking paper sheets and flatten them with a rolling pin to about a fifth of an inch thick. Lay the slices on a clean surface and spread them with the pesto. Top with mozzarella, spinach, and bell pepper.
2. Roll up the slices and secure using a toothpick. Season with salt and pepper. Place the slices in the greased basket and Bake for 15 minutes. Serve immediately!

302.Crunchy Parmesan Pork Chops

Servings: 4
Cooking Time: 10 Minutes
Ingredients:
- 4 pork chops, boneless
- 2 tbsp olive oil
- 1/4 tsp pepper
- 1/2 tsp garlic powder
- 1 tsp dried parsley
- 1/4 tsp smoked paprika
- 2 tbsp breadcrumbs
- 1/4 cup parmesan cheese, grated

Directions:
1. Fit the oven with the rack in position
2. In a shallow dish, mix breadcrumbs, paprika, parmesan cheese, garlic powder, parsley, and pepper.
3. Brush pork chops with oil and coat with breadcrumb mixture.
4. Place coated pork chops into the baking pan.
5. Set to bake at 450 F for 15 minutes. After 5 minutes place the baking pan in the preheated oven.
6. Serve and enjoy.
- **Nutrition Info:** Calories 350 Fat 28.3 g Carbohydrates 3.1 g Sugar 0.3 g Protein 20.4 g Cholesterol 73 mg

303.Golden Chicken Fries

Servings:4 To 6
Cooking Time: 6 Minutes
Ingredients:
- 1 pound (454 g) chicken tenders, cut into about ½-inch-wide strips
- Salt, to taste
- ¼ cup all-purpose flour
- 2 eggs
- ¾ cup panko bread crumbs
- ¾ cup crushed organic nacho cheese tortilla chips
- Cooking spray
- Seasonings:
- ½ teaspoon garlic powder
- 1 tablespoon chili powder
- ½ teaspoon onion powder
- 1 teaspoon ground cumin

Directions:
1. Stir together all seasonings in a small bowl and set aside.
2. Sprinkle the chicken with salt. Place strips in a large bowl and sprinkle with 1 tablespoon of the seasoning mix. Stir well to distribute seasonings.
3. Add flour to chicken and stir well to coat all sides.
4. Beat eggs in a separate bowl.
5. In a shallow dish, combine the panko, crushed chips, and the remaining 2 teaspoons of seasoning mix.
6. Dip chicken strips in eggs, then roll in crumbs. Mist with oil or cooking spray. Arrange the chicken strips in a single layer in the basket.
7. Put the air fryer basket on the baking pan and slide into Rack Position 2, select Air Fry, set the temperature to 400ºF (205ºC) and set the time to 6 minutes.
8. After 4 minutes, remove from the oven. Flip the strips with tongs. Return to the oven and continue cooking.
9. When cooking is complete, the chicken should be crispy and its juices should be run clear.
10. Allow to cool under room temperature before serving.

304.Easy Smothered Chicken

Servings: 4
Cooking Time: 55 Minutes
Ingredients:
- 4 chicken breasts
- 1/2 tsp garlic powder
- 1 tsp dried basil
- 1 tsp dried oregano
- 1 tbsp cornstarch
- 3/4 cup parmesan cheese, grated
- 1 cup sour cream
- 4 mozzarella cheese slices
- 1/4 tsp pepper
- 1/2 tsp salt

Directions:
1. Fit the oven with the rack in position
2. Place chicken breasts into the baking dish and top with mozzarella cheese slices.
3. In a bowl, mix sour cream, parmesan cheese, cornstarch, oregano, basil, garlic powder, pepper, and salt.
4. Pour sour cream mixture over chicken.
5. Set to bake at 375 F for 60 minutes. After 5 minutes place the baking dish in the preheated oven.
6. Serve and enjoy.
- **Nutrition Info:** Calories 545 Fat 31.5 g Carbohydrates 6.5 g Sugar 0.2 g Protein 57.2 g Cholesterol 182 mg

305.Cheesy Chicken With Tomato Sauce

Servings:2
Cooking Time: 20 Minutes
Ingredients:
- 2 chicken breasts, ½-inch thick
- 1 egg, beaten
- ½ cup breadcrumbs
- Salt and black pepper to taste
- 2 tbsp tomato sauce
- 2 tbsp Grana Padano cheese, grated
- ¼ cup mozzarella cheese, shredded

Directions:

1. Preheat on AirFry function to 350 F. Dip the breasts into the egg, then into the crumbs and arrange on the greased basket. Cook for 5 minutes. Turn, drizzle with tomato sauce, sprinkle with Grana Padano and mozzarella cheeses, and cook for 5 more minutes. Serve warm.

306.Mutton French Cuisine Galette

Servings:x
Cooking Time:x
Ingredients:
- 2 tbsp. garam masala
- 1 lb. minced mutton
- 3 tsp ginger finely chopped
- 1-2 tbsp. fresh coriander leaves
- 2 or 3 green chilies finely chopped
- 1 ½ tbsp. lemon juice
- Salt and pepper to taste

Directions:
1. Mix the ingredients in a clean bowl. Mold this mixture into round and flat French Cuisine Galettes. Wet the French Cuisine Galettes slightly with water.
2. Pre heat the oven at 160 degrees Fahrenheit for 5 minutes. Place the French Cuisine Galettes in the fry basket and let them cook for another 25 minutes at the same temperature. Keep rolling them over to get a uniform cook. Serve either with mint sauce or ketchup.

307.Chinese Bbq Pork

Servings: 8
Cooking Time: 40 Minutes
Ingredients:
- ½ cup soy sauce
- 2 tbsp. hoisin sauce
- ½ tsp Chinese five spice
- 1 tsp Sriracha sauce
- 1 cup brown sugar
- 3 lbs. pork shoulder, boneless, cut in 2-3-inch cubes

Directions:
1. In a large bowl, whisk together soy sauce, hoisin, five spice, Sriracha, and sugar until sugar is almost dissolved.
2. Add pork and toss to coat well. Cover and refrigerate overnight, stir occasionally.
3. Place baking pan in position 1 of the oven. Set to convection bake on 325°F for 45 minutes.
4. Add the pork to the fryer basket in a single layer. After oven has preheated for 5 minutes, place basket on baking pan. Cook 40 minutes, or until pork is cooked through, flipping over halfway through cooking time. Use marinade to baste meat occasionally. Serve immediately.

- **Nutrition Info:** Calories 344, Total Fat 6g, Saturated Fat 2g, Total Carbs 30g, Net Carbs 30g, Protein 40g, Sugar 28g, Fiber 0g, Sodium 754mg, Potassium 743mg, Phosphorus 319mg

308.Cheesy Bacon Chicken

Servings: 4
Cooking Time: 30 Minutes
Ingredients:
- 4 chicken breasts, sliced in half
- 1 cup cheddar cheese, shredded
- 8 bacon slices, cooked & chopped
- 6 oz cream cheese
- Pepper
- Salt

Directions:
1. Fit the oven with the rack in position
2. Place season chicken with pepper and salt and place it into the greased baking dish.
3. Add cream cheese and bacon on top of chicken.
4. Sprinkle shredded cheddar cheese on top of chicken.
5. Set to bake at 400 F for 35 minutes. After 5 minutes place the baking dish in the preheated oven.
6. Serve and enjoy.
- **Nutrition Info:** Calories 745 Fat 50.9 g Carbohydrates 2.1 g Sugar 0.2 g Protein 66.6 g Cholesterol 248 mg

309.Teriyaki Pork Ribs In Tomato Sauce

Servings:4
Cooking Time: 20 Minutes
Ingredients:
- 1 pound pork ribs
- Salt and black pepper to taste
- 1 tbsp sugar
- 1 tsp ginger juice
- 1 tsp five-spice powder
- 1 tbsp teriyaki sauce
- 1 tbsp soy sauce
- 1 garlic clove, minced
- 2 tbsp honey
- 1 tbsp water
- 1 tbsp tomato sauce

Directions:
1. In a bowl, mix pepper, sugar, five-spice powder, salt, ginger juice, and teriyaki sauce. Add in the pork ribs and let marinate for 2 hours.
2. Preheat on Bake function to 380 F. Put the marinated pork ribs in a baking tray and place in the oven. Press Start and cook for 8 minutes.
3. In a pan over medium heat, mix soy sauce, garlic, honey, water, and tomato sauce. Stir and cook for 2-3 minutes until the sauce

thickens. Pour the sauce over the pork ribs and serve.

310.Meatballs(14)

Servings: 4
Cooking Time: 25 Minutes
Ingredients:
- 1 lb ground beef
- 1 tsp fresh rosemary, chopped
- 1 tbsp garlic, chopped
- 1/2 tsp pepper
- 1 tsp garlic powder
- 1 tsp onion powder
- 1/4 cup breadcrumbs
- 2 eggs
- 1 lb ground pork
- 1/2 tsp pepper
- 1 tsp sea salt

Directions:
1. Fit the oven with the rack in position
2. Add all ingredients into the mixing bowl and mix until well combined.
3. Make small balls from the meat mixture and place it into the parchment-lined baking pan.
4. Set to bake at 400 F for 30 minutes. After 5 minutes place the baking pan in the preheated oven.
5. Serve and enjoy.
- **Nutrition Info:** Calories 441 Fat 13.7 g Carbohydrates 7.2 g Sugar 1 g Protein 68.1 g Cholesterol 266 mg

FISH & SEAFOOD RECIPES

311.Roasted Scallops With Snow Peas

Servings:4
Cooking Time: 8 Minutes
Ingredients:
- 1 pound (454 g) sea scallops
- 3 tablespoons hoisin sauce
- ½ cup toasted sesame seeds
- 6 ounces (170 g) snow peas, trimmed
- 3 teaspoons vegetable oil, divided
- 1 teaspoon soy sauce
- 1 teaspoon sesame oil
- 1 cup roasted mushrooms

Directions:
1. Brush the scallops with the hoisin sauce. Put the sesame seeds in a shallow dish. Roll the scallops in the sesame seeds until evenly coated.
2. Combine the snow peas with 1 teaspoon of vegetable oil, the sesame oil, and soy sauce in a medium bowl and toss to coat.
3. Grease the baking pan with the remaining 2 teaspoons of vegetable oil. Put the scallops in the middle of the pan and arrange the snow peas around the scallops in a single layer.
4. Slide the baking pan into Rack Position 2, select Roast, set temperature to 375ºF (190ºC), and set time to 8 minutes.
5. After 5 minutes, remove the pan and flip the scallops. Fold in the mushrooms and stir well. Return the pan to the oven and continue cooking.
6. When done, remove from the oven and cool for 5 minutes. Serve warm.

312.Quick Shrimp Bowl

Servings: 4
Cooking Time: 15 Minutes
Ingredients:
- 1 ¼ pounds tiger shrimp
- ¼ tsp cayenne pepper
- ½ tsp old bay seasoning
- ¼ tsp smoked paprika
- A pinch of salt
- 1 tbsp olive oil

Directions:
1. Preheat your oven to 390 F on Air Fry function. In a bowl, mix all the ingredients. Place the mixture in your the cooking basket and fit in the baking tray; cook for 5 minutes, flipping once. Serve drizzled with lemon juice.

313.Shrimp And Cherry Tomato Kebabs

Servings:4
Cooking Time: 5 Minutes
Ingredients:
- 1½ pounds (680 g) jumbo shrimp, cleaned, shelled and deveined
- 1 pound (454 g) cherry tomatoes
- 2 tablespoons butter, melted
- 1 tablespoons Sriracha sauce
- Sea salt and ground black pepper, to taste
- 1 teaspoon dried parsley flakes
- ½ teaspoon dried basil
- ½ teaspoon dried oregano
- ½ teaspoon mustard seeds
- ½ teaspoon marjoram
- Special Equipment:
- 4 to 6 wooden skewers, soaked in water for 30 minutes

Directions:
1. Put all the ingredients in a large bowl and toss to coat well.
2. Make the kebabs: Thread, alternating jumbo shrimp and cherry tomatoes, onto the wooden skewers. Place the kebabs in the air fryer basket.
3. Put the air fryer basket on the baking pan and slide into Rack Position 2, select Air Fry, set temperature to 400ºF (205ºC), and set time to 5 minutes.
4. When cooking is complete, the shrimp should be pink and the cherry tomatoes should be softened. Remove from the oven. Let the shrimp and cherry tomato kebabs cool for 5 minutes and serve hot.

314.Dijon Salmon Fillets

Servings: 4
Cooking Time: 15 Minutes
Ingredients:
- 1 lb salmon fillets
- 2 tbsp Dijon mustard
- 1/4 cup brown sugar
- Pepper
- Salt

Directions:
1. Fit the oven with the rack in position 2.
2. Season salmon fillets with pepper and salt.
3. In a small bowl, mix Dijon mustard and brown sugar.
4. Brush salmon fillets with Dijon mustard mixture.
5. Place salmon fillets in the air fryer basket then place an air fryer basket in the baking pan.
6. Place a baking pan on the oven rack. Set to air fry at 350 F for 15 minutes.
7. Serve and enjoy.
- **Nutrition Info:** Calories 190 Fat 7.3 g Carbohydrates 9.3 g Sugar 8.9 g Protein 22.4 g Cholesterol 50 mg

315.Herbed Scallops With Vegetables

Servings:4
Cooking Time: 9 Minutes
Ingredients:
- 1 cup frozen peas
- 1 cup green beans
- 1 cup frozen chopped broccoli
- 2 teaspoons olive oil
- ½ teaspoon dried oregano
- ½ teaspoon dried basil
- 12 ounces (340 g) sea scallops, rinsed and patted dry

Directions:
1. Put the peas, green beans, and broccoli in a large bowl. Drizzle with the olive oil and toss to coat well. Transfer the vegetables to the air fryer basket.
2. Put the air fryer basket on the baking pan and slide into Rack Position 2, select Air Fry, set temperature to 400ºF (205ºC), and set time to 5 minutes.
3. When cooking is complete, the vegetables should be fork-tender. Transfer the vegetables to a serving bowl. Scatter with the oregano and basil and set aside.
4. Place the scallops in the basket.
5. Put the air fryer basket on the baking pan and slide into Rack Position 2, select Air Fry, set temperature to 400ºF (205ºC), and set time to 4 minutes.
6. When cooking is complete, the scallops should be firm and just opaque in the center. Remove from the oven to the bowl of vegetables and toss well. Serve warm.

316.Mediterranean Sole

Servings: 6
Cooking Time: 20 Minutes
Ingredients:
- Nonstick cooking spray
- 2 tbsp. olive oil
- 8 scallions, sliced thin
- 2 cloves garlic, diced fine
- 4 tomatoes, chopped
- ½ cup dry white wine
- 2 tbsp. fresh parsley, chopped fine
- 1 tsp oregano
- 1 tsp pepper
- 2 lbs. sole, cut in 6 pieces
- 4 oz. feta cheese, crumbled

Directions:
1. Place the rack in position 1 of the oven. Spray an 8x11-inch baking dish with cooking spray.
2. Heat the oil in a medium skillet over medium heat. Add scallions and garlic and cook until tender, stirring frequently.
3. Add the tomatoes, wine, parsley, oregano, and pepper. Stir to mix. Simmer for 5

minutes, or until sauce thickens. Remove from heat.
4. Pour half the sauce on the bottom of the prepared dish. Lay fish on top then pour remaining sauce over the top. Sprinkle with feta.
5. Set the oven to bake on 400°F for 25 minutes. After 5 minutes, place the baking dish on the rack and cook 15-18 minutes or until fish flakes easily with a fork. Serve immediately.
- **Nutrition Info:** Calories 220, Total Fat 12g, Saturated Fat 4g, Total Carbs 6g, Net Carbs 4g, Protein 22g, Sugar 4g, Fiber 2g, Sodium 631mg, Potassium 540mg, Phosphorus 478mg

317.Savory Cod Fish In Soy Sauce

Servings: 4
Cooking Time: 20 Minutes
Ingredients:
- 4 cod fish fillets
- 4 tbsp chopped cilantro
- Salt to taste
- 2 green onions, chopped
- 1 cup water
- 4 slices of ginger
- 4 tbsp light soy sauce
- 3 tbsp oil
- 1 tsp dark soy sauce
- 4 cubes rock sugar

Directions:
1. Sprinkle the cod with salt and cilantro and drizzle with olive oil. Place in the cooking basket and fit in the baking tray; cook for 15 minutes at 360 F on Air Fry function.
2. Place the remaining ingredients in a frying pan over medium heat and cook for 5 minutes until sauce reaches desired consistency. Pour the sauce over the fish and serve.

318.Crusty Scallops

Servings:4
Cooking Time: 20 Minutes
Ingredients:
- 12 fresh scallops
- 3 tbsp flour
- Salt and black pepper to taste
- 1 egg, lightly beaten
- 1 cup breadcrumbs

Directions:
1. Coat the scallops with flour. Dip into the egg, then into the breadcrumbs. Arrange them on the frying basket and spray with cooking spray. Cook for 12 minutes at 360 F on AirFry function.

319.Rosemary & Garlic Prawns

Servings:2
Cooking Time: 15 Minutes + Chilling Time
Ingredients:
- 8 large prawns
- 2 garlic cloves, minced
- 1 rosemary sprig, chopped
- 1 tbsp butter, melted
- Salt and black pepper to taste

Directions:
1. Combine garlic, butter, rosemary, salt, and pepper in a bowl. Add in the prawns and mix to coat. Cover the bowl and refrigerate for 1 hour. Preheat on AirFry function to 350 F. Remove the prawns from the fridge and transfer to the frying basket. Cook for 6-8 minutes.

320.Honey Glazed Salmon

Servings: 4
Cooking Time: 8 Minutes
Ingredients:
- 4 salmon fillets
- 2 tsp soy sauce
- 1 tbsp honey
- Pepper
- Salt

Directions:
1. Fit the oven with the rack in position 2.
2. Brush salmon with soy sauce and season with pepper and salt.
3. Place salmon in the air fryer basket then place an air fryer basket in the baking pan.
4. Place a baking pan on the oven rack. Set to air fry at 375 F for 8 minutes.
5. Brush salmon with honey and serve.
- **Nutrition Info:** Calories 253 Fat 11 g Carbohydrates 4.6 g Sugar 4.4 g Protein 34.7 g Cholesterol 78 mg

321.Delicious Shrimp Casserole

Servings: 10
Cooking Time: 30 Minutes
Ingredients:
- 1 lb shrimp, peeled & tail off
- 2 tsp onion powder
- 2 tsp old bay seasoning
- 2 cups cheddar cheese, shredded
- 10.5 oz can cream of mushroom soup
- 12 oz long-grain rice
- 1 tsp salt

Directions:
1. Fit the oven with the rack in position
2. Cook rice according to the packet instructions.
3. Add shrimp into the boiling water and cook for 4 minutes or until cooked. Drain shrimp.
4. In a bowl, mix rice, shrimp, and remaining ingredients and pour into the greased 13*9-inch casserole dish.
5. Set to bake at 350 F for 35 minutes. After 5 minutes place the casserole dish in the preheated oven.
6. Serve and enjoy.
- **Nutrition Info:** Calories 286 Fat 9 g Carbohydrates 31 g Sugar 1 g Protein 18.8 g Cholesterol 120 mg

322.Spicy Lemon Cod

Servings: 2
Cooking Time: 10 Minutes
Ingredients:
- 1 lb cod fillets
- 1/4 tsp chili powder
- 1 tbsp fresh parsley, chopped
- 1 1/2 tbsp olive oil
- 1 tbsp fresh lemon juice
- 1/8 tsp cayenne pepper
- 1/4 tsp salt

Directions:
1. Fit the oven with the rack in position
2. Arrange fish fillets in a baking dish. Drizzle with oil and lemon juice.
3. Sprinkle with chili powder, salt, and cayenne pepper.
4. Set to bake at 400 F for 15 minutes. After 5 minutes place the baking dish in the preheated oven.
5. Garnish with parsley and serve.
- **Nutrition Info:** Calories 276 Fat 12.7 g Carbohydrates 0.5 g Sugar 0.2 g Protein 40.7 g Cholesterol 111 mg

323.Paprika Cod

Servings: 4
Cooking Time: 15 Minutes
Ingredients:
- 4 cod fillets
- 1 tsp smoked paprika
- 1/2 cup parmesan cheese, grated
- 1/2 tbsp olive oil
- 1 tsp parsley
- Pepper
- Salt

Directions:
1. Fit the oven with the rack in position
2. Brush fish fillets with oil and season with pepper and salt.
3. In a shallow dish, mix parmesan cheese, paprika, and parsley.
4. Coat fish fillets with cheese mixture and place into the baking dish.
5. Set to bake at 400 F for 20 minutes. After 5 minutes place the baking dish in the preheated oven.
6. Serve and enjoy.

- **Nutrition Info:** Calories 125 Fat 5 g Carbohydrates 0.7 g Sugar 0.1 g Protein 19.8 g Cholesterol 52 mg

324.Baked Flounder Fillets

Servings:2
Cooking Time: 12 Minutes
Ingredients:
- 2 flounder fillets, patted dry
- 1 egg
- ½ teaspoon Worcestershire sauce
- ¼ cup almond flour
- ¼ cup coconut flour
- ½ teaspoon coarse sea salt
- ½ teaspoon lemon pepper
- ¼ teaspoon chili powder
- Cooking spray

Directions:
1. In a shallow bowl, beat together the egg with Worcestershire sauce until well incorporated.
2. In another bowl, thoroughly combine the almond flour, coconut flour, sea salt, lemon pepper, and chili powder.
3. Dredge the fillets in the egg mixture, shaking off any excess, then roll in the flour mixture to coat well.
4. Spritz the baking pan with cooking spray. Place the fillets in the pan.
5. Slide the baking pan into Rack Position 1, select Convection Bake, set temperature to 390ºF (199ºC), and set time to 12 minutes.
6. After 7 minutes, remove from the oven and flip the fillets and spray with cooking spray. Return the pan to the oven and continue cooking for 5 minutes, or until the fish is flaky.
7. When cooking is complete, remove from the oven and serve warm.

325.Quick Tuna Patties

Servings: 10
Cooking Time: 10 Minutes
Ingredients:
- 15 oz can tuna, drained and flaked
- 3 tbsp parmesan cheese, grated
- 1/2 cup breadcrumbs
- 1 tbsp lemon juice
- 2 eggs, lightly beaten
- 1/2 tsp dried mixed herbs
- 1/2 tsp garlic powder
- 2 tbsp onion, minced
- 1 celery stalk, chopped
- Pepper
- Salt

Directions:
1. Fit the oven with the rack in position 2.
2. Add all ingredients into the mixing bowl and mix until well combined.

3. Make patties from mixture and place in the air fryer basket then place the air fryer basket in the baking pan.
4. Place a baking pan on the oven rack. Set to air fry at 360 F for 10 minutes.
5. Serve and enjoy.
- **Nutrition Info:** Calories 90 Fat 1.8 g Carbohydrates 4.4 g Sugar 0.6 g Protein 13.2 g Cholesterol 47 mg

326.Spicy Catfish

Servings: 4
Cooking Time: 15 Minutes
Ingredients:
- 1 lb catfish fillets, cut 1/2-inch thick
- 1 tsp crushed red pepper
- 2 tsp onion powder
- 1 tbsp dried oregano, crushed
- 1/2 tsp ground cumin
- 1/2 tsp chili powder
- Pepper
- Salt

Directions:
1. Fit the oven with the rack in position
2. In a small bowl, mix cumin, chili powder, crushed red pepper, onion powder, oregano, pepper, and salt.
3. Rub fish fillets with the spice mixture and place in baking dish.
4. Set to bake at 350 F for 20 minutes. After 5 minutes place the baking dish in the preheated oven.
5. Serve and enjoy.
- **Nutrition Info:** Calories 164 Fat 8.9 g Carbohydrates 2.3 g Sugar 0.6 g Protein 18 g Cholesterol 53 mg

327.Cheesy Tuna Patties

Servings:4
Cooking Time: 17 To 18 Minutes
Ingredients:
- Tuna Patties:
- 1 pound (454 g) canned tuna, drained
- 1 egg, whisked
- 2 tablespoons shallots, minced
- 1 garlic clove, minced
- 1 cup grated Romano cheese
- Sea salt and ground black pepper, to taste
- 1 tablespoon sesame oil
- Cheese Sauce:
- 1 tablespoon butter
- 1 cup beer
- 2 tablespoons grated Colby cheese

Directions:
1. Mix together the canned tuna, whisked egg, shallots, garlic, cheese, salt, and pepper in a large bowl and stir to incorporate.
2. Divide the tuna mixture into four equal portions and form each portion into a patty

with your hands. Refrigerate the patties for 2 hours.
3. When ready, brush both sides of each patty with sesame oil, then place in the baking pan.
4. Slide the baking pan into Rack Position 1, select Convection Bake, set temperature to 360ºF (182ºC), and set time to 14 minutes.
5. Flip the patties halfway through the cooking time.
6. Meanwhile, melt the butter in a saucepan over medium heat.
7. Pour in the beer and whisk constantly, or until it begins to bubble. Add the grated Colby cheese and mix well. Continue cooking for 3 to 4 minutes, or until the cheese melts. Remove from the heat.
8. When cooking is complete, the patties should be lightly browned and cooked through. Remove the patties from the oven to a plate. Drizzle them with the cheese sauce and serve immediately.

328.Salmon Burgers

Servings: 4
Cooking Time: 10 Minutes
Ingredients:
- 14.75 oz. can salmon, drain & flake
- ¼ cup onion, chopped fine
- 1 egg
- ¼ cup multi-grain crackers, crushed
- 2 tsp fresh dill, chopped
- ¼ tsp pepper
- Nonstick cooking spray

Directions:
1. In a medium bowl, combine all ingredients until combined. Form into 4 patties.
2. Lightly spray fryer basket with cooking spray. Place the baking pan in position 2 of the oven.
3. Set oven to air fryer on 350°F.
4. Place the patties in the basket and set on baking pan. Set timer for 8 minutes. Cook until burgers are golden brown, turning over halfway through cooking time. Serve on toasted buns with choice of toppings.
- **Nutrition Info:** Calories 330, Total Fat 10g, Saturated Fat 2g, Total Carbs 11g, Net Carbs 11g, Protein 24g, Sugar 0g, Fiber 0g, Sodium 643mg, Potassium 407mg, Phosphorus 391mg

329.Air Fry Tuna Patties

Servings: 4
Cooking Time: 6 Minutes
Ingredients:
- 1 egg, lightly beaten
- 8 oz can tuna, drained
- 1/4 cup breadcrumbs

- 1 tbsp mustard
- 1/4 tsp garlic powder
- Pepper
- Salt

Directions:
1. Fit the oven with the rack in position 2.
2. Add all ingredients into the large bowl and mix until well combined.
3. Make four equal shapes of patties from the mixture and place in the air fryer basket then place an air fryer basket in the baking pan.
4. Place a baking pan on the oven rack. Set to air fry at 400 F for 6 minutes.
5. Serve and enjoy.
- **Nutrition Info:** Calories 122 Fat 2.7 g Carbohydrates 6.1 g Sugar 0.7 g Protein 17.5 g Cholesterol 58 mg

330.Coconut-crusted Prawns

Servings:4
Cooking Time: 8 Minutes
Ingredients:
- 12 prawns, cleaned and deveined
- 1 teaspoon fresh lemon juice
- ½ teaspoon cumin powder
- Salt and ground black pepper, to taste
- 1 medium egg
- $^1/_3$ cup beer
- ½ cup flour, divided
- 1 tablespoon curry powder
- 1 teaspoon baking powder
- ½ teaspoon grated fresh ginger
- 1 cup flaked coconut

Directions:
1. In a large bowl, toss the prawns with the lemon juice, cumin powder, salt, and pepper until well coated. Set aside.
2. In a shallow bowl, whisk together the egg, beer, ¼ cup of flour, curry powder, baking powder, and ginger until combined.
3. In a separate shallow bowl, put the remaining ¼ cup of flour, and on a plate, place the flaked coconut.
4. Dip the prawns in the flour, then in the egg mixture, finally roll in the flaked coconut to coat well. Transfer the prawns to a baking sheet.
5. Put the air fryer basket on the baking pan and slide into Rack Position 2, select Air Fry, set temperature to 350ºF (180ºC), and set time to 8 minutes.
6. After 5 minutes, remove from the oven and flip the prawns. Return to the oven and continue cooking for 3 minutes more.
7. When cooking is complete, remove from the oven and serve warm.

331.Air-fried Scallops

Servings:2
Cooking Time: 12 Minutes
Ingredients:
- $1/3$ cup shallots, chopped
- 1½ tablespoons olive oil
- 1½ tablespoons coconut aminos
- 1 tablespoon Mediterranean seasoning mix
- ½ tablespoon balsamic vinegar
- ½ teaspoon ginger, grated
- 1 clove garlic, chopped
- 1 pound (454 g) scallops, cleanedCooking spray
- Belgian endive, for garnish

Directions:
1. Place all the ingredients except the scallops and Belgian endive in a small skillet over medium heat and stir to combine. Let this mixture simmer for about 2 minutes.
2. Remove the mixture from the skillet to a large bowl and set aside to cool.
3. Add the scallops, coating them all over, then transfer to the refrigerator to marinate for at least 2 hours.
4. When ready, place the scallops in the air fryer basket in a single layer and spray with cooking spray.
5. Put the air fryer basket on the baking pan and slide into Rack Position 2, select Air Fry, set temperature to 345ºF (174ºC), and set time to 10 minutes.
6. Flip the scallops halfway through the cooking time.
7. When cooking is complete, the scallops should be tender and opaque. Remove from the oven and serve garnished with the Belgian endive.

332.Easy Shrimp Fajitas

Servings: 10
Cooking Time: 20 Minutes
Ingredients:
- 1 lb shrimp
- 1 tbsp olive oil
- 2 bell peppers, diced
- 2 tbsp taco seasoning
- 1/2 cup onion, diced

Directions:
1. Fit the oven with the rack in position 2.
2. Add shrimp and remaining ingredients into the bowl and toss well.
3. Add shrimp mixture to the air fryer basket then place an air fryer basket in baking pan.
4. Place a baking pan on the oven rack. Set to air fry at 390 F for 20 minutes.
5. Serve and enjoy.
- **Nutrition Info:** Calories 76 Fat 2.2 g Carbohydrates 3 g Sugar 1.4 g Protein 10.6 g Cholesterol 96 mg

333.Old Bay Tilapia Fillets

Servings: 4
Cooking Time: 15 Minutes
Ingredients:
- 1 pound tilapia fillets
- 1 tbsp old bay seasoning
- 2 tbsp canola oil
- 2 tbsp lemon pepper
- Salt to taste
- 2-3 butter buds

Directions:
1. Preheat your oven to 400 F on Bake function. Drizzle tilapia fillets with canola oil. In a bowl, mix salt, lemon pepper, butter buds, and seasoning; spread on the fish. Place the fillet on the basket and fit in the baking tray. Cook for 10 minutes, flipping once until tender and crispy.

334.Glazed Tuna And Fruit Kebabs

Servings:4
Cooking Time: 10 Minutes
Ingredients:
- Kebabs:
- 1 pound (454 g) tuna steaks, cut into 1-inch cubes
- ½ cup canned pineapple chunks, drained, juice reserved
- ½ cup large red grapes
- Marinade:
- 1 tablespoon honey
- 1 teaspoon olive oil
- 2 teaspoons grated fresh ginger
- Pinch cayenne pepper
- Special Equipment:
- 4 metal skewers

Directions:
1. Make the kebabs: Thread, alternating tuna cubes, pineapple chunks, and red grapes, onto the metal skewers.
2. Make the marinade: Whisk together the honey, olive oil, ginger, and cayenne pepper in a small bowl. Brush generously the marinade over the kebabs and allow to sit for 10 minutes.
3. When ready, transfer the kebabs to the air fryer basket.
4. Put the air fryer basket on the baking pan and slide into Rack Position 2, select Air Fry, set temperature to 370ºF (188ºC), and set time to 10 minutes.
5. After 5 minutes, remove from the oven and flip the kebabs and brush with the remaining marinade. Return the pan to the oven and continue cooking for an additional 5 minutes.
6. When cooking is complete, the kebabs should reach an internal temperature of 145ºF (63ºC) on a meat thermometer.

Remove from the oven and discard any remaining marinade. Serve hot.

335.Spiced Red Snapper

Servings:4
Cooking Time: 10 Minutes
Ingredients:
- 1 teaspoon olive oil
- 1½ teaspoons black pepper
- ¼ teaspoon garlic powder
- ¼ teaspoon thyme
- ⅛ teaspoon cayenne pepper
- 4 (4-ounce / 113-g) red snapper fillets, skin on
- 4 thin slices lemon
- Nonstick cooking spray

Directions:
1. Spritz the baking pan with nonstick cooking spray.
2. In a small bowl, stir together the olive oil, black pepper, garlic powder, thyme, and cayenne pepper. Rub the mixture all over the fillets until completely coated.
3. Lay the fillets, skin-side down, in the baking pan and top each fillet with a slice of lemon.
4. Slide the baking pan into Rack Position 1, select Convection Bake, set temperature to 390ºF (199ºC), and set time to 10 minutes.
5. Flip the fillets halfway through the cooking time.
6. When cooking is complete, the fish should be cooked through. Let the fish cool for 5 minutes and serve.

336.Crispy Crab And Fish Cakes

Servings:4
Cooking Time: 12 Minutes
Ingredients:
- 8 ounces (227 g) imitation crab meat
- 4 ounces (113 g) leftover cooked fish (such as cod, pollock, or haddock)
- 2 tablespoons minced celery
- 2 tablespoons minced green onion
- 2 tablespoons light mayonnaise
- 1 tablespoon plus 2 teaspoons Worcestershire sauce
- ¾ cup crushed saltine cracker crumbs
- 2 teaspoons dried parsley flakes
- 1 teaspoon prepared yellow mustard
- ½ teaspoon garlic powder
- ½ teaspoon dried dill weed, crushed
- ½ teaspoon Old Bay seasoning
- ½ cup panko bread crumbs
- Cooking spray

Directions:
1. Pulse the crab meat and fish in a food processor until finely chopped.
2. Transfer the meat mixture to a large bowl, along with the celery, green onion, mayo,

Worcestershire sauce, cracker crumbs, parsley flakes, mustard, garlic powder, dill weed, and Old Bay seasoning. Stir to mix well.
3. Scoop out the meat mixture and form into 8 equal-sized patties with your hands.
4. Place the panko bread crumbs on a plate. Roll the patties in the bread crumbs until they are evenly coated on both sides. Put the patties in the baking pan and spritz them with cooking spray.
5. Slide the baking pan into Rack Position 1, select Convection Bake, set temperature to 390ºF (199ºC), and set time to 12 minutes.
6. Flip the patties halfway through the cooking time.
7. When cooking is complete, they should be golden brown and cooked through. Remove the pan from the oven. Divide the patties among four plates and serve.

337.Orange Fish Fillets

Servings: 2
Cooking Time: 25 Minutes
Ingredients:
- 1 lb salmon fillets
- 1 orange juice
- 1 orange zest, grated
- 2 tbsp honey
- 3 tbsp soy sauce

Directions:
1. Fit the oven with the rack in position
2. In a small bowl, whisk together honey, soy sauce, orange juice, and orange zest.
3. Place salmon fillets in a baking dish and pour honey mixture over salmon fillets.
4. Set to bake at 425 F for 30 minutes. After 5 minutes place the baking dish in the preheated oven.
5. Serve and enjoy.
- **Nutrition Info:** Calories 399 Fat 14.1 g Carbohydrates 24.4 g Sugar 21.3 g Protein 45.9 g Cholesterol 100 mg

338.Parmesan Fish Fillets

Servings:4
Cooking Time: 17 Minutes
Ingredients:
- $1/3$ cup grated Parmesan cheese
- ½ teaspoon fennel seed
- ½ teaspoon tarragon
- $1/3$ teaspoon mixed peppercorns
- 2 eggs, beaten
- 4 (4-ounce / 113-g) fish fillets, halved
- 2 tablespoons dry white wine
- 1 teaspoon seasoned salt

Directions:
1. Place the grated Parmesan cheese, fennel seed, tarragon, and mixed peppercorns in a

food processor and pulse for about 20 seconds until well combined. Transfer the cheese mixture to a shallow dish.

2. Place the beaten eggs in another shallow dish.
3. Drizzle the dry white wine over the top of fish fillets. Dredge each fillet in the beaten eggs on both sides, shaking off any excess, then roll them in the cheese mixture until fully coated. Season with the salt.
4. Arrange the fillets in the air fryer basket.
5. Put the air fryer basket on the baking pan and slide into Rack Position 2, select Air Fry, set temperature to 345ºF (174ºC), and set time to 17 minutes.
6. Flip the fillets once halfway through the cooking time.
7. When cooking is complete, the fish should be cooked through no longer translucent. Remove from the oven and cool for 5 minutes before serving.

339.Chili Tuna Casserole

Servings:4
Cooking Time: 16 Minutes
Ingredients:
- ½ tablespoon sesame oil
- $^1/_3$ cup yellow onions, chopped
- ½ bell pepper, deveined and chopped
- 2 cups canned tuna, chopped
- Cooking spray
- 5 eggs, beaten
- ½ chili pepper, deveined and finely minced
- 1½ tablespoons sour cream
- $^1/_3$ teaspoon dried basil
- $^1/_3$ teaspoon dried oregano
- Fine sea salt and ground black pepper, to taste

Directions:
1. Heat the sesame oil in a nonstick skillet over medium heat until it shimmers.
2. Add the onions and bell pepper and sauté for 4 minutes, stirring occasionally, or until tender.
3. Add the canned tuna and keep stirring until the tuna is heated through.
4. Meanwhile, coat the baking pan lightly with cooking spray.
5. Transfer the tuna mixture to the baking pan, along with the beaten eggs, chili pepper, sour cream, basil, and oregano. Stir to combine well. Season with sea salt and black pepper.
6. Slide the baking pan into Rack Position 1, select Convection Bake, set temperature to 325ºF (160ºC), and set time to 12 minutes.
7. When cooking is complete, the eggs should be completely set and the top lightly browned. Remove from the oven and serve on a plate.

340.Piri-piri King Prawns

Servings:2
Cooking Time: 8 Minutes
Ingredients:
- 12 king prawns, rinsed
- 1 tablespoon coconut oil
- Salt and ground black pepper, to taste
- 1 teaspoon onion powder
- 1 teaspoon garlic paste
- 1 teaspoon curry powder
- ½ teaspoon piri piri powder
- ½ teaspoon cumin powder

Directions:
1. Combine all the ingredients in a large bowl and toss until the prawns are completely coated. Place the prawns in the air fryer basket.
2. Put the air fryer basket on the baking pan and slide into Rack Position 2, select Air Fry, set temperature to 360ºF (182ºC), and set time to 8 minutes.
3. Flip the prawns halfway through the cooking time.
4. When cooking is complete, the prawns will turn pink. Remove from the oven and serve hot.

341.Scallops And Spring Veggies

Servings: 4
Cooking Time: 8 Minutes
Ingredients:
- ½ pound asparagus ends trimmed, cut into 2-inch pieces
- 1 cup sugar snap peas
- 1 pound sea scallops
- 1 tablespoon lemon juice
- 2 teaspoons olive oil
- ½ teaspoon dried thyme
- Pinch salt
- Freshly ground black pepper

Directions:
1. Preparing the Ingredients. Place the asparagus and sugar snap peas in the Oven rack/basket. Place the Rack on the middle-shelf of the air fryer oven.
2. Air Frying. Cook for 2 to 3 minutes or until the vegetables are just starting to get tender.
3. Meanwhile, check the scallops for a small muscle attached to the side, and pull it off and discard.
4. In a medium bowl, toss the scallops with the lemon juice, olive oil, thyme, salt, and pepper. Place into the Oven rack/basket on top of the vegetables. Place the Rack on the middle-shelf of the air fryer oven.
5. Air Frying. Steam for 5 to 7 minutes. Until the scallops are just firm, and the vegetables are tender. Serve immediately.

- **Nutrition Info:** CALORIES: 162; CARBS:10G; FAT: 4G; PROTEIN:22G; FIBER:3G

342.Flavorful Baked Halibut

Servings: 4
Cooking Time: 12 Minutes
Ingredients:
- 1 lb halibut fillets
- 1/4 tsp garlic powder
- 1/4 tsp paprika
- 1/4 tsp smoked paprika
- 1/4 tsp pepper
- 1/4 cup olive oil
- 1 lemon juice
- 1/2 tsp salt

Directions:
1. Fit the oven with the rack in position
2. Place fish fillets into the baking dish.
3. In a small bowl, mix lemon juice, oil, paprika, smoked paprika, garlic powder, and salt.
4. Brush lemon juice mixture over fish fillets.
5. Set to bake at 425 F for 17 minutes. After 5 minutes place the baking dish in the preheated oven.
6. Serve and enjoy.
- **Nutrition Info:** Calories 236 Fat 15.3 g Carbohydrates 0.4 g Sugar 0.1 g Protein 24 g Cholesterol 36 mg

343.Garlic-butter Catfish

Servings: 2
Cooking Time: 20 Minutes
Ingredients:
- 2 catfish fillets
- 2 tsp blackening seasoning
- Juice of 1 lime
- 2 tbsp butter, melted
- 1 garlic clove, mashed
- 2 tbsp cilantro

Directions:
1. In a bowl, blend in garlic, lime juice, cilantro, and butter. Pour half of the mixture over the fillets and sprinkle with blackening seasoning. Place the fillets in the basket and fit in the baking tray; cook for 15 minutes at 360 F on Air Fry function. Serve the fish with remaining sauce.

344.Carp Best Homemade Croquette

Servings:x
Cooking Time:x
Ingredients:
- 1 lb. Carp filets
- 3 onions chopped
- 5 green chilies-roughly chopped
- 1 ½ tbsp. ginger paste
- 1 ½ tsp garlic paste
- 1 ½ tsp salt
- 3 tsp lemon juice
- 2 tsp garam masala
- 4 tbsp. chopped coriander
- 3 tbsp. cream
- 2 tbsp. coriander powder
- 4 tbsp. fresh mint chopped
- 3 tbsp. chopped capsicum
- 3 eggs
- 2 ½ tbsp. white sesame seeds

Directions:
1. Take all the ingredients mentioned under the first heading and mix them in a bowl. Grind them thoroughly to make a smooth paste. Take the eggs in a different bowl and beat them. Add a pinch of salt and leave them aside. Mold the fish mixture into small balls and flatten them into round and flat Best Homemade Croquettes. Dip these Best Homemade Croquettes in the egg and salt mixture and then in the mixture of breadcrumbs and sesame seeds.
2. Leave these Best Homemade Croquettes in the fridge for an hour or so to set. Pre heat the oven at 160 degrees Fahrenheit for around 5 minutes. Place the Best Homemade Croquettes in the basket and let them cook for another 25 minutes at the same temperature. Turn the Best Homemade Croquettes over in between the cooking process to get a uniform cook. Serve the Best Homemade Croquettes with mint sauce.

345.Tilapia Meunière With Vegetables

Servings:4
Cooking Time: 20 Minutes
Ingredients:
- 10 ounces (283 g) Yukon Gold potatoes, sliced ¼-inch thick
- 5 tablespoons unsalted butter, melted, divided
- 1 teaspoon kosher salt, divided
- 4 (8-ounce / 227-g) tilapia fillets
- ½ pound (227 g) green beans, trimmed
- Juice of 1 lemon
- 2 tablespoons chopped fresh parsley, for garnish

Directions:
1. In a large bowl, drizzle the potatoes with 2 tablespoons of melted butter and ¼ teaspoon of kosher salt. Transfer the potatoes to the baking pan.
2. Slide the baking pan into Rack Position 2, select Roast, set temperature to 375ºF (190ºC), and set time to 20 minutes.
3. Meanwhile, season both sides of the fillets with ½ teaspoon of kosher salt. Put the green beans in the medium bowl and sprinkle with the remaining ¼ teaspoon of

kosher salt and 1 tablespoon of butter, tossing to coat.
4. After 10 minutes, remove from the oven and push the potatoes to one side. Put the fillets in the middle of the pan and add the green beans on the other side. Drizzle the remaining 2 tablespoons of butter over the fillets. Return the pan to the oven and continue cooking, or until the fish flakes easily with a fork and the green beans are crisp-tender.
5. When cooked, remove from the oven. Drizzle the lemon juice over the fillets and sprinkle the parsley on top for garnish. Serve hot.

346.Butter-wine Baked Salmon

Servings:4
Cooking Time: 10 Minutes
Ingredients:
- 4 tablespoons butter, melted
- 2 cloves garlic, minced
- Sea salt and ground black pepper, to taste
- ¼ cup dry white wine
- 1 tablespoon lime juice
- 1 teaspoon smoked paprika
- ½ teaspoon onion powder
- 4 salmon steaks
- Cooking spray

Directions:
1. Place all the ingredients except the salmon and oil in a shallow dish and stir to mix well.
2. Add the salmon steaks, turning to coat well on both sides. Transfer the salmon to the refrigerator to marinate for 30 minutes.
3. When ready, put the salmon steaks in the air fryer basket, discarding any excess marinade. Spray the salmon steaks with cooking spray.
4. Put the air fryer basket on the baking pan and slide into Rack Position 2, select Air Fry, set temperature to 360ºF (182ºC), and set time to 10 minutes.
5. Flip the salmon steaks halfway through.
6. When cooking is complete, remove from the oven and divide the salmon steaks among four plates. Serve warm.

347.Salmon Tandoor

Servings:x
Cooking Time:x
Ingredients:
- 2 lb. boneless salmon filets
- 1st Marinade:
- 3 tbsp. vinegar or lemon juice
- 2 or 3 tsp. paprika
- 1 tsp. black pepper
- 1 tsp. salt
- 3 tsp. ginger-garlic paste

- 2nd Marinade:
- 1 cup yogurt
- 4 tsp. tandoori masala
- 2 tbsp. dry fenugreek leaves
- 1 tsp. black salt
- 1 tsp. chat masala
- 1 tsp. garam masala powder
- 1 tsp. red chili powder
- 1 tsp. salt
- 3 drops of red color

Directions:
1. Make the first marinade and soak the fileted salmon in it for four hours. While this is happening, make the second marinade and soak the salmon in it overnight to let the flavors blend. Pre heat the oven at 160 degrees Fahrenheit for 5 minutes.
2. Place the Oregano Fingers in the fry basket and close it. Let them cook at the same temperature for another 15 minutes or so. Toss the Oregano Fingers well so that they are cooked uniformly. Serve them with mint sauce.

348.Rosemary Buttered Prawns

Servings: 2
Cooking Time: 15 Minutes + Marinating Time
Ingredients:
- 8 large prawns
- 1 rosemary sprig, chopped
- ½ tbsp melted butter
- Salt and black pepper to taste

Directions:
1. Combine butter, rosemary, salt, and pepper in a bowl. Add in the prawns and mix to coat. Cover the bowl and refrigerate for 1 hour.
2. Preheat on Air Fry function to 350 F Remove the prawns from the fridge and place them in the basket. Fit in the baking tray and cook for 10 minutes, flipping once. Serve.

349.Fired Shrimp With Mayonnaise Sauce

Servings:4
Cooking Time: 7 Minutes
Ingredients:
- Shrimp
- 12 jumbo shrimp
- ½ teaspoon garlic salt
- ¼ teaspoon freshly cracked mixed peppercorns
- Sauce:
- 4 tablespoons mayonnaise
- 1 teaspoon grated lemon rind
- 1 teaspoon Dijon mustard
- 1 teaspoon chipotle powder
- ½ teaspoon cumin powder

Directions:
1. In a medium bowl, season the shrimp with garlic salt and cracked mixed peppercorns.

2. Place the shrimp in the air fryer basket.
3. Put the air fryer basket on the baking pan and slide into Rack Position 2, select Air Fry, set temperature to 395ºF (202ºC), and set time to 7 minutes.
4. After 5 minutes, remove from the oven and flip the shrimp. Return to the oven and continue cooking for 2 minutes more, or until they are pink and no longer opaque.
5. Meanwhile, stir together all the ingredients for the sauce in a small bowl until well mixed.
6. When cooking is complete, remove the shrimp from the oven and serve alongside the sauce.

350.Cajun Red Snapper

Servings: 2
Cooking Time: 12 Minutes
Ingredients:
- 8 oz red snapper fillets
- 2 tbsp parmesan cheese, grated
- 1/4 cup breadcrumbs
- 1/2 tsp Cajun seasoning
- 1/4 tsp Worcestershire sauce
- 1 garlic clove, minced
- 1/4 cup butter

Directions:
1. Fit the oven with the rack in position
2. Melt butter in a pan over low heat. Add Cajun seasoning, garlic, and Worcestershire sauce into the melted butter and stir well.
3. Brush fish fillets with melted butter and place into the baking dish.
4. Mix together parmesan cheese and breadcrumbs and sprinkle over fish fillets.
5. Set to bake at 400 F for 17 minutes. After 5 minutes place the baking dish in the preheated oven.
6. Serve and enjoy.
- **Nutrition Info:** Calories 424 Fat 27 g Carbohydrates 10.6 g Sugar 1 g Protein 33.9 g Cholesterol 119 mg

351.Citrus Cilantro Catfish

Servings:2
Cooking Time: 20 Minutes
Ingredients:
- 2 catfish fillets
- 2 tsp blackening seasoning
- Juice of 1 lime
- 2 tbsp butter, melted
- 1 garlic clove, mashed
- 2 tbsp fresh cilantro, chopped

Directions:
1. In a bowl, blend garlic, lime juice, cilantro, and butter. Pour half of the mixture over the fillets and sprinkle with blackening seasoning. Place the fillets in the basket and press Start. Cook for 15 minutes at 360 F on AirFry function. Serve the fish topped with the remaining sauce.

352.Baked Pesto Salmon

Servings: 4
Cooking Time: 15 Minutes
Ingredients:
- 4 salmon fillets
- 1/3 cup parmesan cheese, grated
- 1/3 cup breadcrumbs
- 6 tbsp pesto

Directions:
1. Fit the oven with the rack in position
2. Place fish fillets into the baking dish.
3. Pour pesto over fish fillets.
4. Mix together breadcrumbs and parmesan cheese and sprinkle over fish.
5. Set to bake at 325 F for 20 minutes. After 5 minutes place the baking dish in the preheated oven.
6. Serve and enjoy.
- **Nutrition Info:** Calories 396 Fat 22.8 g Carbohydrates 8.3 g Sugar 2.1 g Protein 40.4 g Cholesterol 89 mg

353.Garlic-butter Shrimp With Vegetables

Servings:4
Cooking Time: 15 Minutes
Ingredients:
- 1 pound (454 g) small red potatoes, halved
- 2 ears corn, shucked and cut into rounds, 1 to 1½ inches thick
- 2 tablespoons Old Bay or similar seasoning
- ½ cup unsalted butter, melted
- 1 (12- to 13-ounce / 340- to 369-g) package kielbasa or other smoked sausages
- 3 garlic cloves, minced
- 1 pound (454 g) medium shrimp, peeled and deveined

Directions:
1. Place the potatoes and corn in a large bowl.
2. Stir together the butter and Old Bay seasoning in a small bowl. Drizzle half the butter mixture over the potatoes and corn, tossing to coat. Spread out the vegetables in the baking pan.
3. Slide the baking pan into Rack Position 2, select Roast, set temperature to 350ºF (180ºC), and set time to 15 minutes.
4. Meanwhile, cut the sausages into 2-inch lengths, then cut each piece in half lengthwise. Put the sausages and shrimp in a medium bowl and set aside.
5. Add the garlic to the bowl of remaining butter mixture and stir well.
6. After 10 minutes, remove the pan and pour the vegetables into the large bowl. Drizzle with the garlic butter and toss until well coated. Arrange the vegetables, sausages, and shrimp in the pan.
7. Return to the oven and continue cooking. After 5 minutes, check the shrimp for doneness. The shrimp should be pink and opaque. If they are not quite cooked through, roast for an additional 1 minute.

8. When done, remove from the oven and serve on a plate.

354.Sweet And Savory Breaded Shrimp

Servings: 2
Cooking Time: 20 Minutes
Ingredients:
- ½ pound of fresh shrimp, peeled from their shells and rinsed
- 2 raw eggs
- ½ cup of breadcrumbs (we like Panko, but any brand or home recipe will do)
- ½ white onion, peeled and rinsed and finely chopped
- 1 teaspoon of ginger-garlic paste
- ½ teaspoon of turmeric powder
- ½ teaspoon of red chili powder
- ½ teaspoon of cumin powder
- ½ teaspoon of black pepper powder
- ½ teaspoon of dry mango powder
- Pinch of salt

Directions:
1. Preparing the Ingredients. Cover the basket of the air fryer oven with a lining of tin foil, leaving the edges uncovered to allow air to circulate through the basket.
2. Preheat the air fryer oven to 350 degrees.
3. In a large mixing bowl, beat the eggs until fluffy and until the yolks and whites are fully combined.
4. Dunk all the shrimp in the egg mixture, fully submerging.
5. In a separate mixing bowl, combine the bread crumbs with all the dry ingredients until evenly blended.
6. One by one, coat the egg-covered shrimp in the mixed dry ingredients so that fully covered, and place on the foil-lined air-fryer basket.
7. Air Frying. Set the air-fryer timer to 20 minutes.
8. Halfway through the cooking time, shake the handle of the air-fryer so that the breaded shrimp jostles inside and fry-coverage is even.
9. After 20 minutes, when the fryer shuts off, the shrimp will be perfectly cooked and their breaded crust golden-brown and delicious! Using tongs, remove from the air fryer oven and set on a serving dish to cool.

355.Fish Club Classic Sandwich

Servings:x
Cooking Time:x
Ingredients:
- 2 slices of white bread
- 1 tbsp. softened butter
- 1 tin tuna
- 1 small capsicum
- For Barbeque Sauce:
- ¼ tbsp. Worcestershire sauce
- ½ tsp. olive oil
- ½ flake garlic crushed
- ¼ cup chopped onion
- ¼ tsp. mustard powder
- ½ tbsp. sugar
- ¼ tbsp. red chili sauce
- 1 tbsp. tomato ketchup
- ½ cup water.
- A pinch of salt and black pepper to taste

Directions:
1. Take the slices of bread and remove the edges. Now cut the slices horizontally. Cook the ingredients for the sauce and wait till it thickens. Now, add the fish to the sauce and stir till it obtains the flavors. Roast the capsicum and peel the skin off. Cut the capsicum into slices.
2. Mix the ingredients together and apply it to the bread slices. Pre-heat the oven for 5 minutes at 300 Fahrenheit.
3. Open the basket of the Fryer and place the prepared Classic Sandwiches in it such that no two Classic Sandwiches are touching each other. Now keep the fryer at 250 degrees for around 15 minutes. Turn the Classic Sandwiches in between the cooking process to cook both slices. Serve the Classic Sandwiches with tomato ketchup or mint sauce.

356.Delicious Fried Seafood

Servings: 4
Cooking Time: 15 Minutes
Ingredients:
- 1 lb fresh scallops, mussels, fish fillets, prawns, shrimp
- 2 eggs, lightly beaten
- Salt and black pepper to taste
- 1 cup breadcrumbs mixed with zest of 1 lemon

Directions:
1. Dip each piece of the seafood into the eggs and season with salt and pepper. Coat in the crumbs and spray with oil. Arrange into the frying basket and fit in the baking tray; cook for 10 minutes at 400 F on Air Fry function, turning once halfway through. Serve.

357.Healthy Haddock

Servings: 2
Cooking Time: 25 Minutes
Ingredients:
- 1 lb haddock fillets
- 1/4 cup parsley, chopped
- 1 lemon juice
- 1/4 cup brown sugar
- 1/4 cup onion, diced
- 1 tsp ginger, grated
- 3/4 cup soy sauce
- Pepper
- Salt

Directions:
1. Fit the oven with the rack in position

2. Add fish fillets and remaining ingredients into the large bowl and coat well and place in the refrigerator for 1 hour.
3. Place marinated fish fillets into the baking dish.
4. Set to bake at 325 F for 30 minutes. After 5 minutes place the baking dish in the preheated oven.
5. Serve and enjoy.
- **Nutrition Info:** Calories 391 Fat 2.5 g Carbohydrates 28 g Sugar 20.4 g Protein 61.7 g Cholesterol 168 mg

358.Firecracker Shrimp

Servings: 4
Cooking Time: 8 Minutes
Ingredients:
- For the shrimp
- 1 pound raw shrimp, peeled and deveined
- Salt
- Pepper
- 1 egg
- ½ cup all-purpose flour
- ¾ cup panko bread crumbs
- Cooking oil
- For the firecracker sauce
- ⅓ cup sour cream
- 2 tablespoons Sriracha
- ¼ cup sweet chili sauce

Directions:
1. Preparing the Ingredients. Season the shrimp with salt and pepper to taste. In a small bowl, beat the egg. In another small bowl, place the flour. In a third small bowl, add the panko bread crumbs.
2. Spray the Oven rack/basket with cooking oil. Dip the shrimp in the flour, then the egg, and then the bread crumbs. Place the shrimp in the Oven rack/basket. It is okay to stack them. Spray the shrimp with cooking oil. Place the Rack on the middle-shelf of the air fryer oven.
3. Air Frying. Cook for 4 minutes. Open the air fryer oven and flip the shrimp. I recommend flipping individually instead of shaking to keep the breading intact. Cook for an additional 4 minutes or until crisp.
4. While the shrimp is cooking, make the firecracker sauce: In a small bowl, combine the sour cream, Sriracha, and sweet chili sauce. Mix well. Serve with the shrimp.
- **Nutrition Info:** CALORIES: 266; CARBS:23g; FAT:6G; PROTEIN:27G; FIBER:1G

359.Parmesan-crusted Hake With Garlic Sauce

Servings:3
Cooking Time: 10 Minutes
Ingredients:
- Fish:
- 6 tablespoons mayonnaise
- 1 tablespoon fresh lime juice

- 1 teaspoon Dijon mustard
- 1 cup grated Parmesan cheese
- Salt, to taste
- ¼ teaspoon ground black pepper, or more to taste
- 3 hake fillets, patted dry
- Nonstick cooking spray
- Garlic Sauce:
- ¼ cup plain Greek yogurt
- 2 tablespoons olive oil
- 2 cloves garlic, minced
- ½ teaspoon minced tarragon leaves

Directions:
1. Mix the mayo, lime juice, and mustard in a shallow bowl and whisk to combine. In another shallow bowl, stir together the grated Parmesan cheese, salt, and pepper.
2. Dredge each fillet in the mayo mixture, then roll them in the cheese mixture until they are evenly coated on both sides.
3. Spray the air fryer basket with nonstick cooking spray. Place the fillets in the pan.
4. Put the air fryer basket on the baking pan and slide into Rack Position 2, select Air Fry, set temperature to 395ºF (202ºC), and set time to 10 minutes.
5. Flip the fillets halfway through the cooking time.
6. Meanwhile, in a small bowl, whisk all the ingredients for the sauce until well incorporated.
7. When cooking is complete, the fish should flake apart with a fork. Remove the fillets from the oven and serve warm alongside the sauce.

360.Fish Tacos

Servings:6
Cooking Time: 10 To 15 Minutes
Ingredients:
- 1 tablespoon avocado oil
- 1 tablespoon Cajun seasoning
- 4 (5 to 6 ounce / 142 to 170 g) tilapia fillets
- 1 (14-ounce / 397-g) package coleslaw mix
- 12 corn tortillas
- 2 limes, cut into wedges

Directions:
1. Line the baking pan with parchment paper.
2. In a shallow bowl, stir together the avocado oil and Cajun seasoning to make a marinade. Place the tilapia fillets into the bowl, turning to coat evenly.
3. Put the fillets in the baking pan in a single layer.
4. Put the air fryer basket on the baking pan and slide into Rack Position 2, select Air Fry, set temperature to 375ºF (190ºC), and set time to 10 minutes.
5. When cooked, the fish should be flaky. If necessary, continue cooking for 5 minutes more. Remove the fish from the oven to a plate.

6. Assemble the tacos: Spoon some of the coleslaw mix into each tortilla and top each with $1/_3$ of a tilapia fillet. Squeeze some lime juice over the top of each taco and serve immediately.

361.Chili-rubbed Jumbo Shrimp

Servings: 2 To 3
Cooking Time: 10 Minutes
Ingredients:
- 1 lb jumbo shrimp
- Salt to taste
- ¼ tsp old bay seasoning
- ⅓ tsp smoked paprika
- ¼ tsp chili powder
- 1 tbsp olive oil

Directions:
1. Preheat on Air Fry function to 390 F. In a bowl, add the shrimp, paprika, olive oil, salt, old bay seasoning, and chili powder; mix well. Place the shrimp in the basket and fit in the baking tray. Cook for 5 minutes, flipping once. Serve with mayo and rice.

362.Fish Oregano Fingers

Servings:x
Cooking Time:x
Ingredients:
- ½ lb. firm white fish fillet cut into Oregano Fingers
- 1 tbsp. lemon juice
- 2 cups of dry breadcrumbs
- 1 cup oil for frying
- 1 ½ tbsp. ginger-garlic paste
- 3 tbsp. lemon juice
- 2 tsp salt
- 1 ½ tsp pepper powder
- 1 tsp red chili flakes or to taste
- 3 eggs
- 5 tbsp. corn flour
- 2 tsp tomato ketchup

Directions:
1. Rub a little lemon juice on the Oregano Fingers and set aside. Wash the fish after an hour and pat dry. Make the marinade and transfer the Oregano Fingers into the marinade. Leave them on a plate to dry for fifteen minutes. Now cover the Oregano Fingers with the crumbs and set aside to dry for fifteen minutes.
2. Pre heat the oven at 160 degrees Fahrenheit for 5 minutes or so. Keep the fish in the fry basket now and close it properly.
3. Let the Oregano Fingers cook at the same temperature for another 25 minutes. In between the cooking process, toss the fish once in a while to avoid burning the food. Serve either with tomato ketchup or chili sauce. Mint sauce also works well with the fish.

363.Lemon Salmon

Servings:2
Cooking Time: 20 Minutes
Ingredients:
- 2 salmon fillets
- Salt to taste
- Zest of 1 lemon

Directions:
1. Rub the fillets with salt and lemon zest. Place them in the frying basket and spray with cooking spray. Press Start and cook the salmon in the preheated oven for 14 minutes at 360 F on AirFry function. Serve with steamed asparagus and a drizzle of lemon juice.

364.Coconut Shrimp

Servings: 4
Cooking Time: 5 Minutes
Ingredients:
- 1 (8-ounce) can crushed pineapple
- ½ cup sour cream
- ¼ cup pineapple preserves
- 2 egg whites
- ⅔ cup cornstarch
- ⅔ cup sweetened coconut
- 1 cup panko bread crumbs
- 1 pound uncooked large shrimp, thawed if frozen, deveined and shelled
- Olive oil for misting

Directions:
1. Preparing the Ingredients. Drain the crushed pineapple well, reserving the juice. In a small bowl, combine the pineapple, sour cream, and preserves, and mix well. Set aside. In a shallow bowl, beat the egg whites with 2 tablespoons of the reserved pineapple liquid. Place the cornstarch on a plate. Combine the coconut and bread crumbs on another plate. Dip the shrimp into the cornstarch, shake it off, then dip into the egg white mixture and finally into the coconut mixture. Place the shrimp in the air fryer rack/basket and mist with oil.
2. Air Frying. Air-fry for 5 to 7 minutes or until the shrimp are crisp and golden brown.
- **Nutrition Info:** CALORIES: 524; FAT: 14G; PROTEIN:33G; FIBER:4G

365.Salmon Beans & Mushrooms

Servings: 6
Cooking Time: 25 Minutes
Ingredients:
- 4 salmon fillets
- 2 tbsp fresh parsley, minced
- 1/4 cup fresh lemon juice
- 1 tsp garlic, minced
- 1 tbsp olive oil
- 1/2 lb mushrooms, sliced
- 1/2 lb green beans, trimmed
- 1/2 cup parmesan cheese, grated
- Pepper

- Salt

Directions:
1. Fit the oven with the rack in position
2. Heat oil in a small saucepan over medium-high heat.
3. Add garlic and sauté for 30 seconds.
4. Remove from heat and stir in lemon juice, parsley, pepper, and salt.
5. Arrange fish fillets, mushrooms, and green beans in baking pan and drizzle with oil mixture.
6. Sprinkle with grated parmesan cheese.
7. Set to bake at 400 F for 30 minutes. After 5 minutes place the baking pan in the preheated oven.
8. Serve and enjoy.
- **Nutrition Info:** Calories 225 Fat 11.5 g Carbohydrates 4.7 g Sugar 1.4 g Protein 27.5 g Cholesterol 58 mg

366.Easy Salmon Patties

Servings: 6 Patties
Cooking Time: 11 Minutes
Ingredients:
- 1 (14.75-ounce / 418-g) can Alaskan pink salmon, drained and bones removed
- ½ cup bread crumbs
- 1 egg, whisked
- 2 scallions, diced
- 1 teaspoon garlic powder
- Salt and pepper, to taste
- Cooking spray

Directions:
1. Stir together the salmon, bread crumbs, whisked egg, scallions, garlic powder, salt, and pepper in a large bowl until well incorporated.
2. Divide the salmon mixture into six equal portions and form each into a patty with your hands.
3. Arrange the salmon patties in the air fryer basket and spritz them with cooking spray.
4. Put the air fryer basket on the baking pan and slide into Rack Position 2, select Air Fry, set temperature to 400ºF (205ºC), and set time to 10 minutes.
5. Flip the patties once halfway through.
6. When cooking is complete, the patties should be golden brown and cooked through. Remove the patties from the oven and serve on a plate.

367.Prawn Grandma's Easy To Cook Wontons

Servings:x
Cooking Time:x
Ingredients:
- 1 ½ cup all-purpose flour
- ½ tsp. salt
- 5 tbsp. water
- 2 cups minced prawn
- 2 tbsp. oil

- 2 tsp. ginger-garlic paste
- 2 tsp. soya sauce
- 2 tsp. vinegar

Directions:
1. Squeeze the dough and cover it with plastic wrap and set aside. Next, cook the ingredients for the filling and try to ensure that the prawn is covered well with the sauce. Roll the dough and place the filling in the center.
2. Now, wrap the dough to cover the filling and pinch the edges together. Pre heat the oven at 200° F for 5 minutes. Place the wontons in the fry basket and close it. Let them cook at the same temperature for another 20 minutes. Recommended sides are chili sauce or ketchup.

368.Prawn French Cuisine Galette

Servings:x
Cooking Time:x
Ingredients:
- 2 tbsp. garam masala
- 1 lb. minced prawn
- 3 tsp ginger finely chopped
- 1-2 tbsp. fresh coriander leaves
- 2 or 3 green chilies finely chopped
- 1 ½ tbsp. lemon juice
- Salt and pepper to taste

Directions:
1. Mix the ingredients in a clean bowl.
2. Mold this mixture into round and flat French Cuisine Galettes.
3. Wet the French Cuisine Galettes slightly with water.
4. Pre heat the oven at 160 degrees Fahrenheit for 5 minutes. Place the French Cuisine Galettes in the fry basket and let them cook for another 25 minutes at the same temperature. Keep rolling them over to get a uniform cook. Serve either with mint sauce or ketchup.

369.Carp Flat Cakes

Servings:x
Cooking Time:x
Ingredients:
- 2 tbsp. garam masala
- 1 lb. fileted carp
- 3 tsp ginger finely chopped
- 1-2 tbsp. fresh coriander leaves
- 2 or 3 green chilies finely chopped
- 1 ½ tbsp. lemon juice
- Salt and pepper to taste

Directions:
1. Mix the ingredients in a clean bowl and add water to it. Make sure that the paste is not too watery but is enough to apply on the sides of the carp filets.
2. Pre heat the oven at 160 degrees Fahrenheit for 5 minutes. Place the French Cuisine Galettes in the fry basket and let them cook for another 25 minutes at the

same temperature. Keep rolling them over to get a uniform cook. Serve either with mint sauce or ketchup.

370.Speedy Fried Scallops

Servings: 4
Cooking Time: 5 Minutes
Ingredients:
- 12 fresh scallops
- 3 tbsp flour
- Salt and black pepper to taste
- 1 egg, lightly beaten
- 1 cup breadcrumbs

Directions:
1. Coat the scallops with flour. Dip into the egg, then into the breadcrumbs. Spray with olive oil and arrange them on the basket. Fit in the baking tray and cook for 6 minutes at 360 F on Air Fry function, turning once halfway through cooking. Serve.

371.Garlic Shrimp With Parsley

Servings:4
Cooking Time: 5 Minutes
Ingredients:
- 18 shrimp, shelled and deveined
- 2 garlic cloves, peeled and minced
- 2 tablespoons extra-virgin olive oil
- 2 tablespoons freshly squeezed lemon juice
- ½ cup fresh parsley, coarsely chopped
- 1 teaspoon onion powder
- 1 teaspoon lemon-pepper seasoning
- ½ teaspoon hot paprika
- ½ teaspoon salt
- ¼ teaspoon cumin powder

Directions:
1. Toss all the ingredients in a mixing bowl until the shrimp are well coated.
2. Cover and allow to marinate in the refrigerator for 30 minutes.

3. When ready, transfer the shrimp to the air fryer basket.
4. Put the air fryer basket on the baking pan and slide into Rack Position 2, select Air Fry, set temperature to 400ºF (205ºC), and set time to 5 minutes.
5. When cooking is complete, the shrimp should be pink on the outside and opaque in the center. Remove from the oven and serve warm.

372.Spinach Scallops

Servings: 2
Cooking Time: 10 Minutes
Ingredients:
- 8 sea scallops
- 1 tbsp fresh basil, chopped
- 1 tbsp tomato paste
- 3/4 cup heavy cream
- 12 oz frozen spinach, thawed and drained
- 1 tsp garlic, minced
- 1/2 tsp pepper
- 1/2 tsp salt

Directions:
1. Fit the oven with the rack in position
2. Layer spinach in the baking dish.
3. Spray scallops with cooking spray and season with pepper and salt.
4. Place scallops on top of spinach.
5. In a small bowl, mix garlic, basil, tomato paste, whipping cream, pepper, and salt and pour over scallops and spinach.
6. Set to bake at 350 F for 15 minutes. After 5 minutes place the baking dish in the preheated oven.
7. Serve and enjoy.
- **Nutrition Info:** Calories 310 Fat 18.3 g Carbohydrates 12.6 g Sugar 1.7 g Protein 26.5 g Cholesterol 101 mg

MEATLESS RECIPES

373.Fenugreek French Cuisine Galette

Servings:x
Cooking Time:x
Ingredients:

- 2 or 3 green chilies finely chopped
- 1 ½ tbsp. lemon juice
- Salt and pepper to taste
- 2 cups fenugreek
- 2 medium potatoes boiled and mashed
- 3 tsp. ginger finely chopped
- 1-2 tbsp. fresh coriander leaves

Directions:

1. Mix the ingredients in a clean bowl.
2. Mold this mixture into round and flat French Cuisine Galettes.
3. Wet the French Cuisine Galettes slightly with water.
4. Pre heat the oven at 160 degrees Fahrenheit for 5 minutes. Place the French Cuisine Galettes in the fry basket and let them cook for another 25 minutes at the same temperature. Keep rolling them over to get a uniform cook. Serve either with mint sauce or ketchup.

374.Mushroom Fried Baked Pastry

Servings:x
Cooking Time:x
Ingredients:

- 2 capsicum sliced
- 2 carrot sliced
- 2 cabbage sliced
- 2 tbsp. soya sauce
- 2 tsp. vinegar
- 1 cup all-purpose flour
- 2 tbsp. unsalted butter
- A pinch of salt to taste
- Take the amount of water sufficient enough to make a stiff dough
- 3 cups whole mushrooms
- 2 onion sliced
- 2 tbsp. green chilies finely chopped
- 2 tbsp. ginger-garlic paste
- Some salt and pepper to taste

Directions:

1. Mix the dough for the outer covering and make it stiff and smooth. Leave it to rest in a container while making the filling.
2. Cook the ingredients in a pan and stir them well to make a thick paste. Roll the paste out.
3. Roll the dough into balls and flatten them. Cut them in halves and add the filling. Use water to help you fold the edges to create the shape of a cone.
4. Pre-heat the oven for around 5 to 6 minutes at 300 Fahrenheit. Place all the samosas in the fry basket and close the basket properly. Keep the oven at 200 degrees for another 20 to 25 minutes. Around the halfway point, open the basket and turn the samosas over for uniform cooking. After this, fry at 250 degrees for around 10 minutes in order to give them the desired golden-brown color. Serve hot. Recommended sides are tamarind or mint sauce.

375.Vegetable And Cheese Stuffed Tomatoes

Servings:4
Cooking Time: 18 Minutes
Ingredients:

- 4 medium beefsteak tomatoes, rinsed
- ½ cup grated carrot
- 1 medium onion, chopped
- 1 garlic clove, minced
- 2 teaspoons olive oil
- 2 cups fresh baby spinach
- ¼ cup crumbled low-sodium feta cheese
- ½ teaspoon dried basil

Directions:

1. On your cutting board, cut a thin slice off the top of each tomato. Scoop out a ¼- to ½-inch-thick tomato pulp and place the tomatoes upside down on paper towels to drain. Set aside.
2. Stir together the carrot, onion, garlic, and olive oil in the baking pan.
3. Slide the baking pan into Rack Position 1, select Convection Bake, set temperature to 350ºF (180ºC) and set time to 5 minutes.
4. Stir the vegetables halfway through.
5. When cooking is complete, the carrot should be crisp-tender.
6. Remove from the oven and stir in the spinach, feta cheese, and basil.
7. Spoon ¼ of the vegetable mixture into each tomato and transfer the stuffed tomatoes to the oven. Set time to 13 minutes.
8. When cooking is complete, the filling should be hot and the tomatoes should be lightly caramelized.
9. Let the tomatoes cool for 5 minutes and serve.

376.Cottage Cheese Fried Baked Pastry

Servings:x
Cooking Time:x
Ingredients:

- 1 or 2 green chilies that are finely chopped or mashed
- ½ tsp. cumin
- 1 tsp. coarsely crushed coriander
- 1 dry red chili broken into pieces

- A small amount of salt (to taste)
- ½ tsp. dried mango powder
- ½ tsp. red chili power
- 1-2 tbsp. coriander
- 2 tbsp. unsalted butter
- 1 ½ cup all-purpose flour
- A pinch of salt to taste
- Water
- 2 cups mashed cottage cheese
- ¼ cup boiled peas
- 1 tsp. powdered ginger

Directions:
1. Mix the dough for the outer covering and make it stiff and smooth. Leave it to rest in a container while making the filling.
2. Cook the ingredients in a pan and stir them well to make a thick paste. Roll the paste out.
3. Roll the dough into balls and flatten them. Cut them in halves and add the filling. Use water to help you fold the edges to create the shape of a cone.
4. Pre-heat the oven for around 5 to 6 minutes at 300 Fahrenheit. Place all the samosas in the fry basket and close the basket properly. Keep the oven at 200 degrees for another 20 to 25 minutes. Around the halfway point, open the basket and turn the samosas over for uniform cooking. After this, fry at 250 degrees for around 10 minutes in order to give them the desired golden-brown color. Serve hot. Recommended sides are tamarind or mint sauce.

377.Cottage Cheese French Cuisine Galette

Servings:x
Cooking Time:x
Ingredients:
- 1-2 tbsp. fresh coriander leaves
- 2 or 3 green chilies finely chopped
- 1 ½ tbsp. lemon juice
- Salt and pepper to taste
- 2 tbsp. garam masala
- 2 cups grated cottage cheese
- 1 ½ cup coarsely crushed peanuts
- 3 tsp. ginger finely chopped

Directions:
1. Mix the ingredients in a clean bowl.
2. Mold this mixture into round and flat French Cuisine Galettes.
3. Wet the French Cuisine Galettes slightly with water. Coat each French Cuisine Galette with the crushed peanuts.
4. Pre heat the oven at 160 degrees Fahrenheit for 5 minutes. Place the French Cuisine Galettes in the fry basket and let them cook for another 25 minutes at the same temperature. Keep rolling them over

to get a uniform cook. Serve either with mint sauce or ketchup.

378.Macaroni Fried Baked Pastry

Servings:x
Cooking Time:x
Ingredients:
- 2 carrot sliced
- 2 cabbage sliced
- 2 tbsp. soya sauce
- 2 tsp. vinegar
- Some salt and pepper to taste
- 2 tbsp. olive oil
- ½ tsp. axiomata
- 1 cup all-purpose flour
- 2 tbsp. unsalted butter
- A pinch of salt to taste
- Take the amount of water sufficient enough to make a stiff dough
- 3 cups boiled macaroni
- 2 onion sliced
- 2 capsicum sliced
- 2 tbsp. ginger finely chopped
- 2 tbsp. garlic finely chopped
- 2 tbsp. green chilies finely chopped
- 2 tbsp. ginger-garlic paste

Directions:
1. Mix the dough for the outer covering and make it stiff and smooth. Leave it to rest in a container while making the filling. Cook the ingredients in a pan and stir them well to make a thick paste. Roll the paste out.
2. Roll the dough into balls and flatten them. Cut them in halves and add the filling. Use water to help you fold the edges to create the shape of a cone. Pre-heat the oven for around 5 to 6 minutes at 300 Fahrenheit. Place all the samosas in the fry basket and close the basket properly. Keep the oven at 200 degrees for another 20 to 25 minutes.
3. Around the halfway point, open the basket and turn the samosas over for uniform cooking. After this, fry at 250 degrees for around 10 minutes in order to give them the desired golden-brown color. Serve hot. Recommended sides are tamarind or mint sauce.

379.Banana Best Homemade Croquette

Servings:x
Cooking Time:x
Ingredients:
- 2 tsp. garam masala
- 4 tbsp. chopped coriander
- 3 tbsp. cream
- 3 tbsp. chopped capsicum
- 3 eggs
- 2 ½ tbsp. white sesame seeds
- 2 cups sliced banana

- 3 onions chopped
- 5 green chilies-roughly chopped
- 1 ½ tbsp. ginger paste
- 1 ½ tsp. garlic paste
- 1 ½ tsp. salt
- 3 tsp. lemon juice

Directions:
1. Grind the ingredients except for the egg and form a smooth paste. Coat the banana in the paste. Now, beat the eggs and add a little salt to it.
2. Dip the coated bananas in the egg mixture and then transfer to the sesame seeds and coat the vegetables well. Place the vegetables on a stick.
3. Pre heat the oven at 160 degrees Fahrenheit for around 5 minutes. Place the sticks in the basket and let them cook for another 25 minutes at the same temperature. Turn the sticks over in between the cooking process to get a uniform cook.

380.Sweet Baby Carrots

Servings: 4
Cooking Time: 20 Minutes
Ingredients:
- 1 pound baby carrots
- 1 tsp dried dill
- 1 tbsp olive oil
- 1 tbsp honey
- Salt and black pepper to taste

Directions:
1. Preheat your Oven to 300 F on Air Fry function. In a bowl, mix oil, carrots, and honey; gently stir to coat. Season with dill, pepper, and salt. Place the carrots in the cooking basket and fit in the baking tray; cook for 15 minutes, shaking once. Serve.

381.Potato Fried Baked Pastry

Servings:x
Cooking Time:x
Ingredients:
- 1 tsp. powdered ginger
- 1 or 2 green chilies that are finely chopped or mashed
- ½ tsp. cumin
- 1 tsp. coarsely crushed coriander
- 1 dry red chili broken into pieces
- A small amount of salt (to taste)
- 2 tbsp. unsalted butter
- 1 ½ cup all-purpose flour
- A pinch of salt to taste
- Add as much water as required to make the dough stiff and firm
- 2-3 big potatoes boiled and mashed
- ¼ cup boiled peas
- ½ tsp. dried mango powder

- ½ tsp. red chili power.
- 1-2 tbsp. coriander.

Directions:
1. Mix the dough for the outer covering and make it stiff and smooth. Leave it to rest in a container while making the filling. Cook the ingredients in a pan and stir them well to make a thick paste. Roll the paste out.
2. Roll the dough into balls and flatten them. Cut them in halves and add the filling. Use water to help you fold the edges to create the shape of a cone. Pre-heat the oven for around 5 to 6 minutes at 300 Fahrenheit.
3. Place all the samosas in the fry basket and close the basket properly. Keep the oven at 200 degrees for another 20 to 25 minutes. Around the halfway point, open the basket and turn the samosas over for uniform cooking. After this, fry at 250 degrees for around 10 minutes in order to give them the desired golden-brown color. Serve hot. Recommended sides are tamarind or mint sauce.

382.Crispy Potato Lentil Nuggets

Servings: 4
Cooking Time: 10 Minutes
Ingredients:
- Nonstick cooking spray
- 1 cup red lentils
- 1 tbsp. olive oil
- 1 cup onion, grated
- 1 cup carrot, grated
- 1 cup potato, grated
- ½ cup flour
- ½ tsp salt
- ½ tsp garlic powder
- ¾ tsp paprika
- ¼ tsp pepper

Directions:
1. Place baking pan in position 2. Lightly spray fryer basket with cooking spray.
2. Soak lentils in just enough water to cover them for 25 minutes.
3. Heat oil in a large skillet over medium heat. Add onion, carrot, and potato. Cook, stirring frequently until vegetables are tender, 12-15 minutes.
4. Drain the lentils and place them in a food processor. Add flour and spices and pulse to combine, leave some texture to the mixture.
5. Add cooked veggies to the food processor and pulse just until combined. Mixture will be sticky, so oil your hands. Form mixture into nugget shapes and add to the fryer basket in a single layer.
6. Place basket in the oven and set air fry on 350°F for 10 minutes. Turn nuggets over halfway through cooking time. Repeat with

remaining mixture. Serve with your favorite dipping sauce.

- **Nutrition Info:** Calories 317, Total Fat 5g, Saturated Fat 1g, Total Carbs 54g, Net Carbs 46g, Protein 14g, Sugar 3g, Fiber 8g, Sodium 317mg, Potassium 625mg, Phosphorus 197mg

383.Roasted Vegetable Mélange With Herbs

Servings:4
Cooking Time: 16 Minutes
Ingredients:
- 1 (8-ounce / 227-g) package sliced mushrooms
- 1 yellow summer squash, sliced
- 1 red bell pepper, sliced
- 3 cloves garlic, sliced
- 1 tablespoon olive oil
- ½ teaspoon dried basil
- ½ teaspoon dried thyme
- ½ teaspoon dried tarragon

Directions:
1. Toss the mushrooms, squash, and bell pepper with the garlic and olive oil in a large bowl until well coated. Mix in the basil, thyme, and tarragon and toss again.
2. Spread the vegetables evenly in the air fryer basket.
3. Put the air fryer basket on the baking pan and slide into Rack Position 2, select Roast, set temperature to 350ºF (180ºC), and set time to 16 minutes.
4. When cooking is complete, the vegetables should be fork-tender. Remove from the oven and cool for 5 minutes before serving.

384.Fried Root Vegetable Medley With Thyme

Servings:4
Cooking Time: 22 Minutes
Ingredients:
- 2 carrots, sliced
- 2 potatoes, cut into chunks
- 1 rutabaga, cut into chunks
- 1 turnip, cut into chunks
- 1 beet, cut into chunks
- 8 shallots, halved
- 2 tablespoons olive oil
- Salt and black pepper, to taste
- 2 tablespoons tomato pesto
- 2 tablespoons water
- 2 tablespoons chopped fresh thyme

Directions:
1. Toss the carrots, potatoes, rutabaga, turnip, beet, shallots, olive oil, salt, and pepper in a large mixing bowl until the root vegetables are evenly coated.

2. Place the root vegetables in the air fryer basket.
3. Put the air fryer basket on the baking pan and slide into Rack Position 2, select Air Fry, set temperature to 400ºF (205ºC) and set time to 22 minutes.
4. Stir the vegetables twice during cooking.
5. When cooking is complete, the vegetables should be tender.
6. Meanwhile, in a small bowl, whisk together the tomato pesto and water until smooth.
7. When ready, remove the root vegetables from the oven to a platter. Drizzle with the tomato pesto mixture and sprinkle with the thyme. Serve immediately.

385.Maple And Pecan Granola

Servings:4
Cooking Time: 20 Minutes
Ingredients:
- 1½ cups rolled oats
- ¼ cup maple syrup
- ¼ cup pecan pieces
- 1 teaspoon vanilla extract
- ½ teaspoon ground cinnamon

Directions:
1. Line a baking sheet with parchment paper.
2. Mix together the oats, maple syrup, pecan pieces, vanilla, and cinnamon in a large bowl and stir until the oats and pecan pieces are completely coated. Spread the mixture evenly in the baking pan.
3. Slide the baking pan into Rack Position 1, select Convection Bake, set temperature to 300ºF (150ºC), and set time to 20 minutes.
4. Stir once halfway through the cooking time.
5. When done, remove from the oven and cool for 30 minutes before serving. The granola may still be a bit soft right after removing, but it will gradually firm up as it cools.

386.Coconut Vegan Fries

Servings: 2
Cooking Time: 20 Minutes
Ingredients:
- 2 potatoes, spiralized
- 1 tbsp tomato ketchup
- 2 tbsp olive oil
- Salt and black pepper to taste
- 2 tbsp coconut oil

Directions:
1. In a bowl, mix olive oil, coconut oil, salt, and pepper. Add in the potatoes and toss to coat. Place them in the basket and fit in the baking tray; cook for 15 minutes on Air Fry function at 360 F. Serve with ketchup and enjoy!

387.Aloo Patties

Servings:x
Cooking Time:x
Ingredients:
- 1 tbsp. fresh coriander leaves
- ¼ tsp. red chili powder
- ¼ tsp. cumin powder
- 1 cup mashed potato
- A pinch of salt to taste
- ¼ tsp. ginger finely chopped
- 1 green chili finely chopped
- 1 tsp. lemon juice

Directions:
1. Mix the ingredients together and ensure that the flavors are right. You will now make round patties with the mixture and roll them out well.
2. Pre heat the oven at 250 Fahrenheit for 5 minutes. Open the basket of the Fryer and arrange the patties in the basket. Close it carefully. Keep the fryer at 150 degrees for around 10 or 12 minutes. In between the cooking process, turn the patties over to get a uniform cook. Serve hot with mint sauce.

388.Air Fried Carrots, Yellow Squash & Zucchini

Servings: 4
Cooking Time: 35 Minutes
Ingredients:
- 1 tbsp. chopped tarragon leaves
- ½ tsp. white pepper
- 1 tsp. salt
- 1 pound yellow squash
- 1 pound zucchini
- 6 tsp. olive oil
- ½ pound carrots

Directions:
1. Preparing the Ingredients. Stem and root the end of squash and zucchini and cut in ¾-inch half-moons. Peel and cut carrots into 1-inch cubes
2. Combine carrot cubes with 2 teaspoons of olive oil, tossing to combine.
3. Air Frying. Pour into the Oven rack/basket. Place the Rack on the middle-shelf of the air fryer oven. Set temperature to 400°F, and set time to 5 minutes.
4. As carrots cook, drizzle remaining olive oil over squash and zucchini pieces, then season with pepper and salt. Toss well to coat.
5. Add squash and zucchini when the timer for carrots goes off. Cook 30 minutes, making sure to toss 2-3 times during the cooking process.
6. Once done, take out veggies and toss with tarragon. Serve up warm!

- **Nutrition Info:** CALORIES: 122; FAT: 9G; PROTEIN: 6G; SUGAR:0G

389.Cheese And Garlic French Fries

Servings:x
Cooking Time:x
Ingredients:
- 1 cup molten cheese
- 2 tsp. garlic powder
- 1 tbsp. lemon juice
- 2 medium sized potatoes peeled and cut into thick pieces lengthwise
- ingredients for the marinade:
- 1 tbsp. olive oil
- 1 tsp. mixed herbs
- ½ tsp. red chili flakes
- A pinch of salt to taste

Directions:
1. Boil the potatoes and blanch them. Cut the potato into Oregano Fingers. Mix the ingredients for the marinade and add the potato Oregano Fingers to it making sure that they are coated well.
2. Pre heat the oven for around 5 minutes at 300 Fahrenheit. Take out the basket of the fryer and place the potato Oregano Fingers in them. Close the basket.
3. Now keep the fryer at 200 Fahrenheit for 20 or 25 minutes. In between the process, toss the fries twice or thrice so that they get cooked properly.

390.Awesome Sweet Potato Fries

Servings: 4
Cooking Time: 30 Minutes
Ingredients:
- ½ tsp salt
- ½ tsp garlic powder
- ½ tsp chili powder
- ¼ tsp cumin
- 3 tbsp olive oil
- 3 sweet potatoes, cut into thick strips

Directions:
1. In a bowl, mix salt, garlic powder, chili, and cumin, and olive oil. Coat the strips well in this mixture and arrange them in the basket without overcrowding. Fit in the baking tray and cook for 20 minutes at 380 F on Air Fry function or until crispy. Serve.

391.Cheesy Broccoli Tots

Servings:4
Cooking Time: 15 Minutes
Ingredients:
- 12 ounces (340 g) frozen broccoli, thawed, drained, and patted dry
- 1 large egg, lightly beaten
- ½ cup seasoned whole-wheat bread crumbs

- ¼ cup shredded reduced-fat sharp Cheddar cheese
- ¼ cup grated Parmesan cheese
- 1½ teaspoons minced garlic
- Salt and freshly ground black pepper, to taste
- Cooking spray

Directions:
1. Spritz the air fryer basket lightly with cooking spray.
2. Place the remaining ingredients into a food processor and process until the mixture resembles a coarse meal. Transfer the mixture to a bowl.
3. Using a tablespoon, scoop out the broccoli mixture and form into 24 oval "tater tot" shapes with your hands.
4. Put the tots in the prepared basket in a single layer, spacing them 1 inch apart. Mist the tots lightly with cooking spray.
5. Put the air fryer basket on the baking pan and slide into Rack Position 2, select Air Fry, set temperature to 375ºF (190ºC), and set time to 15 minutes.
6. Flip the tots halfway through the cooking time.
7. When done, the tots will be lightly browned and crispy. Remove from the oven and serve on a plate.

392.Yummy Chili Bean Burritos

Servings: 3
Cooking Time: 30 Minutes
Ingredients:
- 6 tortillas
- 1 cup grated cheddar cheese
- 1 can (8 oz) beans
- 1 tsp Italian seasoning

Directions:
1. Preheat on Bake function to 350 F. Season the beans with the seasoning and divide them between the tortillas. Top with cheddar cheese. Roll the burritos and arrange them on a lined baking dish. Cook for 5 minutes. Serve.

393.Cilantro Roasted Carrots With Cumin Seeds

Servings:4
Cooking Time: 15 Minutes
Ingredients:
- 1 lb carrots, julienned
- 1 tbsp olive oil
- 1 tsp cumin seeds
- 2 tbsp fresh cilantro, chopped

Directions:
1. Preheat on AirFry function to 350 F. In a bowl, mix oil, carrots, and cumin seeds. Gently stir to coat the carrots well. Place the carrots in a baking tray and press Star. Cook for 10 minutes. Scatter fresh coriander over the carrots and serve.

394.Chili Cottage Cheese

Servings:x
Cooking Time:x
Ingredients:
- 2 tbsp. olive oil
- 1 capsicum. Cut into thin and long pieces (lengthwise).
- 2 small onions. Cut them into halves.
- 1 ½ tsp. ginger garlic paste.
- ½ tbsp. red chili sauce.
- 2 tbsp. tomato ketchup.
- 1 ½ tbsp. sweet chili sauce.
- 2 tsp. vinegar.
- 2 tsp. soya sauce.
- A few drops of edible red food coloring.
- 1-2 tbsp. honey.
- 2 cups cubed cottage cheese
- 2 ½ tsp. ginger-garlic paste
- 1 tsp. red chili sauce
- ¼ tsp. salt
- ¼ tsp. red chili powder/black pepper
- A few drops of edible orange food coloring
- ¼ tsp. Ajinomoto.
- A pinch of black pepper powder.
- 1-2 tsp. red chili flakes.
- For the garnish, use the greens of spring onions and sesame seeds.

Directions:
1. Create the mix for the cottage cheese cubes and coat the chicken well with it.
2. Pre heat the oven at 250 Fahrenheit for 5 minutes or so. Open the basket of the Fryer. Place the Oregano Fingers inside the basket. Now let the fryer stay at 290 Fahrenheit for another 20 minutes. Keep tossing the Oregano Fingers periodically through the cook to get a uniform cook.
3. Add the ingredients to the sauce and cook it with the vegetables till it thickens. Add the Oregano Fingers to the sauce and cook till the flavors have blended.

395.Cheesy Asparagus And Potato Platter

Servings:5
Cooking Time: 26 Minutes
Ingredients:
- 4 medium potatoes, cut into wedges
- Cooking spray
- 1 bunch asparagus, trimmed
- 2 tablespoons olive oil
- Salt and pepper, to taste
- Cheese Sauce:
- ¼ cup crumbled cottage cheese
- ¼ cup buttermilk

- 1 tablespoon whole-grain mustard
- Salt and black pepper, to taste

Directions:
1. Spritz the air fryer basket with cooking spray.
2. Put the potatoes in the air fryer basket.
3. Put the air fryer basket on the baking pan and slide into Rack Position 2, select Roast, set temperature to 400ºF (205ºC) and set time to 20 minutes.
4. Stir the potatoes halfway through.
5. When cooking is complete, the potatoes should be golden brown.
6. Remove the potatoes from the oven to a platter. Cover the potatoes with foil to keep warm. Set aside.
7. Place the asparagus in the air fryer basket and drizzle with the olive oil. Sprinkle with salt and pepper.
8. Put the air fryer basket on the baking pan and slide into Rack Position 2, select Roast, set temperature to 400ºF (205ºC) and set time to 6 minutes. Stir the asparagus halfway through.
9. When cooking is complete, the asparagus should be crispy.
10. Meanwhile, make the cheese sauce by stirring together the cottage cheese, buttermilk, and mustard in a small bowl. Season as needed with salt and pepper.
11. Transfer the asparagus to the platter of potatoes and drizzle with the cheese sauce. Serve immediately.

396.Roasted Vegetables With Basil

Servings:2
Cooking Time: 20 Minutes
Ingredients:
- 1 small eggplant, halved and sliced
- 1 yellow bell pepper, cut into thick strips
- 1 red bell pepper, cut into thick strips
- 2 garlic cloves, quartered
- 1 red onion, sliced
- 1 tablespoon extra-virgin olive oil
- Salt and freshly ground black pepper, to taste
- ½ cup chopped fresh basil, for garnish
- Cooking spray

Directions:
1. Grease the baking pan with cooking spray.
2. Place the eggplant, bell peppers, garlic, and red onion in the greased baking pan. Drizzle with the olive oil and toss to coat well. Spritz any uncoated surfaces with cooking spray.
3. Slide the baking pan into Rack Position 1, select Convection Bake, set temperature to 350ºF (180ºC), and set time to 20 minutes.
4. Flip the vegetables halfway through the cooking time.

5. When done, remove from the oven and sprinkle with salt and pepper.
6. Sprinkle the basil on top for garnish and serve.

397.Cottage Cheese Spicy Lemon Kebab

Servings:x
Cooking Time:x
Ingredients:
- 3 tsp. lemon juice
- 2 tbsp. coriander powder
- 3 tbsp. chopped capsicum
- 2 tbsp. peanut flour
- 2 cups cubed cottage cheese
- 3 onions chopped
- 5 green chilies-roughly chopped
- 1 ½ tbsp. ginger paste
- 1 ½ tsp. garlic paste
- 1 ½ tsp. salt
- 3 eggs

Directions:
1. Coat the cottage cheese cubes with the corn flour and mix the other ingredients in a bowl. Make the mixture into a smooth paste and coat the cheese cubes with the mixture. Beat the eggs in a bowl and add a little salt to them.
2. Dip the cubes in the egg mixture and coat them with sesame seeds and leave them in the refrigerator for an hour.
3. Pre heat the oven at 290 Fahrenheit for around 5 minutes. Place the kebabs in the basket and let them cook for another 25 minutes at the same temperature. Turn the kebabs over in between the cooking process to get a uniform cook. Serve the kebabs with mint sauce.

398.Baked Turnip And Zucchini

Servings:4
Cooking Time: 18 Minutes
Ingredients:
- 3 turnips, sliced
- 1 large zucchini, sliced
- 1 large red onion, cut into rings
- 2 cloves garlic, crushed
- 1 tablespoon olive oil
- Salt and black pepper, to taste

Directions:
1. Put the turnips, zucchini, red onion, and garlic in the baking pan. Drizzle the olive oil over the top and sprinkle with the salt and pepper.
2. Slide the baking pan into Rack Position 1, select Convection Bake, set temperature to 330ºF (166ºC), and set time to 18 minutes.
3. When cooking is complete, the vegetables should be tender. Remove from the oven and serve on a plate.

399.Carrot & Chickpea Oat Balls With Cashews

Servings:4
Cooking Time: 30 Minutes
Ingredients:
- 2 tbsp olive oil
- 2 tbsp soy sauce
- 1 tbsp flax meal
- 2 cups canned chickpeas, drained
- ½ cup sweet onions, diced
- ½ cup carrots, grated
- ½ cup cashews, toasted
- Juice of 1 lemon
- ½ tsp turmeric
- 1 tsp cumin
- 1 tsp garlic powder
- 1 cup rolled oats

Directions:
1. Preheat on AirFry function to 380 F. Heat olive oil in a skillet and sauté onions and carrots for 5 minutes. Ground the oats and cashews in a food processor. Transfer to a bowl.
2. Place the chickpeas, lemon juice, and soy sauce in the food processor and process until smooth. Add them to the bowl as well. Mix in the onions and carrots.
3. Stir in the remaining ingredients until fully incorporated. Make balls out of the mixture. Place them in the frying basket and press Start. Cook for 12 minutes. Serve warm.

400.Bottle Gourd Flat Cakes

Servings:x
Cooking Time:x
Ingredients:
- 2 or 3 green chilies finely chopped
- 1 ½ tbsp. lemon juice
- Salt and pepper to taste
- 2 tbsp. garam masala
- 2 cups sliced bottle gourd
- 3 tsp. ginger finely chopped
- 1-2 tbsp. fresh coriander leaves

Directions:
1. Mix the ingredients in a clean bowl and add water to it. Make sure that the paste is not too watery but is enough to apply on the bottle gourd slices. Pre heat the oven at 160 degrees Fahrenheit for 5 minutes.
2. Place the French Cuisine Galettes in the fry basket and let them cook for another 25 minutes at the same temperature. Keep rolling them over to get a uniform cook. Serve either with mint sauce or ketchup.

401.Roasted Bell Peppers With Garlic

Servings:4
Cooking Time: 22 Minutes

Ingredients:
- 1 green bell pepper, sliced into 1-inch strips
- 1 red bell pepper, sliced into 1-inch strips
- 1 orange bell pepper, sliced into 1-inch strips
- 1 yellow bell pepper, sliced into 1-inch strips
- 2 tablespoons olive oil, divided
- ½ teaspoon dried marjoram
- Pinch salt
- Freshly ground black pepper, to taste
- 1 head garlic

Directions:
1. Toss the bell peppers with 1 tablespoon of olive oil in a large bowl until well coated. Season with the marjoram, salt, and pepper. Toss again and set aside.
2. Cut off the top of a head of garlic. Place the garlic cloves on a large square of aluminum foil. Drizzle the top with the remaining 1 tablespoon of olive oil and wrap the garlic cloves in foil.
3. Transfer the garlic to the air fryer basket.
4. Put the air fryer basket on the baking pan and slide into Rack Position 2, select Roast, set temperature to 330ºF (166ºC) and set time to 15 minutes.
5. After 15 minutes, remove from the oven and add the bell peppers. Return to the oven and set time to 7 minutes.
6. When cooking is complete or until the garlic is soft and the bell peppers are tender.
7. Transfer the cooked bell peppers to a plate. Remove the garlic and unwrap the foil. Let the garlic rest for a few minutes. Once cooled, squeeze the roasted garlic cloves out of their skins and add them to the plate of bell peppers. Stir well and serve immediately.

402.Jalapeño Cheese Balls

Servings: 12
Cooking Time: 8 Minutes
Ingredients:
- 4 ounces cream cheese
- ⅓ cup shredded mozzarella cheese
- ⅓ cup shredded Cheddar cheese
- 2 jalapeños, finely chopped
- ½ cup bread crumbs
- 2 eggs
- ½ cup all-purpose flour
- Salt
- Pepper
- Cooking oil

Directions:
1. Preparing the Ingredients. In a medium bowl, combine the cream cheese, mozzarella, Cheddar, and jalapeños. Mix well.

2. Form the cheese mixture into balls about an inch thick. Using a small ice cream scoop works well.
3. Arrange the cheese balls on a sheet pan and place in the freezer for 15 minutes. This will help the cheese balls maintain their shape while frying.
4. Spray the Oven rack/basket with cooking oil. Place the bread crumbs in a small bowl. In another small bowl, beat the eggs. In a third small bowl, combine the flour with salt and pepper to taste, and mix well. Remove the cheese balls from the freezer. Dip the cheese balls in the flour, then the eggs, and then the bread crumbs.
5. Air Frying. Place the cheese balls in the Oven rack/basket. Spray with cooking oil. Place the Rack on the middle-shelf of the air fryer oven. Cook for 8 minutes.
6. Open the air fryer oven and flip the cheese balls. I recommend flipping them instead of shaking, so the balls maintain their form. Cook an additional 4 minutes. Cool before serving.
- **Nutrition Info:** CALORIES: 96; FAT: 6G; PROTEIN:4G; SUGAR:

403.Easy Cheesy Vegetable Quesadilla

Servings:1
Cooking Time: 10 Minutes
Ingredients:
- 1 teaspoon olive oil
- 2 flour tortillas
- ¼ zucchini, sliced
- ¼ yellow bell pepper, sliced
- ¼ cup shredded gouda cheese
- 1 tablespoon chopped cilantro
- ½ green onion, sliced

Directions:
1. Coat the air fryer basket with 1 teaspoon of olive oil.
2. Arrange a flour tortilla in the basket and scatter the top with zucchini, bell pepper, gouda cheese, cilantro, and green onion. Place the other flour tortilla on top.
3. Put the air fryer basket on the baking pan and slide into Rack Position 2, select Air Fry, set temperature to 390ºF (199ºC), and set time to 10 minutes.
4. When cooking is complete, the tortillas should be lightly browned and the vegetables should be tender. Remove from the oven and cool for 5 minutes before slicing into wedges.

404.Parsley Feta Triangles

Servings: 4
Cooking Time: 20 Minutes
Ingredients:
- 4 oz feta cheese
- 2 sheets filo pastry
- 1 egg yolk
- 2 tbsp parsley, finely chopped
- 1 scallion, finely chopped
- 2 tbsp olive oil
- salt and black pepper

Directions:
1. In a bowl, beat the yolk and mix with feta cheese, parsley, scallion, salt, and black pepper. Cut each filo sheet in three parts or strips. Put a teaspoon of the feta mixture on the bottom. Roll the strip in a spinning spiral way until the filling of the inside mixture is wrapped in a triangle.
2. Preheat on Bake function to 360 F. Brush the surface of filo with olive oil. Arrange the triangles on a greased baking tray and cook for 5 minutes. Lower the temperature to 330 F and cook for 3 more minutes or until golden brown. Serve chilled.

405.Veggie Mix Fried Chips

Servings:4
Cooking Time: 45 Minutes
Ingredients:
- 1 large eggplant, cut into strips
- 5 potatoes, peeled and cut into strips
- 3 zucchinis, cut into strips
- ½ cup cornstarch
- ½ cup olive oil
- Salt to taste

Directions:
1. Preheat on AirFry function to 390 F. In a bowl, stir cornstarch, ½ cup of water, salt, pepper, olive oil, eggplants, zucchini, and potatoes. Place the veggie mixture in the basket and press Start. Cook for 12 minutes. Serve warm.

406.Roasted Vegetables Salad

Servings: 5
Cooking Time: 85 Minutes
Ingredients:
- 3 eggplants
- 1 tbsp of olive oil
- 3 medium zucchini
- 1 tbsp of olive oil
- 4 large tomatoes, cut them in eighths
- 4 cups of one shaped pasta
- 2 peppers of any color
- 1 cup of sliced tomatoes cut into small cubes
- 2 teaspoon of salt substitute
- 8 tbsp of grated parmesan cheese
- ½ cup of Italian dressing
- Leaves of fresh basil

Directions:

1. Preparing the Ingredients. Wash your eggplant and slice it off then discard the green end. Make sure not to peel.
2. Slice your eggplant into1/2 inch of thick rounds. 1/2 inch)
3. Pour 1tbsp of olive oil on the eggplant round.
4. Air Frying. Put the eggplants in the basket of the air fryer oven and then toss it in the air fryer oven. Cook the eggplants for 40 minutes. Set the heat to 360 ° F
5. Meanwhile, wash your zucchini and slice it then discard the green end. But do not peel it.
6. Slice the Zucchini into thick rounds of ½ inch each. Toss your ingredients
7. Add 1 tbsp of olive oil.
8. Air Frying. Cook the zucchini for 25 minutes on a heat of 360° F and when the time is off set it aside.
9. Wash and cut the tomatoes.
10. Air Frying. Arrange your tomatoes in the basket of the air fryer oven. Set the timer to 30 minutes. Set the heat to 350° F
11. When the time is off, cook your pasta according to the pasta guiding directions, empty it into a colander. Run the cold water on it and wash it and drain the pasta and put it aside.
12. Meanwhile, wash and chop your peppers and place it in a bow
13. Wash and thinly slice your cherry tomatoes and add it to the bowl. Add your roasted veggies.
14. Add the pasta, a pinch of salt, the topping dressing, add the basil and the parm and toss everything together. (It is better to mix with your hands). Set the ingredients together in the refrigerator, and let it chill
15. Serve your salad and enjoy it!

407.Asian Tofu "meatballs"

Servings: 4
Cooking Time: 10 Minutes
Ingredients:
- 3 dried shitake mushrooms
- Nonstick cooking spray
- 14 oz. firm tofu, drained & pressed
- ¼ cup carrots, cooked
- ¼ cup bamboo shoots, sliced thin
- ½ cup Panko bread crumbs
- 2 tbsp. corn starch
- 3 ½ tablespoon soy sauce, divided
- 1 tsp garlic powder
- ¼ tsp salt
- 1/8 tsp pepper
- 1 tbsp. olive oil
- 2 tbsp. garlic, diced fine
- 2 tbsp. ketchup
- 2 tsp sugar

Directions:
1. Place the shitake mushrooms in a bowl and add just enough water to cover. Let soak 20 minutes until soft. Drain well and chop.
2. Place the baking pan in position Lightly spray the fryer basket with cooking spray.
3. Place mushrooms, tofu, carrots, bamboo shoots, bread crumbs, corn starch, 1 ½ tablespoons soy sauce, and seasonings in a food processor. Pulse until thoroughly combined. Form mixture into 1-inch balls.
4. Place balls in fryer basket, these may need to be cooked in batches, and place in oven. Set to air fry on 380°F for 10 minutes. Turn the balls around halfway through cooking time.
5. Heat oil in a saucepan over medium heat. Add garlic and cook 1 minute.
6. Stir in remaining soy sauce, ketchup, and sugar. Bring to a simmer and cook until sauce thickens, 3-5 minutes.
7. When the meatballs are done, add them to sauce and stir to coat. Serve immediately.
- **Nutrition Info:** Calories 305, Total Fat 13g, Saturated Fat 2g, Total Carbs 28g, Net Carbs 24g, Protein 20g, Sugar 5g, Fiber 4g, Sodium 789mg, Potassium 470mg, Phosphorus 260mg

408.Carrots & Shallots With Yogurt

Servings:4
Cooking Time: 25 Minutes
Ingredients:
- 2 tsp olive oil
- 2 shallots, chopped
- 3 carrots, sliced
- Salt to taste
- ¼ cup yogurt
- 2 garlic cloves, minced
- 3 tbsp parsley, chopped

Directions:
1. In a bowl, mix sliced carrots, salt, garlic, shallots, parsley, and yogurt. Sprinkle with oil. Place the veggies in the basket and press Start. Cook for 15 minutes on AirFry function at 370 F. Serve with basil and garlic mayo.

409.Broccoli Momo's Recipe

Servings:x
Cooking Time:x
Ingredients:
- 2 tbsp. oil
- 2 tsp. ginger-garlic paste
- 2 tsp. soya sauce
- 2 tsp. vinegar
- 1 ½ cup all-purpose flour
- ½ tsp. salt

- 5 tbsp. water
- 2 cups grated broccoli

Directions:
1. Squeeze the dough and cover it with plastic wrap and set aside. Next, cook the ingredients for the filling and try to ensure that the broccoli is covered well with the sauce.
2. Roll the dough and cut it into a square. Place the filling in the center. Now, wrap the dough to cover the filling and pinch the edges together.
3. Pre heat the oven at 200° F for 5 minutes. Place the gnocchi's in the fry basket and close it. Let them cook at the same temperature for another 20 minutes. Recommended sides are chili sauce or ketchup.

410.Parmesan Coated Green Beans

Servings:4
Cooking Time: 20 Minutes
Ingredients:
- 1 cup panko breadcrumbs
- 2 whole eggs, beaten
- ½ cup Parmesan cheese, grated
- ½ cup flour
- 1 tsp cayenne pepper powder
- 1 ½ pounds green beans
- Salt to taste

Directions:
1. Preheat on AirFry function to 380 F. In a bowl, mix breadcrumbs, Parmesan cheese, cayenne pepper powder, salt, and pepper. Flour the green beans and dip them in eggs. Dredge beans in the Parmesan-panko mix. Place in the cooking basket and cook for 15 minutes Serve.

411.Cheesy Cabbage Wedges

Servings: 4
Cooking Time: 25 Minutes
Ingredients:
- ½ head cabbage, cut into wedges
- 2 cups Parmesan cheese, chopped
- 4 tbsp melted butter
- Salt and black pepper to taste
- ½ cup blue cheese sauce

Directions:
1. Brush the cabbage wedges with butter and coat with mozzarella cheese. Place the coated wedges in the greased basket and fit in the baking tray; cook for 20 minutes at 380 F on Air Fry setting. Serve with blue cheese sauce.

412.Asian-inspired Broccoli

Servings:2
Cooking Time: 10 Minutes

Ingredients:
- 12 ounces (340 g) broccoli florets
- 2 tablespoons Asian hot chili oil
- 1 teaspoon ground Sichuan peppercorns (or black pepper)
- 2 garlic cloves, finely chopped
- 1 (2-inch) piece fresh ginger, peeled and finely chopped
- Kosher salt and freshly ground black pepper

Directions:
1. Toss the broccoli florets with the chili oil, Sichuan peppercorns, garlic, ginger, salt, and pepper in a mixing bowl until thoroughly coated.
2. Transfer the broccoli florets to the air fryer basket.
3. Put the air fryer basket on the baking pan and slide into Rack Position 2, select Air Fry, set temperature to 375ºF (190ºC), and set time to 10 minutes.
4. Stir the broccoli florets halfway through the cooking time.
5. When cooking is complete, the broccoli florets should be lightly browned and tender. Remove the broccoli from the oven and serve on a plate.

413.Yam Spicy Lemon Kebab

Servings:x
Cooking Time:x
Ingredients:
- 2 tsp. garam masala
- 4 tbsp. chopped coriander
- 3 tbsp. cream
- 3 tbsp. chopped capsicum
- 3 eggs
- 2 ½ tbsp. white sesame seeds
- 2 cups sliced yam
- 3 onions chopped
- 5 green chilies-roughly chopped
- 1 ½ tbsp. ginger paste
- 1 ½ tsp. garlic paste
- 1 ½ tsp. salt
- 3 tsp. lemon juice

Directions:
1. Grind the ingredients except for the egg and form a smooth paste. Coat the yam in the paste. Now, beat the eggs and add a little salt to it.
2. Dip the coated vegetables in the egg mixture and then transfer to the sesame seeds and coat the yam well. Place the vegetables on a stick.
3. Pre heat the oven at 160 degrees Fahrenheit for around 5 minutes. Place the sticks in the basket and let them cook for another 25 minutes at the same temperature. Turn the sticks over in

between the cooking process to get a uniform cook.

414.Stuffed Peppers With Beans And Rice

Servings:4
Cooking Time: 18 Minutes
Ingredients:
- 4 medium red, green, or yellow bell peppers, halved and deseeded
- 4 tablespoons extra-virgin olive oil, divided
- ½ teaspoon kosher salt, divided
- 1 (15-ounce / 425-g) can chickpeas
- 1½ cups cooked white rice
- ½ cup diced roasted red peppers
- ¼ cup chopped parsley
- ½ small onion, finely chopped
- 3 garlic cloves, minced
- ½ teaspoon cumin
- ¼ teaspoon freshly ground black pepper
- ¾ cup panko bread crumbs

Directions:
1. Brush the peppers inside and out with 1 tablespoon of olive oil. Season the insides with ¼ teaspoon of kosher salt. Arrange the peppers in the air fryer basket, cut side up.
2. Place the chickpeas with their liquid into a large bowl. Lightly mash the beans with a potato masher. Sprinkle with the remaining ¼ teaspoon of kosher salt and 1 tablespoon of olive oil. Add the rice, red peppers, parsley, onion, garlic, cumin, and black pepper to the bowl and stir to incorporate.
3. Divide the mixture among the bell pepper halves.
4. Stir together the remaining 2 tablespoons of olive oil and panko in a small bowl. Top the pepper halves with the panko mixture.
5. Put the air fryer basket on the baking pan and slide into Rack Position 2, select Roast, set temperature to 375ºF (190ºC), and set time to 18 minutes.
6. When done, the peppers should be slightly wrinkled, and the panko should be golden brown.
7. Remove from the oven and serve on a plate.

415.Balsamic Eggplant Caviar

Servings:4
Cooking Time: 20 Minutes
Ingredients:
- 3 medium eggplants
- ½ red onion, chopped and blended
- 2 tbsp balsamic vinegar
- 1 tbsp olive oil
- Salt to taste

Directions:
1. Arrange the eggplants on the basket and cook them in the oven for 15 minutes at 380 F on Bake function. Let cool. Cut the eggplants in half, lengthwise and empty their insides.
2. Pulse the onion the inside of the eggplants in a blender. Add in vinegar, olive oil, and salt, then blend again. Serve cool with bread and tomato sauce or ketchup.

416.Cheese Stuffed Green Peppers With Tomato Sauce

Servings:4
Cooking Time: 35 Minutes
Ingredients:
- 2 cans green chili peppers
- 1 cup cheddar cheese, shredded
- 1 cup Monterey Jack cheese, shredded
- 2 tbsp all-purpose flour
- 2 large eggs, beaten
- ½ cup milk
- 1 can tomato sauce

Directions:
1. Preheat on AirFry function to 380 F. Spray a baking dish with cooking spray. Take half of the chilies and arrange them in the baking dish. Top with half of the cheese and cover with the remaining chilies. In a medium bowl, combine eggs, milk, and flour and pour over the chilies.
2. Press Start and cook for 20 minutes. Remove the chilies and pour the tomato sauce over them; cook for 15 more minutes. Top with the remaining cheese and serve.

417.Parmesan Breaded Zucchini Chips

Servings: 5
Cooking Time: 20 Minutes
Ingredients:
- For the zucchini chips:
- 2 medium zucchini
- 2 eggs
- ⅓ cup bread crumbs
- ⅓ cup grated Parmesan cheese
- Salt
- Pepper
- Cooking oil
- For the lemon aioli:
- ½ cup mayonnaise
- ½ tablespoon olive oil
- Juice of ½ lemon
- 1 teaspoon minced garlic
- Salt
- Pepper

Directions:
1. Preparing the Ingredients. To make the zucchini chips:
2. Slice the zucchini into thin chips (about ⅛ inch thick) using a knife or mandoline.
3. In a small bowl, beat the eggs. In another small bowl, combine the bread crumbs,

Parmesan cheese, and salt and pepper to taste.

4. Spray the Oven rack/basket with cooking oil.
5. Dip the zucchini slices one at a time in the eggs and then the bread crumb mixture. You can also sprinkle the bread crumbs onto the zucchini slices with a spoon.
6. Place the zucchini chips in the Oven rack/basket, but do not stack. Place the Rack on the middle-shelf of the air fryer oven.
7. Air Frying. Cook in batches. Spray the chips with cooking oil from a distance (otherwise, the breading may fly off). Cook for 10 minutes.
8. Remove the cooked zucchini chips from the air fryer oven, then repeat step 5 with the remaining zucchini.
9. To make the lemon aioli:
10. While the zucchini is cooking, combine the mayonnaise, olive oil, lemon juice, and garlic in a small bowl, adding salt and pepper to taste. Mix well until fully combined.
11. Cool the zucchini and serve alongside the aioli.

- **Nutrition Info:** CALORIES: 192; FAT: 13G; PROTEIN: 6

418.Vegetable Au Gratin

Servings: 3
Cooking Time: 30 Minutes
Ingredients:
- 1 cup cubed eggplant
- ¼ cup chopped red pepper
- ¼ cup chopped green pepper
- ¼ cup chopped onion
- ⅓ cup chopped tomatoes
- 1 clove garlic, minced
- 1 tbsp sliced pimiento-stuffed olives
- 1 tsp capers
- ¼ tsp dried basil
- ¼ tsp dried marjoram
- Salt and black pepper to taste
- ¼ cup grated mozzarella cheese
- 1 tbsp breadcrumbs

Directions:
1. In a bowl, add eggplant, peppers, onion, tomatoes, olives, garlic, basil, marjoram, capers, salt, and black pepper. Lightly grease a baking tray with cooking spray. Add in the vegetable mixture and spread it evenly. Sprinkle mozzarella cheese on top and cover with breadcrumbs. Cook in your for 20 minutes on Bake function at 360 F. Serve.

419.Panko Green Beans

Servings:4
Cooking Time: 15 Minutes
Ingredients:
- ½ cup flour
- 2 eggs
- 1 cup panko bread crumbs
- ½ cup grated Parmesan cheese
- 1 teaspoon cayenne pepper
- Salt and black pepper, to taste
- 1½ pounds (680 g) green beans

Directions:
1. In a bowl, place the flour. In a separate bowl, lightly beat the eggs. In a separate shallow bowl, thoroughly combine the bread crumbs, cheese, cayenne pepper, salt, and pepper.
2. Dip the green beans in the flour, then in the beaten eggs, finally in the bread crumb mixture to coat well. Transfer the green beans to the air fryer basket.
3. Put the air fryer basket on the baking pan and slide into Rack Position 2, select Air Fry, set temperature to 400ºF (205ºC), and set time to 15 minutes.
4. Stir the green beans halfway through the cooking time.
5. When cooking is complete, remove from the oven to a bowl and serve.

420.Mint French Cuisine Galette

Servings:x
Cooking Time:x
Ingredients:
- 1-2 tbsp. fresh coriander leaves
- 2 or 3 green chilies finely chopped
- 1 ½ tbsp. lemon juice
- Salt and pepper to taste
- 2 cups mint leaves (Sliced fine)
- 2 medium potatoes boiled and mashed
- 1 ½ cup coarsely crushed peanuts
- 3 tsp. ginger finely chopped

Directions:
1. Mix the sliced mint leaves with the rest of the ingredients in a clean bowl.
2. Mold this mixture into round and flat French Cuisine Galettes.
3. Wet the French Cuisine Galettes slightly with water. Coat each French Cuisine Galette with the crushed peanuts.
4. Pre heat the oven at 160 degrees Fahrenheit for 5 minutes. Place the French Cuisine Galettes in the fry basket and let them cook for another 25 minutes at the same temperature. Keep rolling them over to get a uniform cook. Serve either with mint sauce or ketchup.

421.Mushroom Pops

Servings:x
Cooking Time:x
Ingredients:
- 1 tsp. dry basil
- 1 tsp. lemon juice
- 1 tsp. red chili flakes
- 1 cup whole mushrooms
- 1 ½ tsp. garlic paste
- Salt and pepper to taste
- 1 tsp. dry oregano

Directions:
1. Add the ingredients into a separate bowl and mix them well to get a consistent mixture.
2. Dip the mushrooms in the above mixture and leave them aside for some time.
3. Pre heat the oven at 180° C for around 5 minutes. Place the coated cottage cheese pieces in the fry basket and close it properly. Let them cook at the same temperature for 20 more minutes. Keep turning them over in the basket so that they are cooked properly. Serve with tomato ketchup.

422.Yam French Cuisine Galette

Servings:x
Cooking Time:x
Ingredients:
- 1 ½ tbsp. lemon juice
- Salt and pepper to taste
- 2 cups minced yam
- 3 tsp. ginger finely chopped
- 1-2 tbsp. fresh coriander leaves
- 2 or 3 green chilies finely chopped

Directions:
1. Mix the ingredients in a clean bowl.
2. Mold this mixture into round and flat French Cuisine Galettes.
3. Wet the French Cuisine Galettes slightly with water.
4. Pre heat the oven at 160 degrees Fahrenheit for 5 minutes. Place the French Cuisine Galettes in the fry basket and let them cook for another 25 minutes at the same temperature. Keep rolling them over to get a uniform cook. Serve either with mint sauce or ketchup.

423.Masala Potato Wedges

Servings:x
Cooking Time:x
Ingredients:
- 1 tsp. mixed herbs
- ½ tsp. red chili flakes
- A pinch of salt to taste
- 1 tbsp. lemon juice
- 2 medium sized potatoes (Cut into wedges)
- ingredients for the marinade:
- 1 tbsp. olive oil
- 1 tsp. garam masala

Directions:
1. Boil the potatoes and blanch them. Mix the ingredients for the marinade and add the potato Oregano Fingers to it making sure that they are coated well.
2. Pre heat the oven for around 5 minutes at 300 Fahrenheit. Take out the basket of the fryer and place the potato Oregano Fingers in them. Close the basket.
3. Now keep the fryer at 200 Fahrenheit for 20 or 25 minutes. In between the process, toss the fries twice or thrice so that they get cooked properly.

424.Okra Spicy Lemon Kebab

Servings:x
Cooking Time:x
Ingredients:
- 3 tsp. lemon juice
- 2 tsp. garam masala
- 4 tbsp. chopped coriander
- 3 tbsp. cream
- 3 tbsp. chopped capsicum
- 3 eggs
- 2 cups sliced okra
- 3 onions chopped
- 5 green chilies-roughly chopped
- 1 ½ tbsp. ginger paste
- 1 ½ tsp. garlic paste
- 1 ½ tsp. salt
- 2 ½ tbsp. white sesame seeds

Directions:
1. Grind the ingredients except for the egg and form a smooth paste. Coat the okra in the paste. Now, beat the eggs and add a little salt to it.
2. Dip the coated vegetables in the egg mixture and then transfer to the sesame seeds and coat the okra well. Place the vegetables on a stick.
3. Pre heat the oven at 160 degrees Fahrenheit for around 5 minutes. Place the sticks in the basket and let them cook for another 25 minutes at the same temperature. Turn the sticks over in between the cooking process to get a uniform cook.

425.Tofu & Pea Cauli Rice

Servings:4
Cooking Time: 30 Minutes
Ingredients:
- Tofu:
- ½ block tofu
- ½ cup onions, chopped
- 2 tbsp soy sauce
- 1 tsp turmeric

- 1 cup carrots, chopped
- Cauliflower:
- 3 cups cauliflower rice
- 2 tbsp soy sauce
- ½ cup broccoli, chopped
- 2 garlic cloves, minced
- 1 ½ tsp toasted sesame oil
- 1 tbsp fresh ginger, minced
- ½ cup frozen peas
- 1 tbsp rice vinegar

Directions:
1. Preheat on AirFry function to 370 F. Crumble the tofu and combine it with all tofu ingredients. Place in a baking dish and cook for 10 minutes.
2. Meanwhile, place all cauliflower ingredients in a large bowl; mix to combine. Add the cauliflower mixture to the tofu and stir to combine. Press Start and cook for 12 minutes. Serve.

426.Teriyaki Tofu

Servings:3
Cooking Time: 15 Minutes
Ingredients:
- Nonstick cooking spray
- 14 oz. firm or extra firm tofu, pressed & cut in 1-inch cubes
- ¼ cup cornstarch
- ½ tsp salt
- ½ tsp ginger
- ½ tsp white pepper
- 3 tbsp. olive oil
- 12 oz. bottle vegan teriyaki sauce

Directions:
1. Lightly spray baking pan with cooking spray.
2. In a shallow dish, combine cornstarch, salt, ginger, and pepper.
3. Heat oil in a large skillet over med-high heat.
4. Toss tofu cubes in cornstarch mixture then add to skillet. Cook 5 minutes, turning over halfway through, until tofu is nicely seared. Transfer the tofu to the prepared baking pan.
5. Set oven to convection bake on 350°F for 15 minutes.
6. Pour all but ½ cup teriyaki sauce over tofu and stir to coat. After oven has preheated for 5 minutes, place the baking pan in position 2 and bake tofu 10 minutes.
7. Turn tofu over, spoon the sauce in the pan over it and bake another 10 minutes. Serve with reserved sauce for dipping.
- **Nutrition Info:** Calories 469, Total Fat 25g, Saturated Fat 4g, Total Carbs 33g, Net Carbs 30g, Protein 28g, Sugar 16g, Fiber 3g, Sodium 2424mg, Potassium 571mg, Phosphorus 428mg

427.Masala Vegetable Skewers

Servings:4
Cooking Time: 20 Minutes
Ingredients:
- 2 tbsp cornflour
- 1 cup canned white beans, drained
- ⅓ cup carrots, grated
- 2 potatoes, boiled and mashed
- ¼ cup fresh mint leaves, chopped
- ½ tsp garam masala powder
- ½ cup paneer
- 1 green chili
- 1-inch piece of fresh ginger
- 3 garlic cloves
- Salt to taste

Directions:
1. Preheat on AirFry function to 390 F. Place the beans, carrots, garlic, ginger, chili, paneer, and mint in a food processor and blend until smooth. Transfer to a bowl.
2. Add in the mashed potatoes, cornflour, salt, and garam masala powder and mix until fully incorporated. Divide the mixture into 12 equal pieces. Thread each of the pieces onto a skewer. Press Start and cook skewers for 10 minutes. Serve.

428.Roasted Brussels Sprouts With Parmesan

Servings:4
Cooking Time: 20 Minutes
Ingredients:
- 1 pound (454 g) fresh Brussels sprouts, trimmed
- 1 tablespoon olive oil
- ½ teaspoon salt
- ⅛ teaspoon pepper
- ¼ cup grated Parmesan cheese

Directions:
1. In a large bowl, combine the Brussels sprouts with olive oil, salt, and pepper and toss until evenly coated.
2. Spread the Brussels sprouts evenly in the air fryer basket.
3. Put the air fryer basket on the baking pan and slide into Rack Position 2, select Air Fry, set temperature to 330ºF (166ºC), and set time to 20 minutes.
4. Stir the Brussels sprouts twice during cooking.
5. When cooking is complete, the Brussels sprouts should be golden brown and crisp. Sprinkle the grated Parmesan cheese on top and serve warm.

429.Cottage Cheese Fingers

Servings:x
Cooking Time:x
Ingredients:

- 2 tsp. salt
- 1 tsp. pepper powder
- 1 tsp. red chili powder
- 6 tbsp. corn flour
- 4 eggs
- 2 cups cottage cheese Oregano Fingers
- 2 cup dry breadcrumbs
- 2 tsp. oregano
- 1 ½ tbsp. ginger-garlic paste
- 4 tbsp. lemon juice

Directions:
1. Mix all the ingredients for the marinade and put the chicken Oregano Fingers inside and let it rest overnight.
2. Mix the breadcrumbs, oregano and red chili flakes well and place the marinated Oregano Fingers on this mixture. Cover it with plastic wrap and leave it till right before you serve to cook.
3. Pre heat the oven at 160 degrees Fahrenheit for 5 minutes. Place the Oregano Fingers in the fry basket and close it. Let them cook at the same temperature for another 15 minutes or so. Toss the Oregano Fingers well so that they are cooked uniformly.

430.Veggie Delight

Servings:2
Cooking Time: 30 Minutes
Ingredients:
- 1 parsnip, sliced in a 2-inch thickness
- 1 cup chopped butternut squash
- 2 small red onions, cut in wedges
- 1 cup celery, chopped
- 1 tbsp fresh thyme, chopped
- Salt and black pepper to taste
- 2 tsp olive oil

Directions:
1. Preheat on AirFry function to 350 F. In a bowl, add turnip, squash, red onions, celery, thyme, pepper, salt, and olive oil and mix well. Add the veggies to the frying basket and press Start. Cook for 16 minutes, tossing once halfway through. Serve warm.

431.Baked Chickpea Stars

Servings:x
Cooking Time:x
Ingredients:
- 4 tbsp. roasted sesame seeds
- 2 small onion finely chopped
- ½ tsp. coriander powder
- ½ tsp. cumin powder
- Use olive oil for greasing purposes
- 1 cup white chick peas soaked overnight
- 1 tsp. ginger-garlic paste
- 4 tbsp. chopped coriander leaves
- 2 green chilies finely chopped

- 4 tbsp. thick curd
- Pinches of salt and pepper to taste
- 1 tsp. dry mint

Directions:
1. Since the chickpeas have been soaked you will first have to drain them. Add a pinch of salt and pour water until the chickpeas are submerged. Put this container in a pressure cooker and let the chickpeas cook for around 25 minutes until they turn soft. Remove the cooker from the flame. Now mash the chickpeas.
2. Take another container. Into it add the ginger garlic paste, onions, coriander leaves, coriander powder, cumin powder, green chili, salt and pepper, and 1 tbsp. Use your hands to mix these ingredients Pour this mixture into the container with the mashed chickpeas and mix. Spread this mixture over a flat surface to about a half-inch thickness.
3. Cut star shapes out of this layer. Make a mixture of curd and mint leaves and spread this over the surface of the star shaped cutlets. Coat all the sides with sesame seeds. Pre heat the oven at 200-degree Fahrenheit for 5 minutes. Open the basket of the Fryer and put the stars inside. Close the basket properly. Continue to cook the stars for around half an hour. Periodically turn over the stars in the basket in order to prevent overcooking one side. Serve either with mint sauce or tomato ketchup.

432.Cheddar & Bean Burritos

Servings:4
Cooking Time: 30 Minutes
Ingredients:
- 4 flour tortillas
- 1 cup grated cheddar cheese
- 1 (8 oz) can black beans, drained
- 1 tsp taco seasoning

Directions:
1. Preheat on Bake function to 350 F. Mix the black beans with the taco seasoning. Divide the bean mixture between the tortillas and top with cheddar cheese. Roll the burritos and arrange them on a lined baking dish. Place in the oven and press Start. Cook for 5 minutes.

433.Beetroot Chips

Servings: 3
Cooking Time: 25 Minutes
Ingredients:
- 1lb golden beetroots, sliced
- 2 tbsp olive oil
- 1 tbsp yeast flakes
- 1 tsp vegan seasoning
- Salt to taste

Directions:

1. In a bowl, add the olive oil, beetroots, vegan seasoning, and yeast and mix well. Dump the coated chips in the basket.
2. Fit in the baking tray and cook in your for 15 minutes at 370 F on Air Fry function, shaking once halfway through. Serve.

434.Barbeque Corn Sandwich

Servings:x
Cooking Time:x

Ingredients:

- ½ flake garlic crushed
- ¼ cup chopped onion
- ¼ tbsp. red chili sauce
- ½ cup water
- 2 slices of white bread
- 1 tbsp. softened butter
- 1 cup sweet corn kernels
- 1 small capsicum
- ¼ tbsp. Worcestershire sauce
- ½ tsp. olive oil

Directions:

1. Take the slices of bread and remove the edges. Now cut the slices horizontally.
2. Cook the ingredients for the sauce and wait till it thickens. Now, add the corn to the sauce and stir till it obtains the flavors. Roast the capsicum and peel the skin off. Cut the capsicum into slices. Apply the sauce on the slices.
3. Pre-heat the oven for 5 minutes at 300 Fahrenheit. Open the basket of the Fryer and place the prepared Classic Sandwiches in it such that no two Classic Sandwiches are touching each other. Now keep the fryer at 250 degrees for around 15 minutes. Turn the Classic Sandwiches in between the cooking process to cook both slices. Serve the Classic Sandwiches with tomato ketchup or mint sauce.

SNACKS AND DESSERTS RECIPES

435.Black And White Brownies

Servings: 8
Cooking Time: 20 Minutes
Ingredients:
- 1 egg
- ¼ cup brown sugar
- 2 tablespoons white sugar
- 2 tablespoons safflower oil
- 1 teaspoon vanilla
- ¼ cup cocoa powder
- ⅓ cup all-purpose flour
- ¼ cup white chocolate chips
- Nonstick baking spray with flour

Directions:
1. Preparing the Ingredients. In a medium bowl, beat the egg with the brown sugar and white sugar. Beat in the oil and vanilla.
2. Add the cocoa powder and flour, and stir just until combined. Fold in the white chocolate chips.
3. Spray a 6-by-6-by-2-inch baking pan with nonstick spray. Spoon the brownie batter into the pan.
4. Air Frying. Bake for 20 minutes or until the brownies are set when lightly touched with a finger. Let cool for 30 minutes before slicing to serve.
- **Nutrition Info:** CALORIES: 81; FAT:4G; PROTEIN:1G; FIBER:1G

436.Sweet Potato Croquettes

Servings: 6
Cooking Time: 55 Minutes
Ingredients:
- 2 cups cooked quinoa
- 1/4 cup parsley, chopped
- 1/4 cup flour
- 2 cups sweet potatoes, mashed
- 2 tsp Italian seasoning
- 1 garlic clove, minced
- 1/4 cup celery, diced
- 1/4 cup scallions, chopped
- Pepper
- Salt

Directions:
1. Fit the oven with the rack in position
2. Add all ingredients into the mixing bowl and mix until well combined.
3. Make 1-inch round croquettes from mixture and place in baking pan.
4. Set to bake at 375 F for 60 minutes. After 5 minutes place the baking pan in the preheated oven.
5. Serve and enjoy.
- **Nutrition Info:** Calories 295 Fat 4.1 g Carbohydrates 55.2 g Sugar 0.6 g Protein 9.5 g Cholesterol 1 mg

437.Peanut Butter-chocolate Bread Pudding

Servings:8
Cooking Time: 10 Minutes
Ingredients:
- 1 egg
- 1 egg yolk
- ¾ cup chocolate milk
- 3 tablespoons brown sugar
- 3 tablespoons peanut butter
- 2 tablespoons cocoa powder
- 1 teaspoon vanilla
- 5 slices firm white bread, cubed
- Nonstick cooking spray

Directions:
1. Spritz the baking pan with nonstick cooking spray.
2. Whisk together the egg, egg yolk, chocolate milk, brown sugar, peanut butter, cocoa powder, and vanilla until well combined.
3. Fold in the bread cubes and stir to mix well. Allow the bread soak for 10 minutes.
4. When ready, transfer the egg mixture to the prepared baking pan.
5. Slide the baking pan into Rack Position 1, select Convection Bake, set temperature to 330ºF (166ºC), and set time to 10 minutes.
6. When done, the pudding should be just firm to the touch.
7. Serve at room temperature.

438.Garlic Edamame

Servings:4
Cooking Time: 9 Minutes
Ingredients:
- 1 (16-ounce / 454-g) bag frozen edamame in pods
- 2 tablespoon olive oil, divided
- ½ teaspoon garlic salt
- ½ teaspoon salt
- ¼ teaspoon freshly ground black pepper
- ½ teaspoon red pepper flakes (optional)

Directions:
1. Place the edamame in a medium bowl and drizzle with 1 tablespoon of olive oil. Toss to coat well.
2. Stir together the garlic salt, salt, pepper, and red pepper flakes (if desired) in a small bowl. Pour the mixture into the bowl of edamame and toss until the edamame is fully coated.
3. Grease the air fryer basket with the remaining 1 tablespoon of olive oil.
4. Place the edamame in the greased basket.
5. Put the air fryer basket on the baking pan and slide into Rack Position 2, select Air Fry,

set temperature to 375ºF (190ºC), and set time to 9 minutes.

6. Stir the edamame once halfway through the cooking time.
7. When cooking is complete, the edamame should be crisp. Remove from the oven to a plate and serve warm.

439.Cheese Artichoke Spinach Dip

Servings: 10
Cooking Time: 17 Minutes
Ingredients:
- 1/2 cup mozzarella cheese, shredded
- 3 cups spinach, chopped
- 2 garlic cloves, minced
- 1/3 cup sour cream
- 1/3 can artichoke hearts, drained and chopped
- 1/2 cup mayonnaise
- 7 oz brie cheese
- 1/3 tsp dried basil
- 1/3 tsp pepper
- 1 tsp sea salt

Directions:
1. Fit the oven with the rack in position 2.
2. Add all ingredients except mozzarella cheese into the air fryer baking dish and mix until well combined.
3. Spread mozzarella cheese on top.
4. Set to bake at 325 F for 22 minutes. After 5 minutes place the baking dish in the preheated oven.
5. Serve and enjoy.
- **Nutrition Info:** Calories 138 Fat 11.3 g Carbohydrates 4.3 g Sugar 0.9 g Protein 5.3 g Cholesterol 27 mg

440.Chocolate Ramekins

Servings: 4
Cooking Time: 12 Minutes
Ingredients:
- ½ cup butter
- 2/3 cup dark chocolate, chopped
- ¼ cup caster sugar
- 2 medium eggs
- 2 teaspoons fresh orange rind, finely grated
- ¼ cup fresh orange juice
- 2 tablespoons self-rising flour

Directions:
1. In a microwave-safe bowl, add the butter, and chocolate and microwave on high heat for about 2 minutes or until melted completely, stirring after every 30 seconds.
2. Remove from microwave and stir the mixture until smooth.
3. Add the sugar, and eggs and whisk until frothy.
4. Add the orange rind and juice, followed by flour and mix until well combined.

5. Divide mixture into 4 greased ramekins about ¾ full.
6. Press "Power Button" of Air Fry Oven and turn the dial to select the "Air Fry" mode.
7. Press the Time button and again turn the dial to set the cooking time to 12 minutes.
8. Now push the Temp button and rotate the dial to set the temperature at 355 degrees F.
9. Press "Start/Pause" button to start.
10. When the unit beeps to show that it is preheated, open the lid.
11. Arrange the ramekins in "Air Fry Basket" and insert in the oven.
12. Place the ramekins set aside to cool completely before serving.
- **Nutrition Info:** Calories 454 Total Fat 33.6 g Saturated Fat 21.1 g Cholesterol 149 mg Sodium 217 mg Total Carbs 34.2 g Fiber 1.2 g Sugar 28.4g Protein 5.7 g

441.Keto Mixed Berry Crumble Pots

Servings: 6
Cooking Time: 15 Minutes
Ingredients:
- 2 ounces unsweetened mixed berries
- 1/2 cup granulated swerve
- 2 tablespoons golden flaxseed meal
- 1/4 teaspoon ground star anise
- 1/2 teaspoon ground cinnamon
- 1 teaspoon xanthan gum
- 2/3 cup almond flour
- 1 cup powdered swerve
- 1/2 teaspoon baking powder
- 1/3 cup unsweetened coconut, finely shredded
- 1/2 stick butter, cut into small pieces

Directions:
1. Toss the mixed berries with the granulated swerve, golden flaxseed meal, star anise, cinnamon, and xanthan gum. Divide between six custard cups coated with cooking spray.
2. In a mixing dish, thoroughly combine the remaining ingredients. Sprinkle over the berry mixture.
3. Bake in the preheated Air Fryer at 330 degrees F for 35 minutes. Work in batches if needed.
- **Nutrition Info:** 155 Calories; 13g Fat; 1g Carbs; 1g Protein; 8g Sugars; 6g Fiber

442.Olive Tarts With Mushrooms

Servings:x
Cooking Time:x
Ingredients:
- ½ cup sliced black olives
- ½ cup sliced green olives
- ½ teaspoon dried thyme leaves
- 2 sheets frozen puff pastry, thawed

- 1 cup shredded Gouda cheese
- 1 onion, chopped
- 2 cloves garlic, minced
- ½ cup chopped mushrooms
- 1 tablespoon olive oil

Directions:
1. Preheat oven to 400ºF. In heavy skillet, sauté onion, garlic, and mushrooms in olive oil until tender. Remove from heat and add olives and thyme.
2. Gently roll puff pastry dough with rolling pin until ¼-inch thick. Using a 3-inch cookie cutter, cut 24 circles from pastry. Line muffin cups with dough.
3. Place a spoonful of filling in each pastry-lined cup. Bake at 400ºF for 10 to 12 minutes or until crust is golden brown and filling is set.
4. Remove from muffin cups and cool on wire rack. Flash freeze; when frozen solid, pack tarts into zipper-lock bags. Attach zipper-lock bag filled with shredded cheese; label and freeze.
5. To thaw and reheat: Thaw tarts in single layer overnight in refrigerator. Top each tart with cheese and bake at 400ºF for 5 to 6 minutes or until hot and cheese is melted.

443.Cheesy Roasted Jalapeño Poppers

Servings:8
Cooking Time: 15 Minutes
Ingredients:
- 6 ounces (170 g) cream cheese, at room temperature
- 4 ounces (113 g) shredded Cheddar cheese
- 1 teaspoon chili powder
- 12 large jalapeño peppers, deseeded and sliced in half lengthwise
- 2 slices cooked bacon, chopped
- ¼ cup panko bread crumbs
- 1 tablespoon butter, melted

Directions:
1. In a medium bowl, whisk together the cream cheese, Cheddar cheese and chili powder. Spoon the cheese mixture into the jalapeño halves and arrange them in the baking pan.
2. In a small bowl, stir together the bacon, bread crumbs and butter. Sprinkle the mixture over the jalapeño halves.
3. Slide the baking pan into Rack Position 2, select Roast, set temperature to 375ºF (190ºC) and set time to 15 minutes.
4. When cooking is complete, remove from the oven. Let the poppers cool for 5 minutes before serving.

444.Easy Bacon Bites

Servings: 4

Cooking Time: 10 Minutes
Ingredients:
- 4 bacon strips, cut into small pieces
- 1/4 cup hot sauce
- 1/2 cup pork rinds, crushed

Directions:
1. Fit the oven with the rack in position 2.
2. Add bacon pieces in a bowl.
3. Add hot sauce and toss well.
4. Add crushed pork rinds and toss until bacon pieces are well coated.
5. Transfer bacon pieces in the air fryer basket then place an air fryer basket in the baking pan.
6. Place a baking pan on the oven rack. Set to air fry at 350 F for 10 minutes.
7. Serve and enjoy.
- **Nutrition Info:** Calories 123 Fat 10.4 g Carbohydrates 0.3 g Sugar 0.2 g Protein 6.5 g Cholesterol 5 mg

445.Carrot, Raisin & Walnut Bread

Servings: 8
Cooking Time: 35 Minutes
Ingredients:
- 2 cups all-purpose flour
- 1½ teaspoons ground cinnamon
- 2 teaspoons baking soda
- ½ teaspoon salt
- 3 eggs
- ½ cup sunflower oil
- ½ cup applesauce
- ¼ cup honey
- ¼ cup plain yogurt
- 2 teaspoons vanilla essence
- 2½ cups carrots, peeled and shredded
- ½ cup raisins
- ½ cup walnuts

Directions:
1. Line the bottom of a greased baking pan with parchment paper.
2. In a medium bowl, sift together the flour, baking soda, cinnamon and salt.
3. In a large bowl, add the eggs, oil, applesauce, honey and yogurt and with a hand-held mixer, mix on medium speed until well combined.
4. Add the eggs, one at a time and whisk well.
5. Add the vanilla and mix well.
6. Add the flour mixture and mix until just combined.
7. Fold in the carrots, raisins and walnuts.
8. Place the mixture into a lightly greased baking pan.
9. With a piece of foil, cover the pan loosely.
10. Press "Power Button" of Air Fry Oven and turn the dial to select the "Air Crisp" mode.
11. Press the Time button and again turn the dial to set the cooking time to 30 minutes.

12. Now push the Temp button and rotate the dial to set the temperature at 347 degrees F.
13. Press "Start/Pause" button to start.
14. When the unit beeps to show that it is preheated, open the lid.
15. Arrange the pan in "Air Fry Basket" and insert in the oven.
16. After 25 minutes of cooking, remove the foil.
17. Place the pan onto a wire rack to cool for about 10 minutes.
18. Carefully, invert the bread onto wire rack to cool completely before slicing.
19. Cut the bread into desired-sized slices and serve.
- **Nutrition Info:** Calories 441 Total Fat 20.3 g Saturated Fat 2.2 g Cholesterol 62mg Sodium 592 mg Total Carbs 57.6 g Fiber 5.7 g Sugar 23.7 g Protein 9.2 g

446.Air Fried Lemon-pepper Wings

Servings:10
Cooking Time: 24 Minutes
Ingredients:
- 2 pounds (907 g) chicken wings
- 4½ teaspoons salt-free lemon pepper seasoning
- 1½ teaspoons baking powder
- 1½ teaspoons kosher salt

Directions:
1. In a large bowl, toss together all the ingredients until well coated. Place the wings in the air fryer basket, making sure they don't crowd each other too much.
2. Put the air fryer basket on the baking pan and slide into Rack Position 2, select Air Fry, set temperature to 375ºF (190ºC) and set time to 24 minutes.
3. After 12 minutes, remove from the oven. Use tongs to turn the wings over. Return to the oven to continue cooking.
4. When cooking is complete, the wings should be dark golden brown and a bit charred in places. Remove from the oven and let rest for 5 minutes before serving.

447.Apple-toffee Upside-down Cake

Servings: 9
Cooking Time: 30 Minutes
Ingredients:
- Almond butter, ¼ cup
- Sunflower oil, ¼ cup
- Chopped walnuts, ½ cup
- Coconut sugar, 1 cup
- Water, ¾ cup
- Mixed spice, 1 ½ tsps.
- Plain flour, 1 cup
- Zest from 1 lemon
- Baking soda, 1 tsp.
- Vinegar, 1 tsp.
- Cored and sliced, 3

Directions:
1. Preheat the air fryer to 3900 F.
2. In a skillet, melt the almond butter and 3 tablespoons sugar. Pour mixture over a baking dish that will fit in the air fryer. Arrange the slices of apples on top. Set aside.
3. In a mixing bowl, combine flour, ¾ cup sugar, and baking soda. Add the mixed spice.
4. In another bowl, mix the oil, water, vinegar, and lemon zest. Stir in the chopped walnuts.
5. Combine the wet ingredients to dry ingredients until well combined.
6. Pour over the tin with apple slices.
7. Leave to cook for 30 minutes.
- **Nutrition Info:** Calories: 335 Carbs: 39.6g Protein: 3.8g Fat: 17.9g

448.Handmade Donuts

Servings:4
Cooking Time: 25 Minutes
Ingredients:
- 8 oz self-rising flour
- 1 tsp baking powder
- ½ cup milk
- 2 ½ tbsp butter
- 1 egg
- 2 oz brown sugar

Directions:
1. Preheat on Bake function to 350 F. In a bowl, beat the butter with sugar until smooth. Whisk in egg and milk. In another bowl, combine the flour with the baking powder.
2. Fold the flour into the butter mixture. Form donut shapes and cut off the center with cookie cutters. Arrange on a lined baking sheet and cook for 15 minutes. Serve with whipped cream.

449.Delicious Raspberry Cobbler

Servings: 6
Cooking Time: 10 Minutes
Ingredients:
- 1 egg, lightly beaten
- 1 cup raspberries, sliced
- 2 tsp swerve
- 1/2 tsp vanilla
- 1 tbsp butter, melted
- 1 cup almond flour

Directions:
1. Fit the oven with the rack in position
2. Add raspberries into the baking dish.
3. Sprinkle sweetener over raspberries.
4. Mix together almond flour, vanilla, and butter in the bowl.
5. Add egg in almond flour mixture and stir well to combine.

6. Spread almond flour mixture over sliced raspberries.
7. Set to bake at 350 F for 15 minutes. After 5 minutes place the baking dish in the preheated oven.
8. Serve and enjoy.
- **Nutrition Info:** Calories 66 Fat 5 g Carbohydrates 3 g Sugar 1 g Protein 2 g Cholesterol 32 mg

450.Cinnamon Fried Bananas

Servings: 2-3
Cooking Time: 10 Minutes
Ingredients:
- 1 C. panko breadcrumbs
- 3 tbsp. cinnamon
- ½ C. almond flour
- 3 egg whites
- 8 ripe bananas
- 3 tbsp. vegan coconut oil

Directions:
1. Preparing the Ingredients. Heat coconut oil and add breadcrumbs. Mix around 2-3 minutes until golden. Pour into bowl.
2. Peel and cut bananas in half. Roll each bananas half into flour, eggs, and crumb mixture.
3. Air Frying. Place into the air fryer oven. Cook 10 minutes at 280 degrees.
4. A great addition to a healthy banana split!
- **Nutrition Info:** CALORIES: 219; FAT:10G; PROTEIN:3G; SUGAR:5G

451.Pumpkin Bread

Servings: 10
Cooking Time: 40 Minutes
Ingredients:
- 1 1/3 cups all-purpose flour
- 1 cup sugar
- ¾ teaspoon baking soda
- 1 teaspoon pumpkin pie spice
- 1/3 teaspoon ground cinnamon
- ¼ teaspoon salt
- 2 eggs
- ½ cup pumpkin puree
- 1/3 cup vegetable oil
- ¼ cup water

Directions:
1. In a bowl, mix together the flour, sugar, baking soda, spices and salt
2. In another large bowl, add the eggs, pumpkin, oil and water and beat until well combined.
3. In a large mixing bowl or stand mixer.
4. Add the flour mixture and mix until just combined.
5. Place the mixture into a lightly greased loaf pan.
6. With a piece of foil, cover the pan loosely.

7. Press "Power Button" of Air Fry Oven and turn the dial to select the "Air Bake" mode.
8. Press the Time button and again turn the dial to set the cooking time to 40 minutes.
9. Now push the Temp button and rotate the dial to set the temperature at 325 degrees F.
10. Press "Start/Pause" button to start.
11. When the unit beeps to show that it is preheated, open the lid.
12. Arrange the pan in "Air Fry Basket" and insert in the oven.
13. After 25 minutes of cooking, remove the foil.
14. Place the pan onto a wire rack to cool for about 10 minutes.
15. Carefully, invert the bread onto wire rack to cool completely before slicing.
16. Cut the bread into desired-sized slices and serve.
- **Nutrition Info:** Calories 217 Total Fat 8.4 g Saturated Fat 1.4 g Cholesterol 33 mg Sodium 167 mg Total Carbs 34 g Fiber 0.9 g Sugar 20.5g Protein 3 g

452.Air Fryer Walnuts

Servings: 6
Cooking Time: 5 Minutes
Ingredients:
- 2 cups walnuts
- 1 tsp olive oil
- Pepper
- Salt

Directions:
1. Fit the oven with the rack in position 2.
2. Add walnuts, oil, pepper, and salt into the bowl and toss well.
3. Add walnuts to the air fryer basket then place an air fryer basket in baking pan.
4. Place a baking pan on the oven rack. Set to air fry at 350 F for 5 minutes.
5. Serve and enjoy.
- **Nutrition Info:** Calories 264 Fat 25.4 g Carbohydrates 4.1 g Sugar 0.5 g Protein 10 g Cholesterol 0 mg

453.Easy Air Fryer Tofu

Servings: 4
Cooking Time: 15 Minutes
Ingredients:
- 16 oz extra firm tofu, cut into bite-sized pieces
- 1 tbsp olive oil
- 1 garlic clove, minced

Directions:
1. Fit the oven with the rack in position 2.
2. Add tofu, garlic, and oil in a mixing bowl and toss well. Let it sit for 15 minutes.
3. Arrange tofu in the air fryer basket then place an air fryer basket in the baking pan.
4. Place a baking pan on the oven rack. Set to air fry at 370 F for 15 minutes.

5. Serve and enjoy.
- **Nutrition Info:** Calories 111 Fat 8.2 g Carbohydrates 2.2 g Sugar 0.7 g Protein 9.3 g Cholesterol 0 mg

454.Tangy Fried Pickle Spears

Servings:6
Cooking Time: 15 Minutes
Ingredients:
- 2 jars sweet and sour pickle spears, patted dry
- 2 medium-sized eggs
- $^1/_3$ cup milk
- 1 teaspoon garlic powder
- 1 teaspoon sea salt
- ½ teaspoon shallot powder
- $^1/_3$ teaspoon chili powder
- $^1/_3$ cup all-purpose flour
- Cooking spray

Directions:
1. Spritz the air fryer basket with cooking spray.
2. In a bowl, beat together the eggs with milk. In another bowl, combine garlic powder, sea salt, shallot powder, chili powder and all-purpose flour until well blended.
3. One by one, roll the pickle spears in the powder mixture, then dredge them in the egg mixture. Dip them in the powder mixture a second time for additional coating.
4. Place the coated pickles in the basket.
5. Put the air fryer basket on the baking pan and slide into Rack Position 2, select Air Fry, set temperature to 385ºF (196ºC), and set time to 15 minutes.
6. Stir the pickles halfway through the cooking time.
7. When cooking is complete, they should be golden and crispy. Transfer to a plate and let cool for 5 minutes before serving.

455.Mushroom Platter

Servings: 4
Cooking Time: 15 Minutes
Ingredients:
- 12 oz. Portobello mushrooms; sliced
- 2 tbsp. olive oil
- 2 tbsp. balsamic vinegar
- ½ tsp. rosemary; dried
- ½ tsp. thyme; dried
- ½ tsp. basil; dried
- ½ tsp. tarragon; dried
- A pinch of salt and black pepper

Directions:
1. Take a bowl and mix all the ingredients and toss well.
2. Arrange the mushroom slices in your air fryer's basket and cook at 380°F for 12 minutes. Arrange the mushroom slices on a platter and serve
- **Nutrition Info:** Calories: 147; Fat: 8g; Fiber: 2g; Carbs: 3g; Protein: 3g

456.Crispy Pineapple Rings

Servings:6
Cooking Time: 7 Minutes
Ingredients:
- 1 cup rice milk
- $^2/_3$ cup flour
- ½ cup water
- ¼ cup unsweetened flaked coconut
- 4 tablespoons sugar
- ½ teaspoon baking soda
- ½ teaspoon baking powder
- ½ teaspoon vanilla essence
- ½ teaspoon ground cinnamon
- ¼ teaspoon ground anise star
- Pinch of kosher salt
- 1 medium pineapple, peeled and sliced

Directions:
1. In a large bowl, stir together all the ingredients except the pineapple.
2. Dip each pineapple slice into the batter until evenly coated.
3. Arrange the pineapple slices in the air fryer basket.
4. Put the air fryer basket on the baking pan and slide into Rack Position 2, select Air Fry, set temperature to 380ºF (193ºC), and set time to 7 minutes.
5. When cooking is complete, the pineapple rings should be golden brown.
6. Remove from the oven to a plate and cool for 5 minutes before serving.

457.Ruderal Swiss Fondue

Servings:x
Cooking Time:x
Ingredients:
- 1 cup dry white wine
- 1 Tbsp Kirshwasser
- 2 cups grated Emmen haler cheese
- 2 cups grated Gruyere cheese
- 2 Tbsp cornstarch
- Sliced apples and cubed bread, for serving

Directions:
1. In a bowl, mix the two cheeses and the cornstarch with a wooden spoon.
2. Pour the wine and kirshwasser into a 2-quart oven and bring to a gentle simmer over medium-low heat.
3. Add the cheese mixture to the liquid, a handful at a time, and stir until all the cheese is melted.
4. Serve fondue in a bowl over the fire. With a fondue fork, stab a slice of apple or a cube of bread and dip into the melted cheese.

458.Oats Muffins

Servings:x
Cooking Time:x
Ingredients:
- 1 cup sugar
- 3 tsp. vinegar
- 1 cup oats
- ½ tsp. vanilla essence
- Muffin cups or butter paper cups.
- 2 cups All-purpose flour
- 1 ½ cup milk
- ½ tsp. baking powder
- ½ tsp. baking soda
- 2 tbsp. butter

Directions:
1. Mix the ingredients together and use your Oregano Fingers to get a crumbly mixture. You will need to divide the milk into two parts and add one part to the baking soda and the other to the vinegar. Now, mix both the milk mixtures together and wait till the milk begins to foam. Add this to the crumbly mixture and begin to whisk the ingredients very fast. Once you have obtained a smooth batter, you will need to transfer the mixture into a muffin cup and set aside.
2. Preheat the fryer to 300 Fahrenheit for five minutes. You will need to place the muffin cups in the basket and cover it. Cook the muffins for fifteen minutes and check whether or not the muffins are cooked using a toothpick. Remove the cups and serve hot.

459.Tomato Bites

Servings: 6
Cooking Time: 15 Minutes
Ingredients:
- 6 tomatoes; halved
- 2 oz. watercress
- 3 oz. cheddar cheese; grated
- 1 tbsp. olive oil
- 3 tsp. sugar-free apricot jam
- 2 tsp. oregano; dried
- A pinch of salt and black pepper

Directions:
1. Spread the jam on each tomato half, sprinkle oregano, salt and pepper and drizzle the oil all over them
2. Introduce them in the fryer's basket, sprinkle the cheese on top and cook at 360°F for 20 minutes
3. Arrange the tomatoes on a platter, top each half with some watercress and serve as an appetizer.
- **Nutrition Info:** Calories: 131; Fat: 7g; Fiber: 2g; Carbs: 4g; Protein: 7g

460.Chocolate Tarts

Servings:x
Cooking Time:x
Ingredients:
- 1 tbsp. sliced cashew
- For Truffle filling:
- 1 ½ melted chocolate
- 1 cup fresh cream
- 3 tbsp. butter
- 1 ½ cup plain flour
- ½ cup cocoa powder
- 3 tbsp. unsalted butter
- 2 tbsp. powdered sugar
- 2 cups cold water

Directions:
1. In a large bowl, mix the flour, cocoa powder, butter and sugar with your Oregano Fingers. The mixture should resemble breadcrumbs. Squeeze the dough using the cold milk and wrap it and leave it to cool for ten minutes. Roll the dough out into the pie and prick the sides of the pie.
2. Mix the ingredients for the filling in a bowl. Make sure that it is a little thick. Add the filling to the pie and cover it with the second round.
3. Preheat the fryer to 300 Fahrenheit for five minutes. You will need to place the tin in the basket and cover it. When the pastry has turned golden brown, you will need to remove the tin and let it cool. Cut into slices and serve with a dollop of cream.

461.Parmesan Zucchini Fries

Servings: 4
Cooking Time: 10 Minutes
Ingredients:
- 2 medium zucchini, cut into fries shape
- 1/2 cup breadcrumbs
- 1 egg, lightly beaten
- 1/2 tsp garlic powder
- 1 tsp Italian seasoning
- 1/2 cup parmesan cheese, grated
- Pepper
- Salt

Directions:
1. Fit the oven with the rack in position 2.
2. Add egg in a bowl and whisk well.
3. In a shallow bowl, mix together breadcrumbs, spices, parmesan cheese, pepper, and salt.
4. Dip zucchini in egg then coat with breadcrumb mixture and place in air fryer basket then place air fryer basket in baking pan.
5. Place a baking pan on the oven rack. Set to air fry at 400 F for 10 minutes.
6. Serve and enjoy.

- **Nutrition Info:** Calories 126 Fat 4.8 g Carbohydrates 13.9 g Sugar 2.8 g Protein 8.1 g Cholesterol 50 mg

462.Coconut Cookies With Pecans

Servings:10
Cooking Time: 25 Minutes
Ingredients:
- 1½ cups coconut flour
- 1½ cups extra-fine almond flour
- ½ teaspoon baking powder
- $^1/_3$ teaspoon baking soda
- 3 eggs plus an egg yolk, beaten
- ¾ cup coconut oil, at room temperature
- 1 cup unsalted pecan nuts, roughly chopped
- ¾ cup monk fruit
- ¼ teaspoon freshly grated nutmeg
- $^1/_3$ teaspoon ground cloves
- ½ teaspoon pure vanilla extract
- ½ teaspoon pure coconut extract
- ⅛ teaspoon fine sea salt

Directions:
1. Line the baking pan with parchment paper.
2. Mix the coconut flour, almond flour, baking powder, and baking soda in a large mixing bowl.
3. In another mixing bowl, stir together the eggs and coconut oil. Add the wet mixture to the dry mixture.
4. Mix in the remaining ingredients and stir until a soft dough forms.
5. Drop about 2 tablespoons of dough on the parchment paper for each cookie and flatten each biscuit until it's 1 inch thick.
6. Slide the baking pan into Rack Position 1, select Convection Bake, set temperature to 370ºF (188ºC), and set time to 25 minutes.
7. When cooking is complete, the cookies should be golden and firm to the touch.
8. Remove from the oven to a plate. Let the cookies cool to room temperature and serve.

463.Moist Chocolate Brownies

Servings: 16
Cooking Time: 20 Minutes
Ingredients:
- 1 1/3 cups all-purpose flour
- 1/2 tsp baking powder
- 1/3 cup cocoa powder
- 1 cup of sugar
- 1/2 tsp vanilla
- 1/2 cup vegetable oil
- 1/2 cup water
- 1/2 tsp salt

Directions:
1. Fit the oven with the rack in position
2. In a large mixing bowl, mix together flour, baking powder, cocoa powder, sugar, and salt.

3. In a small bowl, whisk together oil, water, and vanilla.
4. Pour oil mixture into the flour mixture and mix until well combined.
5. Pour batter into the greased baking dish.
6. Set to bake at 350 F for 25 minutes. After 5 minutes place the baking dish in the preheated oven.
7. Slice and serve.
- **Nutrition Info:** Calories 150 Fat 7.1 g Carbohydrates 21.5 g Sugar 12.6 g Protein 1.4 g Cholesterol 0 mg

464.Cheesy Zucchini Tots

Servings:8
Cooking Time: 6 Minutes
Ingredients:
- 2 medium zucchini (about 12 ounces / 340 g), shredded
- 1 large egg, whisked
- ½ cup grated pecorino romano cheese
- ½ cup panko bread crumbs
- ¼ teaspoon black pepper
- 1 clove garlic, minced
- Cooking spray

Directions:
1. Using your hands, squeeze out as much liquid from the zucchini as possible. In a large bowl, mix the zucchini with the remaining ingredients except the oil until well incorporated.
2. Make the zucchini tots: Use a spoon or cookie scoop to place tablespoonfuls of the zucchini mixture onto a lightly floured cutting board and form into 1-inch logs.
3. Spritz the air fryer basket with cooking spray. Place the zucchini tots in the pan.
4. Put the air fryer basket on the baking pan and slide into Rack Position 2, select Air Fry, set temperature to 375ºF (190ºC), and set time to 6 minutes.
5. When cooking is complete, the tots should be golden brown. Remove from the oven to a serving plate and serve warm.

465.Mini Crab Cakes

Servings:x
Cooking Time:x
Ingredients:
- ½ cup dried bread crumbs
- ½ cup mayonnaise
- ¼ cup minced green onions
- 3 tablespoons olive oil
- 1-pound canned lump crabmeat
- 1 cup fresh cilantro leaves
- ½ cup chopped walnuts
- ½ cup grated Romano cheese
- 2 tablespoons olive oil

Directions:

1. Drain crabmeat well and pick over to remove any cartilage. Set aside in large bowl. In food processor or blender, combine cilantro, walnuts, cheese, and 2 tablespoons olive oil (6 tablespoons for triple batch). Process or blend until mixture forms a paste. Stir into crabmeat.
2. Add bread crumbs, mayonnaise, and green onions to crab mixture. Stir to combine. Form into 2- inch patties about ½-inch thick. Flash freeze on baking sheet. When frozen solid, pack crab cakes in rigid containers, with waxed paper between the layers. Label crab cakes and freeze. Reserve remaining olive oil in pantry.
3. To thaw and reheat: Thaw crab cakes in refrigerator overnight. Heat 3 tablespoons olive oil (9 for triple batch) in large, heavy skillet over medium heat. Fry crab cakes until golden and hot, turning once, about 3 to 5 minutes on each side.

466.Cinnamon Cheesecake Bars

Servings: 12
Cooking Time: 30 Minutes
Ingredients:
- Nonstick cooking spray
- 16 oz. cream cheese, soft
- 1 tsp vanilla
- 1 ¼ cups sugar, divided
- 2 tubes refrigerated crescent rolls
- 1 tsp cinnamon
- ¼ cup butter

Directions:
1. Place the rack in position Spray the bottom of an 8x11-inch pan with cooking spray.
2. In a medium bowl, beat cream cheese, vanilla, and ¾ cup sugar until smooth.
3. Roll out one can of crescent rolls on the bottom of prepared pan, sealing the perforations and pressing partway up the sides.
4. Spread cream cheese mixture evenly over crescents.
5. Roll out second can of crescents over the top of cheese mixture, sealing the perforations.
6. In a small bowl, stir together cinnamon and remaining sugar. Melt the butter.
7. Set oven to bake on 375°F for 35 minutes.
8. Sprinkle the cinnamon sugar over the top of the crescents and drizzle with melted butter.
9. After the oven has preheated for 5 minutes, place the pan in the oven and bake 30 minutes until the top is golden brown.
10. Cool completely. Cover and refrigerate at least 2 hours before slicing and serving.
- **Nutrition Info:** Calories 332, Total Fat 18g, Saturated Fat 10g, Total Carbs 35g, Net Carbs 35g, Protein 5g, Sugar 23g, Fiber 0g,

Sodium 278mg, Potassium 87mg, Phosphorus 70mg

467.Apple Pastries

Servings: 6
Cooking Time: 10 Minutes
Ingredients:
- ½ of large apple, peeled, cored and chopped
- 1 teaspoon fresh orange zest, grated finely
- ½ tablespoon white sugar
- ½ teaspoon ground cinnamon
- 7.05 oz. prepared frozen puff pastry

Directions:
1. In a bowl, mix together all ingredients except puff pastry.
2. Cut the pastry in 16 squares.
3. Place about a teaspoon of the apple mixture in the center of each square.
4. Fold each square into a triangle and press the edges slightly with wet fingers.
5. Then with a fork, press the edges firmly.
6. Press "Power Button" of Air Fry Oven and turn the dial to select the "Air Fry" mode.
7. Press the Time button and again turn the dial to set the cooking time to 10 minutes.
8. Now push the Temp button and rotate the dial to set the temperature at 390 degrees F.
9. Press "Start/Pause" button to start.
10. When the unit beeps to show that it is preheated, open the lid.
11. Arrange the pastries in greased "Air Fry Basket" and insert in the oven.
12. Serve warm.
- **Nutrition Info:** Calories 198 Total Fat 12.7 g Saturated Fat 3.2 g Cholesterol 0 mg Sodium 83 mg Total Carbs 18.8 g Fiber 1.1 g Sugar 3.2 g Protein 2.5 g

468.Choco Lava Cakes

Servings:4
Cooking Time: 20 Minutes
Ingredients:
- 3 ½ oz butter, melted
- 3 ½ tbsp sugar
- 1 ½ tbsp self-rising flour
- 3 ½ oz dark chocolate, melted
- 2 eggs

Directions:
1. Preheat on Bake function to 375 F. Beat eggs and sugar until frothy. Stir in butter and chocolate; gently fold in the flour.
2. Divide the mixture between 4 buttered ramekins and press Start. Bake in the fryer for 10 minutes. Let cool for 2 minutes before turning the cakes upside down onto serving plates.

469.Delicious Cauliflower Hummus

Servings: 8

Cooking Time: 35 Minutes

Ingredients:

- 1 cauliflower head, cut into florets
- 3 tbsp olive oil
- 1/2 tsp ground cumin
- 2 tbsp fresh lemon juice
- 1/3 cup tahini
- 1 tsp garlic, chopped
- Pepper
- Salt

Directions:

1. Fit the oven with the rack in position
2. Spread cauliflower florets in baking pan.
3. Set to bake at 400 F for 40 minutes. After 5 minutes place the baking dish in the preheated oven.
4. Transfer roasted cauliflower into the food processor along with remaining ingredients and process until smooth.
5. Serve and enjoy.
- **Nutrition Info:** Calories 115 Fat 10.7 g Carbohydrates 4.2 g Sugar 0.9 g Protein 2.4 g Cholesterol 0 mg

470.Ultimate Coconut Chocolate Cake

Servings:10
Cooking Time: 15 Minutes

Ingredients:

- 1¼ cups unsweetened bakers' chocolate
- 1 stick butter
- 1 teaspoon liquid stevia
- $^1/_3$ cup shredded coconut
- 2 tablespoons coconut milk
- 2 eggs, beaten
- Cooking spray

Directions:

1. Lightly spritz the baking pan with cooking spray.
2. Place the chocolate, butter, and stevia in a microwave-safe bowl. Microwave for about 30 seconds until melted. Let the chocolate mixture cool to room temperature.
3. Add the remaining ingredients to the chocolate mixture and stir until well incorporated. Pour the batter into the prepared baking pan.
4. Slide the baking pan into Rack Position 1, select Convection Bake, set temperature to 330ºF (166ºC), and set time to 15 minutes.
5. When cooking is complete, a toothpick inserted in the center should come out clean.
6. Remove from the oven and allow to cool for about 10 minutes before serving.

471.Cinnamon Apple Crisp

Servings: 4
Cooking Time: 35 Minutes

Ingredients:

- 1/8 tsp ground clove
- 1/8 tsp ground nutmeg
- 2 tbsp honey
- 4 1/2 cups apples, diced
- 1 tsp ground cinnamon
- 1 tbsp cornstarch
- 1 tsp vanilla
- 1/2 lemon juice
- For topping:
- 1 cup rolled oats
- 1/3 cup coconut oil, melted
- 1 tsp cinnamon
- 1/3 cup honey
- 1/2 cup almond flour

Directions:

1. Fit the oven with the rack in position
2. In a medium bowl, mix apples, vanilla, lemon juice, and honey. Sprinkle spices and cornstarch on top and stir well.
3. Pour apple mixture into the greased baking dish.
4. In a small bowl, mix together coconut oil, cinnamon, almond flour, oats, and honey and spread on top of apple mixture.
5. Set to bake at 350 F for 40 minutes. After 5 minutes place the baking dish in the preheated oven.
6. Serve and enjoy.
- **Nutrition Info:** Calories 450 Fat 21 g Carbohydrates 65 g Sugar 40 g Protein 4 g Cholesterol 0 mg

472.Cinnamon Maple Glazed Carrot Fries

Servings: 4
Cooking Time: 12 Minutes

Ingredients:

- 1 teaspoon of olive oil
- 1/2 teaspoon of ground cinnamon
- 1 teaspoon of maple syrup
- Salt, to taste
- 1 pound of carrots, cut into sticks

Directions:

1. Set the Instant Vortex on Air fryer to 400 degrees F for 12 minutes. Mix carrots with olive oil, cinnamon, maple syrup, and salt in a bowl. Place the carrots on the cooking tray. Insert the cooking tray in the Vortex when it displays "Add Food". Flip the sides when it displays "Turn Food". Remove from the oven when cooking time is complete. Serve warm.
- **Nutrition Info:** Calories: 62 Cal Total Fat: 1 g Saturated Fat: 0 g Cholesterol: 0 mg Sodium: 0 mg Total Carbs: 12 g Fiber: 0 g Sugar: 0 g Protein: 1 g

473.Carrot Chips

Servings:4
Cooking Time: 10 Minutes

Ingredients:
- 4 to 5 medium carrots, trimmed and thinly sliced
- 1 tablespoon olive oil, plus more for greasing
- 1 teaspoon seasoned salt

Directions:
1. Toss the carrot slices with 1 tablespoon of olive oil and salt in a medium bowl until thoroughly coated.
2. Grease the air fryer basket with the olive oil. Place the carrot slices in the greased pan.
3. Put the air fryer basket on the baking pan and slide into Rack Position 2, select Air Fry, set temperature to 390ºF (199ºC), and set time to 10 minutes.
4. Stir the carrot slices halfway through the cooking time.
5. When cooking is complete, the chips should be crisp-tender. Remove from the oven and allow to cool for 5 minutes before serving.

474.Deluxe Cheese Sandwiches

Servings:4 To 8
Cooking Time: 6 Minutes
Ingredients:
- 8 ounces (227 g) Brie
- 8 slices oat nut bread
- 1 large ripe pear, cored and cut into ½-inch-thick slices
- 2 tablespoons butter, melted

Directions:
1. Make the sandwiches: Spread each of 4 slices of bread with ¼ of the Brie. Top the Brie with the pear slices and remaining 4 bread slices.
2. Brush the melted butter lightly on both sides of each sandwich.
3. Arrange the sandwiches in the baking pan.
4. Slide the baking pan into Rack Position 1, select Convection Bake, set temperature to 360ºF (182ºC), and set time to 6 minutes.
5. When cooking is complete, the cheese should be melted. Remove the pan from the oven and serve warm.

475.Lemon Butter Cake

Servings: 10
Cooking Time: 55 Minutes
Ingredients:
- 4 eggs
- 1/2 cup butter softened
- 2 tsp baking powder
- 1/4 cup coconut flour
- 2 cups almond flour
- 2 tbsp lemon zest
- 1/2 cup fresh lemon juice
- 1/4 cup erythritol
- 1 tbsp vanilla

Directions:
1. Fit the oven with the rack in position
2. In a large bowl, whisk all ingredients until a smooth batter is formed.
3. Pour batter into the loaf pan.
4. Set to bake at 300 F for 60 minutes. After 5 minutes place the loaf pan in the preheated oven.
5. Slice and serve.
- **Nutrition Info:** Calories 85 Fat 5.7 g Carbohydrates 5 g Sugar 0.9 g Protein 3.8 g Cholesterol 65 mg

476.Flavors Pumpkin Custard

Servings: 6
Cooking Time: 40 Minutes
Ingredients:
- 4 egg yolks
- 1/2 tsp cinnamon
- 1 tsp liquid stevia
- 15 oz pumpkin puree
- 3/4 cup coconut cream
- 1/8 tsp cloves
- 1/8 tsp ginger

Directions:
1. Fit the oven with the rack in position
2. In a large bowl, mix together pumpkin puree, cloves, ginger, cinnamon, and swerve.
3. Add egg yolks and beat until well combined.
4. Add coconut cream and stir well.
5. Pour mixture into the six ramekins.
6. Set to bake at 350 F for 45 minutes. After 5 minutes place ramekins in the preheated oven.
7. Serve chilled and enjoy.
- **Nutrition Info:** Calories 130 Fat 10.4 g Carbohydrates 8 g Sugar 3.4 g Protein 3.3 g Cholesterol 140 mg

477.Shrimp Toasts With Sesame Seeds

Servings:4 To 6
Cooking Time: 8 Minutes
Ingredients:
- ½ pound (227 g) raw shrimp, peeled and deveined
- 1 egg, beaten
- 2 scallions, chopped, plus more for garnish
- 2 tablespoons chopped fresh cilantro
- 2 teaspoons grated fresh ginger
- 1 to 2 teaspoons sriracha sauce
- 1 teaspoon soy sauce
- ½ teaspoon toasted sesame oil
- 6 slices thinly sliced white sandwich bread
- ½ cup sesame seeds
- Cooking spray
- Thai chili sauce, for serving

Directions:
1. In a food processor, add the shrimp, egg, scallions, cilantro, ginger, sriracha sauce, soy sauce and sesame oil, and pulse until chopped finely. You'll need to stop the food processor occasionally to scrape down the

sides. Transfer the shrimp mixture to a bowl.
2. On a clean work surface, cut the crusts off the sandwich bread. Using a brush, generously brush one side of each slice of bread with shrimp mixture.
3. Place the sesame seeds on a plate. Press bread slices, shrimp-side down, into sesame seeds to coat evenly. Cut each slice diagonally into quarters.
4. Spritz the air fryer basket with cooking spray. Spread the coated slices in a single layer in the basket.
5. Put the air fryer basket on the baking pan and slide into Rack Position 2, select Air Fry, set temperature to 400ºF (205ºC), and set time to 8 minutes.
6. Flip the bread slices halfway through.
7. When cooking is complete, they should be golden and crispy. Remove from the oven to a plate and let cool for 5 minutes. Top with the chopped scallions and serve warm with Thai chili sauce.

478.Lemon Ricotta Cake

Servings:6
Cooking Time: 25 Minutes
Ingredients:
- 17.5 ounces (496 g) ricotta cheese
- 5.4 ounces (153 g) sugar
- 3 eggs, beaten
- 3 tablespoons flour
- 1 lemon, juiced and zested
- 2 teaspoons vanilla extract

Directions:
1. In a large mixing bowl, stir together all the ingredients until the mixture reaches a creamy consistency.
2. Pour the mixture into the baking pan.
3. Slide the baking pan into Rack Position 1, select Convection Bake, set temperature to 320ºF (160ºC), and set time to 25 minutes.
4. When cooking is complete, a toothpick inserted in the center should come out clean.
5. Allow to cool for 10 minutes on a wire rack before serving.

479.Fruity Oreo Muffins

Servings: 6
Cooking Time: 10 Minutes
Ingredients:
- 1 cup milk
- 1 pack Oreo biscuits, crushed
- ¾ teaspoon baking powder
- 1 banana, peeled and chopped
- 1 apple, peeled, cored and chopped
- 1 teaspoon cocoa powder
- 1 teaspoon honey
- 1 teaspoon fresh lemon juice
- A pinch of ground cinnamon

Directions:

1. Preheat the Air fryer to 320 degree F and grease 6 muffin cups lightly.
2. Mix milk, biscuits, cocoa powder, baking soda, and baking powder in a bowl until well combined.
3. Transfer the mixture into the muffin cups and cook for about 10 minutes.
4. Remove from the Air fryer and invert the muffin cups onto a wire rack to cool.
5. Meanwhile, mix the banana, apple, honey, lemon juice, and cinnamon in another bowl.
6. Scoop some portion of muffins from the center and fill with fruit mixture to serve.
- **Nutrition Info:** Calories: 182, Fat: 3.1g, Carbohydrates: 31.4g, Sugar: 19.5g, Protein: 3.1g, Sodium: 196mg

480.Pork Taquitos

Servings: 4
Cooking Time: 10 Minutes
Ingredients:
- Small whole-wheat tortillas, 10.
- Shredded mozzarella cheese, 2 ½ cup
- Cooked and shredded pork tenderloin, 30 oz.
- Lime juice, 1 lime

Directions:
1. Preheat your air fryer to 380 degrees Fahrenheit.
2. Stir the lime juice over the shredded pork tenderloins.
3. Soften the tortillas in your air fryer by microwaving it for 10 seconds.
4. For each tortilla, add 3-ounces of the shredded pork and ¼ cup of the mozzarella cheese.
5. Lightly roll up the tortillas.
6. Then spray a nonstick cooking spray over the tortillas and place it inside your air fryer.
7. Cook it for 10 minutes or until it gets a golden brown color, as you flip after 5 minutes then serve and enjoy.
- **Nutrition Info:** Calories: 210 Fat: 29g Protein: 7g Carbs: 15g

481.Strawberry Pudding

Servings:x
Cooking Time:x
Ingredients:
- 3 tbsp. powdered sugar
- 3 tbsp. unsalted butter
- 1 cup strawberry slices
- 1 cup strawberry juice
- 2 cups milk
- 2 tbsp. custard powder

Directions:
1. Boil the milk and the sugar in a pan and add the custard powder followed by the strawberry juice and stir till you get a thick mixture.
2. Preheat the fryer to 300 Fahrenheit for five minutes. Place the dish in the basket and reduce the temperature to 250 Fahrenheit.

Cook for ten minutes and set aside to cool. Garnish with strawberry.

482.Cripsy Artichoke Bites

Servings:4
Cooking Time: 8 Minutes
Ingredients:
- 14 whole artichoke hearts packed in water
- ½ cup all-purpose flour
- 1 egg
- $^1/_3$ cup panko bread crumbs
- 1 teaspoon Italian seasoning
- Cooking spray

Directions:
1. Drain the artichoke hearts and dry thoroughly with paper towels.
2. Place the flour on a plate. Beat the egg in a shallow bowl until frothy. Thoroughly combine the bread crumbs and Italian seasoning in a separate shallow bowl.
3. Dredge the artichoke hearts in the flour, then in the beaten egg, and finally roll in the bread crumb mixture until evenly coated.
4. Place the artichoke hearts in the air fryer basket and mist them with cooking spray.
5. Put the air fryer basket on the baking pan and slide into Rack Position 2, select Air Fry, set temperature to 375ºF (190ºC), and set time to 8 minutes.
6. Flip the artichoke hearts halfway through the cooking time.
7. When cooking is complete, the artichoke hearts should start to brown and the edges should be crispy. Remove from the oven and let the artichoke hearts sit for 5 minutes before serving.

483.Sausage And Onion Rolls

Servings:12
Cooking Time: 15 Minutes
Ingredients:
- 1 pound (454 g) bulk breakfast sausage
- ½ cup finely chopped onion
- ½ cup fresh bread crumbs
- ½ teaspoon dried mustard
- ½ teaspoon dried sage
- ¼ teaspoon cayenne pepper
- 1 large egg, beaten
- 1 garlic clove, minced
- 2 sheets (1 package) frozen puff pastry, thawed
- All-purpose flour, for dusting

Directions:
1. In a medium bowl, break up the sausage. Stir in the onion, bread crumbs, mustard, sage, cayenne pepper, egg and garlic. Divide the sausage mixture in half and tightly wrap each half in plastic wrap. Refrigerate for 5 to 10 minutes.
2. Lay the pastry sheets on a lightly floured work surface. Using a rolling pin, lightly roll out the pastry to smooth out the dough. Take out one of the sausage packages and

form the sausage into a long roll. Remove the plastic wrap and place the sausage on top of the puff pastry about 1 inch from one of the long edges. Roll the pastry around the sausage and pinch the edges of the dough together to seal. Repeat with the other pastry sheet and sausage.
3. Slice the logs into lengths about 1½ inches long. Place the sausage rolls in the baking pan, cut-side down.
4. Slide the baking pan into Rack Position 2, select Roast, set temperature to 350ºF (180ºC) and set time to 15 minutes.
5. When cooking is complete, the rolls will be golden brown and sizzling. Remove from the oven and let cool for 5 minutes.

484.Paprika Deviled Eggs

Servings:12
Cooking Time: 16 Minutes
Ingredients:
- 3 cups ice
- 12 large eggs
- ½ cup mayonnaise
- 10 hamburger dill pickle chips, diced
- ¼ cup diced onion
- 2 teaspoons salt
- 2 teaspoons yellow mustard
- 1 teaspoon freshly ground black pepper
- ½ teaspoon paprika

Directions:
1. Put the ice in a large bowl and set aside. Carefully place the eggs in the baking pan.
2. Slide the baking pan into Rack Position 1, select Convection Bake, set temperature to 250ºF (121ºC), and set time to 16 minutes.
3. When cooking is complete, transfer the eggs to the large bowl of ice to cool.
4. When cool enough to handle, peel the eggs. Slice them in half lengthwise and scoop out yolks into a small bowl. Stir in the mayonnaise, pickles, onion, salt, mustard, and pepper. Mash the mixture with a fork until well combined.
5. Fill each egg white half with 1 to 2 teaspoons of the egg yolk mixture.
6. Sprinkle the paprika on top and serve immediately.

485.Currant Pudding

Servings: 6
Cooking Time: 15 Minutes
Ingredients:
- 1 cup red currants, blended
- 1 cup coconut cream
- 1 cup black currants, blended
- 3 tbsp. stevia

Directions:
1. In a bowl, combine all the ingredients and stir well.
2. Divide into ramekins, put them in the fryer and cook at 340°F for 20 minutes
3. Serve the pudding cold.

- **Nutrition Info:** Calories: 200; Fat: 4g; Fiber: 2g; Carbs: 4g; Protein: 6g

486.Green Chiles Nachos

Servings:6
Cooking Time: 10 Minutes
Ingredients:
- 8 ounces (227 g) tortilla chips
- 3 cups shredded Monterey Jack cheese, divided
- 2 (7-ounce / 198-g) cans chopped green chiles, drained
- 1 (8-ounce / 227-g) can tomato sauce
- ¼ teaspoon dried oregano
- ¼ teaspoon granulated garlic
- ¼ teaspoon freshly ground black pepper
- Pinch cinnamon
- Pinch cayenne pepper

Directions:
1. Arrange the tortilla chips close together in a single layer in the baking pan. Sprinkle 1½ cups of the cheese over the chips. Arrange the green chiles over the cheese as evenly as possible. Top with the remaining 1½ cups of the cheese.
2. Slide the baking pan into Rack Position 2, select Roast, set temperature to 375ºF (190ºC) and set time to 10 minutes.
3. Meanwhile, stir together the remaining ingredients in a bowl.
4. When cooking is complete, the cheese will be melted and starting to crisp around the edges of the pan. Remove from the oven. Drizzle the sauce over the nachos and serve warm.

487.Garlicky-lemon Zucchini

Servings:x
Cooking Time:x
Ingredients:
- Coarse salt and black pepper, to taste
- ½ tsp thyme, minced
- ½ lemon
- 4 small green zucchinis, any color, sliced about ¼-inch thick
- 1½ Tbsp extra virgin olive oil
- 1 Tbsp garlic, minced

Directions:
1. Heat oven over medium-low heat. Add oil and let heat for 1 minute.
2. Sprinkle zucchini with salt and pepper.
3. Add to the pan in a single layer. When zucchini is nicely browned, flip
4. and brown on other side.
5. Add garlic and saute for 1 minute.
6. Sprinkle thyme and additional salt if necessary.
7. Remove from pan and squeeze lemon juice on zucchini.

488.Brownies

Servings:x

Cooking Time:x
Ingredients:
- ½ cup condensed milk
- 1 tbsp. unsalted butter
- 2 tbsp. water
- ½ cup chopped nuts
- 3 tbsp. melted dark chocolate
- 1 cup all-purpose flour

Directions:
1. Add the ingredients together and whisk till you get a smooth mixture.
2. Prepare a tin by greasing it with butter. Transfer the mixture into the tin.
3. Preheat the fryer to 300 Fahrenheit for five minutes. You will need to place the tin in the basket and cover it. Check whether the brownies have been cooked using a knife or a toothpick and remove the tray. When the brownies have cooled, cut them and serve with a dollop of ice cream.

489.Apple Cake

Servings: 12
Cooking Time: 45 Minutes
Ingredients:
- 2 cups apples, peeled and chopped
- 1/4 cup sugar
- 1/4 cup butter, melted
- 12 oz apple juice
- 3 cups all-purpose flour
- 3 tsp baking powder
- 1 1/2 tbsp ground cinnamon
- 1 tsp Salt

Directions:
1. Fit the oven with the rack in position
2. In a large bowl, mix together flour, salt, sugar, cinnamon, and baking powder.
3. Add melted butter and apple juice and mix until well combined.
4. Add apples and fold well.
5. Pour batter into the greased baking dish.
6. Set to bake at 350 F for 45 minutes. After 5 minutes place the baking dish in the preheated oven.
7. Serve and enjoy.
- **Nutrition Info:** Calories 200 Fat 4 g Carbohydrates 38 g Sugar 11 g Protein 3 g Cholesterol 10 mg

490.Walnut Carrot Cake

Servings: 4
Cooking Time: 25 Minutes
Ingredients:
- 1 egg
- 1/2 cup sugar
- 1/4 cup canola oil
- 1/4 cup walnuts, chopped
- 1/2 tsp baking powder
- 1/2 cup flour
- 1/4 cup grated carrot
- 1/2 tsp vanilla
- 1/2 tsp cinnamon

Directions:

1. Fit the oven with the rack in position
2. In a medium bowl, beat sugar and oil for 1 minute. Add vanilla, cinnamon, and egg and beat for 30 seconds.
3. Add remaining ingredients and stir everything well until just combined.
4. Pour batter into the greased baking dish.
5. Set to bake at 350 F for 30 minutes. After 5 minutes place the baking dish in the preheated oven.
6. Serve and enjoy.
- **Nutrition Info:** Calories 340 Fat 20 g Carbohydrates 40 g Sugar 25 g Protein 5 g Cholesterol 41 mg

491.Strawberry Muffins

Servings: 12
Cooking Time: 20 Minutes
Ingredients:
- 4 eggs
- 1/4 cup water
- 1/2 cup butter, melted
- 2 tsp baking powder
- 2 cups almond flour
- 2/3 cup strawberries, chopped
- 2 tsp vanilla
- 1/4 cup erythritol
- Pinch of salt

Directions:

1. Fit the oven with the rack in position
2. Line 12-cups muffin tin with cupcake liners and set aside.
3. In a medium bowl, mix together almond flour, baking powder, and salt.
4. In a separate bowl, whisk eggs, sweetener, vanilla, water, and butter.
5. Add almond flour mixture into the egg mixture and mix until well combined.
6. Add strawberries and stir well.
7. Pour batter into the prepared muffin tin.
8. Set to bake at 350 F for 25 minutes. After 5 minutes place muffin tin in the preheated oven.
9. Serve and enjoy.
- **Nutrition Info:** Calories 201 Fat 18.5 g Carbohydrates 5.2 g Sugar 1.3 g Protein 6 g Cholesterol 75 mg

492.Seafood Turnovers

Servings:x
Cooking Time:x
Ingredients:
- ½ teaspoon dried dill weed
- 1 sheet frozen puff pastry, thawed
- 1 egg yolk, beaten
- 1 tablespoon water
- 1 (6-ounce) can small shrimp, drained
- ½ cup ricotta cheese
- 3 green onions, finely chopped
- 1 cup shredded Havarti cheese

Directions:

1. In medium bowl, combine shrimp, ricotta, green onions, Havarti, and dill weed and mix well.
2. Gently roll puff pastry into 12-inch by 18-inch rectangle. Cut into 24 3-inch squares. Place 2 teaspoons shrimp mixture in center of each square. Beat egg yolk with water in small bowl. Brush edges of pastry with egg yolk mixture. Fold puff pastry over filling, forming triangles; press edges with fork to seal.
3. Flash freeze turnovers in single layer on baking sheet. Then pack in rigid containers, with waxed paper separating the layers. Label containers and freeze.
4. To reheat: Preheat oven to 450ºF. Place frozen turnovers on baking sheet. Bake at 450ºF for 4 minutes; then turn oven down to 400ºF and bake for 12 to 15 minutes longer or until pastry is golden and filling is hot.

493.Peanut Butter Muffins

Servings: 12
Cooking Time: 20 Minutes
Ingredients:
- 1 cup peanut butter
- 1/2 cup maple syrup
- 1/2 cup of cocoa powder
- 1 cup applesauce
- 1 tsp baking soda
- 1 tsp vanilla

Directions:

1. Fit the oven with the rack in position
2. Line 12-cups muffin tin with cupcake liners and set aside.
3. Add all ingredients into the blender and blend until smooth.
4. Pour blended mixture into the prepared muffin tin.
5. Set to bake at 350 F for 25 minutes. After 5 minutes place muffin tin in the preheated oven.
6. Serve and enjoy.
- **Nutrition Info:** Calories 178 Fat 11.3 g Carbohydrates 17.3 g Sugar 12 g Protein 6.1 g Cholesterol 0 mg

494.Shrimp Cheese Quiches

Servings:x
Cooking Time:x
Ingredients:
- 1 (6-ounce) can tiny shrimp, drained
- ½ teaspoon dried marjoram leaves
- ½ teaspoon salt
- ½ teaspoon pepper
- ¾ cup shredded Havarti cheese
- 2 9-inch Pie Crusts
- ½ cup chopped leek, rinsed
- 1 tablespoon olive oil
- 2 eggs
- ½ cup cream

Directions:

1. Using a 2-inch cookie cutter, cut 36 rounds from pie crusts. Place each in a 1¾-inch mini muffin cup, pressing to bottom and sides. Set aside.
2. Sauté leek in olive oil until tender. Beat eggs with cream in medium bowl. Add drained shrimp, cooked leek, marjoram, salt, and pepper, and mix well.
3. Sprinkle 1 teaspoon cheese into each muffin cup and fill cups with shrimp mixture. Bake at 375ºF for 15 to 18 minutes or until pastry is golden and filling is set. Cool in refrigerator until cold, then freeze.
4. Freeze in single layer on baking sheet. When frozen solid, pack in rigid containers, using waxed paper to separate layers. Label and freeze.
5. To reheat: Place frozen quiches on baking sheet and bake at 375ºF for 8 to 11 minutes or until hot.

495.Crunchy Chickpeas

Servings:4
Cooking Time: 18 Minutes
Ingredients:
- ½ teaspoon chili powder
- ½ teaspoon ground cumin
- ¼ teaspoon cayenne pepper
- ¼ teaspoon salt
- 1 (19-ounce / 539-g) can chickpeas, drained and rinsed
- Cooking spray

Directions:
1. Lina the air fryer basket with parchment paper and lightly spritz with cooking spray.
2. Mix the chili powder, cumin, cayenne pepper, and salt in a small bowl.
3. Place the chickpeas in a medium bowl and lightly mist with cooking spray.
4. Add the spice mixture to the chickpeas and toss until evenly coated. Transfer the chickpeas to the parchment.
5. Put the air fryer basket on the baking pan and slide into Rack Position 2, select Air Fry, set temperature to 390ºF (199ºC), and set time to 18 minutes.
6. Stir the chickpeas twice during cooking.
7. When cooking is complete, the chickpeas should be crunchy. Remove from the oven and let the chickpeas cool for 5 minutes before serving.

496.Coconut Bars

Servings: 12
Cooking Time: 40 Minutes
Ingredients:
- 1 and ¼ cups almond flour
- 1 cup swerve
- 1 cup butter, melted
- ½ cup coconut cream
- 1 and ½ cups coconut, flaked
- 1 egg yolk
- ¾ cup walnuts, chopped
- ½ teaspoon vanilla extract

Directions:
1. In a bowl, mix the flour with half of the swerve and half of the butter, stir well and press this on the bottom of a baking pan that fits the air fryer.
2. Introduce this in the air fryer and cook at 350 degrees F for 15 minutes.
3. Meanwhile, heat up a pan with the rest of the butter over medium heat, add the remaining swerve and the rest of the Ingredients:, whisk, cook for 1-2 minutes, take off the heat and cool down.
4. Spread this well over the crust, put the pan in the air fryer again and cook at 350 degrees F for 25 minutes.
5. Cool down, cut into bars and serve.
- **Nutrition Info:** Calories 182, fat 12, fiber 2, carbs 4, protein 4

OTHER FAVORITE RECIPES

497.Shrimp Spinach Frittata

Servings:4
Cooking Time: 14 Minutes
Ingredients:
- 4 whole eggs
- 1 teaspoon dried basil
- ½ cup shrimp, cooked and chopped
- ½ cup baby spinach
- ½ cup rice, cooked
- ½ cup Monterey Jack cheese, grated
- Salt, to taste
- Cooking spray

Directions:
1. Spritz the baking pan with cooking spray.
2. Whisk the eggs with basil and salt in a large bowl until bubbly, then mix in the shrimp, spinach, rice, and cheese.
3. Pour the mixture into the baking pan.
4. Slide the baking pan into Rack Position 1, select Convection Bake, set temperature to 360ºF (182ºC) and set time to 14 minutes.
5. Stir the mixture halfway through.
6. When cooking is complete, the eggs should be set and the frittata should be golden brown.
7. Slice to serve.

498.Classic Churros

Servings: 12 Churros
Cooking Time: 10 Minutes
Ingredients:
- 4 tablespoons butter
- ¼ teaspoon salt
- ½ cup water
- ½ cup all-purpose flour
- 2 large eggs
- 2 teaspoons ground cinnamon
- ¼ cup granulated white sugar
- Cooking spray

Directions:
1. Put the butter, salt, and water in a saucepan. Bring to a boil until the butter is melted on high heat. Keep stirring.
2. Reduce the heat to medium and fold in the flour to form a dough. Keep cooking and stirring until the dough is dried out and coat the pan with a crust.
3. Turn off the heat and scrape the dough in a large bowl. Allow to cool for 15 minutes.
4. Break and whisk the eggs into the dough with a hand mixer until the dough is sanity and firm enough to shape.
5. Scoop up 1 tablespoon of the dough and roll it into a ½-inch-diameter and 2-inch-long cylinder. Repeat with remaining dough to make 12 cylinders in total.
6. Combine the cinnamon and sugar in a large bowl and dunk the cylinders into the cinnamon mix to coat.
7. Arrange the cylinders on a plate and refrigerate for 20 minutes.
8. Spritz the air fryer basket with cooking spray. Place the cylinders in the basket and spritz with cooking spray.
9. Put the air fryer basket on the baking pan and slide into Rack Position 2, select Air Fry, set temperature to 375ºF (190ºC) and set time to 10 minutes.
10. Flip the cylinders halfway through the cooking time.
11. When cooked, the cylinders should be golden brown and fluffy.
12. Serve immediately.

499.Simple Baked Green Beans

Servings: 2 Cups
Cooking Time: 10 Minutes
Ingredients:
- ½ teaspoon lemon pepper
- 2 teaspoons granulated garlic
- ½ teaspoon salt
- 1 tablespoon olive oil
- 2 cups fresh green beans, trimmed and snapped in half

Directions:
1. Combine the lemon pepper, garlic, salt, and olive oil in a bowl. Stir to mix well.
2. Add the green beans to the bowl of mixture and toss to coat well.
3. Arrange the green beans in the the baking pan.
4. Slide the baking pan into Rack Position 1, select Convection Bake, set temperature to 370ºF (188ºC) and set time to 10 minutes.
5. Stir the green beans halfway through the cooking time.
6. When cooking is complete, the green beans will be tender and crispy. Remove from the oven and serve immediately.

500.Parsnip Fries With Garlic-yogurt Dip

Servings:4
Cooking Time: 10 Minutes
Ingredients:
- 3 medium parsnips, peeled, cut into sticks
- ¼ teaspoon kosher salt
- 1 teaspoon olive oil
- 1 garlic clove, unpeeled
- Cooking spray
- Dip:
- ¼ cup plain Greek yogurt
- ⅛ teaspoon garlic powder
- 1 tablespoon sour cream
- ¼ teaspoon kosher salt

- Freshly ground black pepper, to taste

Directions:
1. Spritz the air fryer basket with cooking spray.
2. Put the parsnip sticks in a large bowl, then sprinkle with salt and drizzle with olive oil.
3. Transfer the parsnip into the basket and add the garlic.
4. Put the air fryer basket on the baking pan and slide into Rack Position 2, select Air Fry, set temperature to 360ºF (182ºC) and set time to 10 minutes.
5. Stir the parsnip halfway through the cooking time.
6. Meanwhile, peel the garlic and crush it. Combine the crushed garlic with the ingredients for the dip. Stir to mix well.
7. When cooked, the parsnip sticks should be crisp. Remove the parsnip fries from the oven and serve with the dipping sauce.

501.Chocolate Buttermilk Cake

Servings:8
Cooking Time: 20 Minutes
Ingredients:
- 1 cup all-purpose flour
- $^2/_3$ cup granulated white sugar
- ¼ cup unsweetened cocoa powder
- ¾ teaspoon baking soda
- ¼ teaspoon salt
- $^2/_3$ cup buttermilk
- 2 tablespoons plus 2 teaspoons vegetable oil
- 1 teaspoon vanilla extract
- Cooking spray

Directions:
1. Spritz the baking pan with cooking spray.
2. Combine the flour, cocoa powder, baking soda, sugar, and salt in a large bowl. Stir to mix well.
3. Mix in the buttermilk, vanilla, and vegetable oil. Keep stirring until it forms a grainy and thick dough.
4. Scrape the chocolate batter from the bowl and transfer to the pan, level the batter in an even layer with a spatula.
5. Slide the baking pan into Rack Position 1, select Convection Bake, set temperature to 325ºF (163ºC) and set time to 20 minutes.
6. After 15 minutes, remove the pan from the oven. Check the doneness. Return the pan to the oven and continue cooking.
7. When done, a toothpick inserted in the center should come out clean.
8. Invert the cake on a cooling rack and allow to cool for 15 minutes before slicing to serve.

502.Ritzy Chicken And Vegetable Casserole

Servings:4
Cooking Time: 15 Minutes
Ingredients:
- 4 boneless and skinless chicken breasts, cut into cubes
- 2 carrots, sliced
- 1 yellow bell pepper, cut into strips
- 1 red bell pepper, cut into strips
- 15 ounces (425 g) broccoli florets
- 1 cup snow peas
- 1 scallion, sliced
- Cooking spray
- Sauce:
- 1 teaspoon Sriracha
- 3 tablespoons soy sauce
- 2 tablespoons oyster sauce
- 1 tablespoon rice wine vinegar
- 1 teaspoon cornstarch
- 1 tablespoon grated ginger
- 2 garlic cloves, minced
- 1 teaspoon sesame oil
- 1 tablespoon brown sugar

Directions:
1. Spritz the baking pan with cooking spray.
2. Combine the chicken, carrot, and bell peppers in a large bowl. Stir to mix well.
3. Combine the ingredients for the sauce in a separate bowl. Stir to mix well.
4. Pour the chicken mixture into the baking pan, then pour the sauce over. Stir to coat well.
5. Slide the baking pan into Rack Position 1, select Convection Bake, set temperature to 370ºF (188ºC) and set time to 13 minutes.
6. Add the broccoli and snow peas to the pan halfway through.
7. When cooking is complete, the vegetables should be tender.
8. Remove from the oven and sprinkle with sliced scallion before serving.

503.Kale Frittata

Servings:2
Cooking Time: 11 Minutes
Ingredients:
- 1 cup kale, chopped
- 1 teaspoon olive oil
- 4 large eggs, beaten
- Kosher salt, to taste
- 2 tablespoons water
- 3 tablespoons crumbled feta
- Cooking spray

Directions:
1. Spritz the baking pan with cooking spray.
2. Add the kale to the baking pan and drizzle with olive oil.

3. Slide the baking pan into Rack Position 2, select Convection Broil, set temperature to 360ºF (182ºC) and set time to 3 minutes.
4. Stir the kale halfway through.
5. When cooking is complete, the kale should be wilted.
6. Meanwhile, combine the eggs with salt and water in a large bowl. Stir to mix well.
7. Make the frittata: When broiling is complete, pour the eggs into the baking pan and spread with feta cheese.
8. Slide the baking pan into Rack Position 1, select Convection Bake, set temperature to 300ºF (150ºC) and set time to 8 minutes.
9. When cooking is complete, the eggs should be set and the cheese should be melted.
10. Remove from the oven and serve the frittata immediately.

504.Asian Dipping Sauce

Servings: About 1 Cup
Cooking Time: 0 Minutes
Ingredients:
- ¼ cup rice vinegar
- ¼ cup hoisin sauce
- ¼ cup low-sodium chicken or vegetable stock
- 3 tablespoons soy sauce
- 1 tablespoon minced or grated ginger
- 1 tablespoon minced or pressed garlic
- 1 teaspoon chili-garlic sauce or sriracha (or more to taste)

Directions:
1. Stir together all the ingredients in a small bowl, or place in a jar with a tight-fitting lid and shake until well mixed.
2. Use immediately.

505.Garlicky Olive Stromboli

Servings:8
Cooking Time: 25 Minutes
Ingredients:
- 4 large cloves garlic, unpeeled
- 3 tablespoons grated Parmesan cheese
- ½ cup packed fresh basil leaves
- ½ cup marinated, pitted green and black olives
- ¼ teaspoon crushed red pepper
- ½ pound (227 g) pizza dough, at room temperature
- 4 ounces (113 g) sliced provolone cheese (about 8 slices)
- Cooking spray

Directions:
1. Spritz the air fryer basket with cooking spray. Put the unpeeled garlic in the basket.
2. Put the air fryer basket on the baking pan and slide into Rack Position 2, select Air Fry,

set temperature to 370ºF (188ºC) and set time to 10 minutes.
3. When cooked, the garlic will be softened completely. Remove from the oven and allow to cool until you can handle.
4. Peel the garlic and place into a food processor with 2 tablespoons of Parmesan, basil, olives, and crushed red pepper. Pulse to mix well. Set aside.
5. Arrange the pizza dough on a clean work surface, then roll it out with a rolling pin into a rectangle. Cut the rectangle in half.
6. Sprinkle half of the garlic mixture over each rectangle half, and leave ½-inch edges uncover. Top them with the provolone cheese.
7. Brush one long side of each rectangle half with water, then roll them up. Spritz the basket with cooking spray. Transfer the rolls to the basket. Spritz with cooking spray and scatter with remaining Parmesan.
8. Select Air Fry and set time to 15 minutes.
9. Flip the rolls halfway through the cooking time. When done, the rolls should be golden brown.
10. Remove the rolls from the oven and allow to cool for a few minutes before serving.

506.Baked Cherry Tomatoes With Basil

Servings:2
Cooking Time: 5 Minutes
Ingredients:
- 2 cups cherry tomatoes
- 1 clove garlic, thinly sliced
- 1 teaspoon olive oil
- ⅛ teaspoon kosher salt
- 1 tablespoon freshly chopped basil, for topping
- Cooking spray

Directions:
1. Spritz the baking pan with cooking spray and set aside.
2. In a large bowl, toss together the cherry tomatoes, sliced garlic, olive oil, and kosher salt. Spread the mixture in an even layer in the prepared pan.
3. Slide the baking pan into Rack Position 1, select Convection Bake, set temperature to 360ºF (182ºC) and set time to 5 minutes.
4. When cooking is complete, the tomatoes should be the soft and wilted.
5. Transfer to a bowl and rest for 5 minutes. Top with the chopped basil and serve warm.

507.Cheesy Green Bean Casserole

Servings:4
Cooking Time: 6 Minutes
Ingredients:
- 1 tablespoon melted butter
- 1 cup green beans

- 6 ounces (170 g) Cheddar cheese, shredded
- 7 ounces (198 g) Parmesan cheese, shredded
- ¼ cup heavy cream
- Sea salt, to taste

Directions:
1. Grease the baking pan with the melted butter.
2. Add the green beans, Cheddar, salt, and black pepper to the prepared baking pan. Stir to mix well, then spread the Parmesan and cream on top.
3. Slide the baking pan into Rack Position 1, select Convection Bake, set temperature to 400ºF (205ºC) and set time to 6 minutes.
4. When cooking is complete, the beans should be tender and the cheese should be melted.
5. Serve immediately.

508.Potato Chips With Lemony Cream Dip

Servings:2 To 4
Cooking Time: 15 Minutes
Ingredients:
- 2 large russet potatoes, sliced into ⅛-inch slices, rinsed
- Sea salt and freshly ground black pepper, to taste
- Cooking spray
- Lemony Cream Dip:
- ½ cup sour cream
- ¼ teaspoon lemon juice
- 2 scallions, white part only, minced
- 1 tablespoon olive oil
- ¼ teaspoon salt
- Freshly ground black pepper, to taste

Directions:
1. Soak the potato slices in water for 10 minutes, then pat dry with paper towels.
2. Transfer the potato slices in the air fryer basket. Spritz the slices with cooking spray.
3. Put the air fryer basket on the baking pan and slide into Rack Position 2, select Air Fry, set temperature to 300ºF (150ºC) and set time to 15 minutes.
4. Stir the potato slices three times during cooking. Sprinkle with salt and ground black pepper in the last minute.
5. Meanwhile, combine the ingredients for the dip in a small bowl. Stir to mix well.
6. When cooking is complete, the potato slices will be crispy and golden brown. Remove from the oven and serve the potato chips immediately with the dip.

509.Milky Pecan Tart

Servings:8
Cooking Time: 26 Minutes
Ingredients:
- Tart Crust:

- ¼ cup firmly packed brown sugar
- ¹/₃ cup butter, softened
- 1 cup all-purpose flour
- ¼ teaspoon kosher salt
- Filling:
- ¼ cup whole milk
- 4 tablespoons butter, diced
- ½ cup packed brown sugar
- ¼ cup pure maple syrup
- 1½ cups finely chopped pecans
- ¼ teaspoon pure vanilla extract
- ¼ teaspoon sea salt

Directions:
1. Line the baking pan with aluminum foil, then spritz the pan with cooking spray.
2. Stir the brown sugar and butter in a bowl with a hand mixer until puffed, then add the flour and salt and stir until crumbled.
3. Pour the mixture in the prepared baking pan and tilt the pan to coat the bottom evenly.
4. Slide the baking pan into Rack Position 1, select Convection Bake, set temperature to 350ºF (180ºC) and set time to 13 minutes.
5. When done, the crust will be golden brown.
6. Meanwhile, pour the milk, butter, sugar, and maple syrup in a saucepan. Stir to mix well. Bring to a simmer, then cook for 1 more minute. Stir constantly.
7. Turn off the heat and mix the pecans and vanilla into the filling mixture.
8. Pour the filling mixture over the golden crust and spread with a spatula to coat the crust evenly.
9. Select Bake and set time to 12 minutes. When cooked, the filling mixture should be set and frothy.
10. Remove the baking pan from the oven and sprinkle with salt. Allow to sit for 10 minutes or until cooled.
11. Transfer the pan to the refrigerator to chill for at least 2 hours, then remove the aluminum foil and slice to serve.

510.Apple Fritters With Sugary Glaze

Servings: 15 Fritters
Cooking Time: 8 Minutes
Ingredients:
- Apple Fritters:
- 2 firm apples, peeled, cored, and diced
- ½ teaspoon cinnamon
- Juice of 1 lemon
- 1 cup all-purpose flour
- 1½ teaspoons baking powder
- ½ teaspoon kosher salt
- 2 eggs
- ¼ cup milk
- 2 tablespoons unsalted butter, melted
- 2 tablespoons granulated sugar

- Cooking spray
- Glaze:
- ½ teaspoon vanilla extract
- 1¼ cups powdered sugar, sifted
- ¼ cup water

Directions:
1. Line the air fryer basket with parchment paper.
2. Combine the apples with cinnamon and lemon juice in a small bowl. Toss to coat well.
3. Combine the flour, baking powder, and salt in a large bowl. Stir to mix well.
4. Whisk the egg, milk, butter, and sugar in a medium bowl. Stir to mix well.
5. Make a well in the center of the flour mixture, then pour the egg mixture into the well and stir to mix well. Mix in the apple until a dough forms.
6. Use an ice cream scoop to scoop 15 balls from the dough onto the pan. Spritz with cooking spray.
7. Put the air fryer basket on the baking pan and slide into Rack Position 2, select Air Fry, set temperature to 360ºF (182ºC) and set time to 8 minutes.
8. Flip the apple fritters halfway through the cooking time.
9. Meanwhile, combine the ingredients for the glaze in a separate small bowl. Stir to mix well.
10. When cooking is complete, the apple fritters will be golden brown. Serve the fritters with the glaze on top or use the glaze for dipping.

511.Sweet Cinnamon Chickpeas

Servings:2
Cooking Time: 10 Minutes
Ingredients:
- 1 tablespoon cinnamon
- 1 tablespoon sugar
- 1 cup chickpeas, soaked in water overnight, rinsed and drained

Directions:
1. Combine the cinnamon and sugar in a bowl. Stir to mix well.
2. Add the chickpeas to the bowl, then toss to coat well.
3. Pour the chickpeas in the air fryer basket.
4. Put the air fryer basket on the baking pan and slide into Rack Position 2, select Air Fry, set temperature to 390ºF (199ºC) and set time to 10 minutes.
5. Stir the chickpeas three times during cooking.
6. When cooked, the chickpeas should be golden brown and crispy. Remove from the oven and serve immediately.

512.Smoked Trout And Crème Fraiche Frittata

Servings:4
Cooking Time: 17 Minutes
Ingredients:
- 2 tablespoons olive oil
- 1 onion, sliced
- 1 egg, beaten
- ½ tablespoon horseradish sauce
- 6 tablespoons crème fraiche
- 1 cup diced smoked trout
- 2 tablespoons chopped fresh dill
- Cooking spray

Directions:
1. Spritz the baking pan with cooking spray.
2. Heat the olive oil in a nonstick skillet over medium heat until shimmering.
3. Add the onion and sauté for 3 minutes or until translucent.
4. Combine the egg, horseradish sauce, and crème fraiche in a large bowl. Stir to mix well, then mix in the sautéed onion, smoked trout, and dill.
5. Pour the mixture in the prepared baking pan.
6. Slide the baking pan into Rack Position 1, select Convection Bake, set temperature to 350ºF (180ºC) and set time to 14 minutes.
7. Stir the mixture halfway through.
8. When cooking is complete, the egg should be set and the edges should be lightly browned.
9. Serve immediately.

513.Cauliflower And Pumpkin Casserole

Servings:6
Cooking Time: 50 Minutes
Ingredients:
- 1 cup chicken broth
- 2 cups cauliflower florets
- 1 cup canned pumpkin purée
- ¼ cup heavy cream
- 1 teaspoon vanilla extract
- 2 large eggs, beaten
- $1/_3$ cup unsalted butter, melted, plus more for greasing the pan
- ¼ cup sugar
- 1 teaspoon fine sea salt
- Chopped fresh parsley leaves, for garnish
- TOPPING:
- ½ cup blanched almond flour
- 1 cup chopped pecans
- $1/_3$ cup unsalted butter, melted
- ½ cup sugar

Directions:
1. Pour the chicken broth in the baking pan, then add the cauliflower.

2. Slide the baking pan into Rack Position 1, select Convection Bake, set temperature to 350ºF (180ºC) and set time to 20 minutes.
3. When cooking is complete, the cauliflower should be soft.
4. Meanwhile, combine the ingredients for the topping in a large bowl. Stir to mix well.
5. Pat the cauliflower dry with paper towels, then place in a food processor and pulse with pumpkin purée, heavy cream, vanilla extract, eggs, butter, sugar, and salt until smooth.
6. Clean the baking pan and grease with more butter, then pour the purée mixture in the pan. Spread the topping over the mixture.
7. Put the baking pan back to the oven. Select Bake and set time to 30 minutes.
8. When baking is complete, the topping of the casserole should be lightly browned.
9. Remove the casserole from the oven and serve with fresh parsley on top.

514.Broccoli, Carrot, And Tomato Quiche

Servings:4
Cooking Time: 14 Minutes
Ingredients:
- 4 eggs
- 1 teaspoon dried thyme
- 1 cup whole milk
- 1 steamed carrots, diced
- 2 cups steamed broccoli florets
- 2 medium tomatoes, diced
- ¼ cup crumbled feta cheese
- 1 cup grated Cheddar cheese
- 1 teaspoon chopped parsley
- Salt and ground black pepper, to taste
- Cooking spray

Directions:
1. Spritz the baking pan with cooking spray.
2. Whisk together the eggs, thyme, salt, and ground black pepper in a bowl and fold in the milk while mixing.
3. Put the carrots, broccoli, and tomatoes in the prepared baking pan, then spread with feta cheese and ½ cup Cheddar cheese. Pour the egg mixture over, then scatter with remaining Cheddar on top.
4. Slide the baking pan into Rack Position 1, select Convection Bake, set temperature to 350ºF (180ºC) and set time to 14 minutes.
5. When cooking is complete, the egg should be set and the quiche should be puffed.
6. Remove the quiche from the oven and top with chopped parsley, then slice to serve.

515.Simple Air Fried Edamame

Servings:6
Cooking Time: 7 Minutes
Ingredients:
- 1½ pounds (680 g) unshelled edamame
- 2 tablespoons olive oil
- 1 teaspoon sea salt

Directions:
1. Place the edamame in a large bowl, then drizzle with olive oil. Toss to coat well. Transfer the edamame to the air fryer basket.
2. Put the air fryer basket on the baking pan and slide into Rack Position 2, select Air Fry, set temperature to 400ºF (205ºC) and set time to 7 minutes.
3. Stir the edamame at least three times during cooking.
4. When done, the edamame will be tender and warmed through.
5. Transfer the cooked edamame onto a plate and sprinkle with salt. Toss to combine well and set aside for 3 minutes to infuse before serving.

516.Crispy Cheese Wafer

Servings:2
Cooking Time: 5 Minutes
Ingredients:
- 1 cup shredded aged Manchego cheese
- 1 teaspoon all-purpose flour
- ½ teaspoon cumin seeds
- ¼ teaspoon cracked black pepper

Directions:
1. Line the air fryer basket with parchment paper.
2. Combine the cheese and flour in a bowl. Stir to mix well. Spread the mixture in the pan into a 4-inch round.
3. Combine the cumin and black pepper in a small bowl. Stir to mix well. Sprinkle the cumin mixture over the cheese round.
4. Put the air fryer basket on the baking pan and slide into Rack Position 2, select Air Fry, set temperature to 375ºF (190ºC) and set time to 5 minutes.
5. When cooked, the cheese will be lightly browned and frothy.
6. Use tongs to transfer the cheese wafer onto a plate and slice to serve.

517.Classic Marinara Sauce

Servings: About 3 Cups
Cooking Time: 30 Minutes
Ingredients:
- ¼ cup extra-virgin olive oil
- 3 garlic cloves, minced
- 1 small onion, chopped (about ½ cup)
- 2 tablespoons minced or puréed sun-dried tomatoes (optional)
- 1 (28-ounce / 794-g) can crushed tomatoes
- ½ teaspoon dried basil
- ½ teaspoon dried oregano

- ¼ teaspoon red pepper flakes

Directions:
1. 1 teaspoon kosher salt or ½ teaspoon fine salt, plus more as needed
2. Heat the oil in a medium saucepan over medium heat.
3. Add the garlic and onion and sauté for 2 to 3 minutes, or until the onion is softened. Add the sun-dried tomatoes (if desired) and cook for 1 minute until fragrant. Stir in the crushed tomatoes, scraping any brown bits from the bottom of the pot. Fold in the basil, oregano, red pepper flakes, and salt. Stir well.
4. Bring to a simmer. Cook covered for about 30 minutes, stirring occasionally.
5. Turn off the heat and allow the sauce to cool for about 10 minutes.
6. Taste and adjust the seasoning, adding more salt if needed.
7. Use immediately.

518.Riced Cauliflower Casserole

Servings:4
Cooking Time: 12 Minutes
Ingredients:
- 1 head cauliflower, cut into florets
- 1 cup okra, chopped
- 1 yellow bell pepper, chopped
- 2 eggs, beaten
- ½ cup chopped onion
- 1 tablespoon soy sauce
- 2 tablespoons olive oil
- Salt and ground black pepper,
- to taste Spritz the baking pan with cooking spray.

Directions:
1. Put the cauliflower in a food processor and pulse to rice the cauliflower.
2. Pour the cauliflower rice in the baking pan and add the remaining ingredients. Stir to mix well.
3. Slide the baking pan into Rack Position 1, select Convection Bake, set temperature to 380ºF (193ºC) and set time to 12 minutes.
4. When cooking is complete, the eggs should be set.
5. Remove from the oven and serve immediately.

519.Sweet Air Fried Pecans

Servings: 4 Cups
Cooking Time: 10 Minutes
Ingredients:
- 2 egg whites
- 1 tablespoon cumin
- 2 teaspoons smoked paprika
- ½ cup brown sugar
- 2 teaspoons kosher salt

- 1 pound (454 g) pecan halves
- Cooking spray

Directions:
1. Spritz the air fryer basket with cooking spray.
2. Combine the egg whites, cumin, paprika, sugar, and salt in a large bowl. Stir to mix well. Add the pecans to the bowl and toss to coat well.
3. Transfer the pecans to the basket.
4. Put the air fryer basket on the baking pan and slide into Rack Position 2, select Air Fry, set temperature to 300ºF (150ºC) and set time to 10 minutes.
5. Stir the pecans at least two times during the cooking.
6. When cooking is complete, the pecans should be lightly caramelized. Remove from the oven and serve immediately.

520.Lush Seafood Casserole

Servings:2
Cooking Time: 22 Minutes
Ingredients:
- 1 tablespoon olive oil
- 1 small yellow onion, chopped
- 2 garlic cloves, minced
- 4 ounces (113 g) tilapia pieces
- 4 ounces (113 g) rockfish pieces
- ½ teaspoon dried basil
- Salt and ground white pepper, to taste
- 4 eggs, lightly beaten
- 1 tablespoon dry sherry
- 4 tablespoons cheese, shredded

Directions:
1. Heat the olive oil in a nonstick skillet over medium-high heat until shimmering.
2. Add the onion and garlic and sauté for 2 minutes or until fragrant.
3. Add the tilapia, rockfish, basil, salt, and white pepper to the skillet. Sauté to combine well and transfer them into the baking pan.
4. Combine the eggs, sherry and cheese in a large bowl. Stir to mix well. Pour the mixture in the baking pan over the fish mixture.
5. Slide the baking pan into Rack Position 1, select Convection Bake, set temperature to 360ºF (182ºC) and set time to 20 minutes.
6. When cooking is complete, the eggs should be set and the casserole edges should be lightly browned.
7. Serve immediately.

521.Lemony And Garlicky Asparagus

Servings: 10 Spears
Cooking Time: 10 Minutes
Ingredients:

- 10 spears asparagus (about ½ pound / 227 g in total), snap the ends off
- 1 tablespoon lemon juice
- 2 teaspoons minced garlic
- ½ teaspoon salt
- ¼ teaspoon ground black pepper
- Cooking spray

Directions:
1. Line the air fryer basket with parchment paper.
2. Put the asparagus spears in a large bowl. Drizzle with lemon juice and sprinkle with minced garlic, salt, and ground black pepper. Toss to coat well.
3. Transfer the asparagus to the basket and spritz with cooking spray.
4. Put the air fryer basket on the baking pan and slide into Rack Position 2, select Air Fry, set temperature to 400ºF (205ºC) and set time to 10 minutes.
5. Flip the asparagus halfway through cooking.
6. When cooked, the asparagus should be wilted and soft. Remove from the oven and serve immediately.

522.Simple Cheesy Shrimps

Servings:4 To 6
Cooking Time: 8 Minutes
Ingredients:
- ²/₃ cup grated Parmesan cheese
- 4 minced garlic cloves
- 1 teaspoon onion powder
- ½ teaspoon oregano
- 1 teaspoon basil
- 1 teaspoon ground black pepper
- 2 tablespoons olive oil
- 2 pounds (907 g) cooked large shrimps, peeled and deveined
- Lemon wedges, for topping
- Cooking spray

Directions:
1. Spritz the air fryer basket with cooking spray.
2. Combine all the ingredients, except for the shrimps, in a large bowl. Stir to mix well.
3. Dunk the shrimps in the mixture and toss to coat well. Shake the excess off. Arrange the shrimps in the basket.
4. Put the air fryer basket on the baking pan and slide into Rack Position 2, select Air Fry, set temperature to 350ºF (180ºC) and set time to 8 minutes.
5. Flip the shrimps halfway through the cooking time.
6. When cooking is complete, the shrimps should be opaque. Transfer the cooked shrimps onto a large plate and squeeze the lemon wedges over before serving.

523.Spicy Air Fried Old Bay Shrimp

Servings: 2 Cups
Cooking Time: 10 Minutes
Ingredients:
- ½ teaspoon Old Bay Seasoning
- 1 teaspoon ground cayenne pepper
- ½ teaspoon paprika
- 1 tablespoon olive oil
- ⅛ teaspoon salt
- ½ pound (227 g) shrimps, peeled and deveined
- Juice of half a lemon

Directions:
1. Combine the Old Bay Seasoning, cayenne pepper, paprika, olive oil, and salt in a large bowl, then add the shrimps and toss to coat well.
2. Put the shrimps in the air fryer basket.
3. Put the air fryer basket on the baking pan and slide into Rack Position 2, select Air Fry, set temperature to 390ºF (199ºC) and set time to 10 minutes.
4. Flip the shrimps halfway through the cooking time.
5. When cooking is complete, the shrimps should be opaque. Serve the shrimps with lemon juice on top.

524.Air Fried Crispy Brussels Sprouts

Servings:4
Cooking Time: 20 Minutes
Ingredients:
- ¼ teaspoon salt
- ⅛ teaspoon ground black pepper
- 1 tablespoon extra-virgin olive oil
- 1 pound (454 g) Brussels sprouts, trimmed and halved
- Lemon wedges, for garnish

Directions:
1. Combine the salt, black pepper, and olive oil in a large bowl. Stir to mix well.
2. Add the Brussels sprouts to the bowl of mixture and toss to coat well. Arrange the Brussels sprouts in the air fryer basket.
3. Put the air fryer basket on the baking pan and slide into Rack Position 2, select Air Fry, set temperature to 350ºF (180ºC) and set time to 20 minutes.
4. Stir the Brussels sprouts two times during cooking.
5. When cooked, the Brussels sprouts will be lightly browned and wilted. Transfer the cooked Brussels sprouts to a large plate and squeeze the lemon wedges on top to serve.

525.Ritzy Pimento And Almond Turkey Casserole

Servings:4
Cooking Time: 32 Minutes

Ingredients:
- 1 pound (454 g) turkey breasts
- 1 tablespoon olive oil
- 2 boiled eggs, chopped
- 2 tablespoons chopped pimentos
- ¼ cup slivered almonds, chopped
- ¼ cup mayonnaise
- ½ cup diced celery
- 2 tablespoons chopped green onion
- ¼ cup cream of chicken soup
- ¼ cup bread crumbs
- Salt and ground black pepper, to taste

Directions:
1. Put the turkey breasts in a large bowl. Sprinkle with salt and ground black pepper and drizzle with olive oil. Toss to coat well.
2. Transfer the turkey to the air fryer basket.
3. Put the air fryer basket on the baking pan and slide into Rack Position 2, select Air Fry, set temperature to 390ºF (199ºC) and set time to 12 minutes.
4. Flip the turkey halfway through.
5. When cooking is complete, the turkey should be well browned.
6. Remove the turkey breasts from the oven and cut into cubes, then combine the chicken cubes with eggs, pimentos, almonds, mayo, celery, green onions, and chicken soup in a large bowl. Stir to mix.
7. Pour the mixture into the baking pan, then spread with bread crumbs.
8. Slide the baking pan into Rack Position 1, select Convection Bake, set time to 20 minutes.
9. When cooking is complete, the eggs should be set.
10. Remove from the oven and serve immediately.

526.Pão De Queijo

Servings: 12 Balls
Cooking Time: 12 Minutes
Ingredients:
- 2 tablespoons butter, plus more for greasing
- ½ cup milk
- 1½ cups tapioca flour
- ½ teaspoon salt
- 1 large egg
- ²/₃ cup finely grated aged Asiago cheese

Directions:
1. Put the butter in a saucepan and pour in the milk, heat over medium heat until the liquid boils. Keep stirring.
2. Turn off the heat and mix in the tapioca flour and salt to form a soft dough. Transfer the dough in a large bowl, then wrap the bowl in plastic and let sit for 15 minutes.
3. Break the egg in the bowl of dough and whisk with a hand mixer for 2 minutes or until a sanity dough forms. Fold the cheese in the dough. Cover the bowl in plastic again and let sit for 10 more minutes.
4. Grease the baking pan with butter.
5. Scoop 2 tablespoons of the dough into the baking pan. Repeat with the remaining dough to make dough 12 balls. Keep a little distance between each two balls.
6. Slide the baking pan into Rack Position 1, select Convection Bake, set temperature to 375ºF (190ºC) and set time to 12 minutes.
7. Flip the balls halfway through the cooking time.
8. When cooking is complete, the balls should be golden brown and fluffy.
9. Remove the balls from the oven and allow to cool for 5 minutes before serving.

527.Golden Salmon And Carrot Croquettes

Servings:6
Cooking Time: 10 Minutes
Ingredients:
- 2 egg whites
- 1 cup almond flour
- 1 cup panko bread crumbs
- 1 pound (454 g) chopped salmon fillet
- ²/₃ cup grated carrots
- 2 tablespoons minced garlic cloves
- ½ cup chopped onion
- 2 tablespoons chopped chives
- Cooking spray

Directions:
1. Spritz the air fryer basket with cooking spray.
2. Whisk the egg whites in a bowl. Put the flour in a second bowl. Pour the bread crumbs in a third bowl. Set aside.
3. Combine the salmon, carrots, garlic, onion, and chives in a large bowl. Stir to mix well.
4. Form the mixture into balls with your hands. Dredge the balls into the flour, then egg, and then bread crumbs to coat well.
5. Arrange the salmon balls on the basket and spritz with cooking spray.
6. Put the air fryer basket on the baking pan and slide into Rack Position 2, select Air Fry, set temperature to 350ºF (180ºC) and set time to 10 minutes.
7. Flip the salmon balls halfway through cooking.
8. When cooking is complete, the salmon balls will be crispy and browned. Remove from the oven and serve immediately.

528.Dehydrated Bananas With Coconut Sprnikles

Servings:x

Cooking Time:x
Ingredients:
- 5 very ripe bananas, peeled
- 1 cup shredded coconut

Directions:
1. Place coconut in a large shallow dish. Cut Press banana wedges in the coconut and organize in one layer on the dehydrating basket.
2. Hours Put basket in rack place 4 and then press START.
3. Dehydrate for 26 hours or until peanuts are Dry to the touch but still garnish with a sweet, intense banana taste.
4. Let bananas cool completely before storing in an Airtight container for up to 5 months.

529.Classic Worcestershire Poutine

Servings:2
Cooking Time: 33 Minutes
Ingredients:
- 2 russet potatoes, scrubbed and cut into ½-inch sticks
- 2 teaspoons vegetable oil
- 2 tablespoons butter
- ¼ onion, minced
- ¼ teaspoon dried thyme
- 1 clove garlic, smashed
- 3 tablespoons all-purpose flour
- 1 teaspoon tomato paste
- 1½ cups beef stock
- 2 teaspoons Worcestershire sauce
- Salt and freshly ground black pepper, to taste
- $^2/_3$ cup chopped string cheese

Directions:
1. Bring a pot of water to a boil, then put in the potato sticks and blanch for 4 minutes.
2. Drain the potato sticks and rinse under running cold water, then pat dry with paper towels.
3. Transfer the sticks in a large bowl and drizzle with vegetable oil. Toss to coat well. Place the potato sticks in the air fryer basket.
4. Put the air fryer basket on the baking pan and slide into Rack Position 2, select Air Fry, set temperature to 400ºF (205ºC) and set time to 25 minutes.
5. Stir the potato sticks at least three times during cooking.
6. Meanwhile, make the gravy: Heat the butter in a saucepan over medium heat until melted.
7. Add the onion, thyme, and garlic and sauté for 5 minutes or until the onion is translucent.
8. Add the flour and sauté for an additional 2 minutes. Pour in the tomato paste and beef stock and cook for 1 more minute or until lightly thickened.
9. Drizzle the gravy with Worcestershire sauce and sprinkle with salt and ground black pepper. Reduce the heat to low to keep the gravy warm until ready to serve.
10. When done, the sticks should be golden brown. Remove from the oven. Transfer the fried potato sticks onto a plate, then sprinkle with salt and ground black pepper. Scatter with string cheese and pour the gravy over. Serve warm.

530.Air Fried Bacon Pinwheels

Servings: 8 Pinwheels
Cooking Time: 10 Minutes
Ingredients:
- 1 sheet puff pastry
- 2 tablespoons maple syrup
- ¼ cup brown sugar
- 8 slices bacon
- Ground black pepper, to taste
- Cooking spray

Directions:
1. Spritz the air fryer basket with cooking spray.
2. Roll the puff pastry into a 10-inch square with a rolling pin on a clean work surface, then cut the pastry into 8 strips.
3. Brush the strips with maple syrup and sprinkle with sugar, leaving a 1-inch far end uncovered.
4. Arrange each slice of bacon on each strip, leaving a ⅛-inch length of bacon hang over the end close to you. Sprinkle with black pepper.
5. From the end close to you, roll the strips into pinwheels, then dab the uncovered end with water and seal the rolls.
6. Arrange the pinwheels in the basket and spritz with cooking spray.
7. Put the air fryer basket on the baking pan and slide into Rack Position 2, select Air Fry, set temperature to 360ºF (182ºC) and set time to 10 minutes.
8. Flip the pinwheels halfway through.
9. When cooking is complete, the pinwheels should be golden brown. Remove from the oven and serve immediately.

531.Simple Butter Cake

Servings:8
Cooking Time: 20 Minutes
Ingredients:
- 1 cup all-purpose flour
- 1¼ teaspoons baking powder
- ¼ teaspoon salt
- ½ cup plus 1½ tablespoons granulated white sugar

- 9½ tablespoons butter, at room temperature
- 2 large eggs
- 1 large egg yolk
- 2½ tablespoons milk
- 1 teaspoon vanilla extract
- Cooking spray

Directions:
1. Spritz the baking pan with cooking spray.
2. Combine the flour, baking powder, and salt in a large bowl. Stir to mix well.
3. Whip the sugar and butter in a separate bowl with a hand mixer on medium speed for 3 minutes.
4. Whip the eggs, egg yolk, milk, and vanilla extract into the sugar and butter mix with a hand mixer.
5. Pour in the flour mixture and whip with hand mixer until sanity and smooth.
6. Scrape the batter into the baking pan and level the batter with a spatula.
7. Slide the baking pan into Rack Position 1, select Convection Bake, set temperature to 325ºF (163ºC) and set time to 20 minutes.
8. After 15 minutes, remove the pan from the oven. Check the doneness. Return the pan to the oven and continue cooking.
9. When done, a toothpick inserted in the center should come out clean.
10. Invert the cake on a cooling rack and allow to cool for 15 minutes before slicing to serve.

532.Hot Wings

Servings: 16 Wings
Cooking Time: 15 Minutes
Ingredients:
- 16 chicken wings
- 3 tablespoons hot sauce
- Cooking spray

Directions:
1. Spritz the air fryer basket with cooking spray.
2. Arrange the chicken wings in the basket.
3. Put the air fryer basket on the baking pan and slide into Rack Position 2, select Air Fry, set temperature to 360ºF (182ºC) and set time to 15 minutes.
4. Flip the wings at lease three times during cooking.
5. When cooking is complete, the chicken wings will be well browned. Remove from the oven.
6. Transfer the air fried wings to a plate and serve with hot sauce.

533.Butternut Squash With Hazelnuts

Servings: 3 Cups
Cooking Time: 23 Minutes
Ingredients:
- 2 tablespoons whole hazelnuts

- 3 cups butternut squash, peeled, deseeded and cubed
- ¼ teaspoon kosher salt
- ¼ teaspoon freshly ground black pepper
- 2 teaspoons olive oil
- Cooking spray

Directions:
1. Spritz the air fryer basket with cooking spray. Spread the hazelnuts in the pan.
2. Put the air fryer basket on the baking pan and slide into Rack Position 2, select Air Fry, set temperature to 300ºF (150ºC) and set time to 3 minutes.
3. When done, the hazelnuts should be soft. Remove from the oven. Chopped the hazelnuts roughly and transfer to a small bowl. Set aside.
4. Put the butternut squash in a large bowl, then sprinkle with salt and pepper and drizzle with olive oil. Toss to coat well. Transfer the squash to the lightly greased basket.
5. Put the air fryer basket on the baking pan and slide into Rack Position 2, select Air Fry, set temperature to 360ºF (182ºC) and set time to 20 minutes.
6. Flip the squash halfway through the cooking time.
7. When cooking is complete, the squash will be soft. Transfer the squash to a plate and sprinkle with the chopped hazelnuts before serving.

534.Roasted Carrot Chips

Servings: 3 Cups
Cooking Time: 15 Minutes
Ingredients:
- 3 large carrots, peeled and sliced into long and thick chips diagonally
- 1 tablespoon granulated garlic
- 1 teaspoon salt
- ¼ teaspoon ground black pepper
- 1 tablespoon olive oil
- 1 tablespoon finely chopped fresh parsley

Directions:
1. Toss the carrots with garlic, salt, ground black pepper, and olive oil in a large bowl to coat well. Place the carrots in the air fryer basket.
2. Put the air fryer basket on the baking pan and slide into Rack Position 2, select Roast, set temperature to 360ºF (182ºC) and set time to 15 minutes.
3. Stir the carrots halfway through the cooking time.
4. When cooking is complete, the carrot chips should be soft. Remove from the oven. Serve the carrot chips with parsley on top.

535.Oven Baked Rice

Servings: About 4 Cups
Cooking Time: 35 Minutes
Ingredients:

- 1 cup long-grain white rice, rinsed and drained
- 1 tablespoon unsalted butter, melted, or 1 tablespoon extra-virgin olive oil
- 2 cups water
- 1 teaspoon kosher salt or ½ teaspoon fine salt

Directions:
1. Add the butter and rice to the baking pan and stir to coat. Pour in the water and sprinkle with the salt. Stir until the salt is dissolved.
2. Select Bake, set the temperature to 325ºF (163ºC), and set the time for 35 minutes. Select Start to begin preheating.
3. Once the unit has preheated, place the pan in the oven.
4. After 20 minutes, remove the pan from the oven. Stir the rice. Transfer the pan back to the oven and continue cooking for 10 to 15 minutes, or until the rice is mostly cooked through and the water is absorbed.
5. When done, remove the pan from the oven and cover with aluminum foil. Let stand for 10 minutes. Using a fork, gently fluff the rice.
6. Serve immediately.

536.Enchilada Sauce

Servings: 2 Cups
Cooking Time: 0 Minutes
Ingredients:
- 3 large ancho chiles, stems and seeds removed, torn into pieces
- 1½ cups very hot water
- 2 garlic cloves, peeled and lightly smashed
- 2 tablespoons wine vinegar
- 1½ teaspoons sugar
- ½ teaspoon dried oregano
- ½ teaspoon ground cumin
- 2 teaspoons kosher salt or 1 teaspoon fine salt

Directions:
1. Mix together the chile pieces and hot water in a bowl and let stand for 10 to 15 minutes.
2. Pour the chiles and water into a blender jar. Fold in the garlic, vinegar, sugar, oregano, cumin, and salt and blend until smooth.
3. Use immediately.

537.Dehydrated Crackers With Oats

Servings:x
Cooking Time:x
Ingredients:
- 3 tablespoons (20g) psyllium husk powder
- 2 teaspoons fine sea salt
- 1 teaspoon freshly ground black pepper
- 2 teaspoons ground turmeric, divided
- 3 tablespoons melted coconut oil
- 1 cup (125g) sunflower seeds
- ½ cup (75g) flaxseeds
- ¾ cup (50g) pumpkin seeds
- ¼ cup (35g) sesame seeds

- 2 tablespoons (30g) chia seeds
- 1½ cups (150g) rolled oats
- 1½ cups (360ml) water
- 1 large parsnip (10 ounces/300g), finely Grated

Directions:
1. In a large bowl Blend All of the seeds, Oats, psyllium husk, pepper, salt and 1 teaspoon ground turmeric.
2. Whisk coconut water and oil together in a measuring Cup. Add to the dry ingredients and blend well until all is totally saturated and dough becomes very thick.
3. Mix grated parsnip using 1 tsp turmeric and stir to blend.
4. Shape the first half to a disc and place it with a rolling pin, firmly roll dough to a thin sheet that the size of this dehydrate basket.
5. Put dough and parchment paper at the dehydrate basket.
6. Repeat steps 4 with remaining dough.
7. Hours and allow Rotate Remind. Place dehydrate baskets in rack positions 5 and 3. Press START.
8. Dehydrate crackers until tender. When prompted By Rotate Remind, rotate the baskets leading to back and change rack amounts.
9. Eliminate baskets out of oven and let rest for 10 minutes. Split crackers into shards.
10. Container for up to two months.

538.Mediterranean Quiche

Servings:4
Cooking Time: 30 Minutes
Ingredients:
- 4 eggs
- ¼ cup chopped Kalamata olives
- ½ cup chopped tomatoes
- ¼ cup chopped onion
- ½ cup milk
- 1 cup crumbled feta cheese
- ½ tablespoon chopped oregano
- ½ tablespoon chopped basil
- Salt and ground black pepper, to taste
- Cooking spray

Directions:
1. Spritz the baking pan with cooking spray.
2. Whisk the eggs with remaining ingredients in a large bowl. Stir to mix well.
3. Pour the mixture into the prepared baking pan.
4. Slide the baking pan into Rack Position 1, select Convection Bake, set temperature to 340ºF (171ºC) and set time to 30 minutes.
5. When cooking is complete, the eggs should be set and a toothpick inserted in the center should come out clean.
6. Serve immediately.

539.Hillbilly Broccoli Cheese Casserole

Servings:6
Cooking Time: 30 Minutes

Ingredients:
- 4 cups broccoli florets
- ¼ cup heavy whipping cream
- ½ cup sharp Cheddar cheese, shredded
- ¼ cup ranch dressing
- Kosher salt and ground black pepper, to taste

Directions:
1. Combine all the ingredients in a large bowl. Toss to coat well broccoli well.
2. Pour the mixture into the baking pan.
3. Slide the baking pan into Rack Position 1, select Convection Bake, set temperature to 375ºF (190ºC) and set time to 30 minutes.
4. When cooking is complete, the broccoli should be tender.
5. Remove the baking pan from the oven and serve immediately.

540.Buttery Knots With Parsley

Servings: 8 Knots
Cooking Time: 5 Minutes
Ingredients:
- 1 teaspoon dried parsley
- ¼ cup melted butter
- 2 teaspoons garlic powder

Directions:
1. 1 (11-ounce / 312-g) tube refrigerated French bread dough, cut into 8 slices
2. Combine the parsley, butter, and garlic powder in a bowl. Stir to mix well.
3. Place the French bread dough slices on a clean work surface, then roll each slice into a 6-inch long rope. Tie the ropes into knots and arrange them on a plate.
4. Transfer the knots into the baking pan. Brush the knots with butter mixture.
5. Put the air fryer basket on the baking pan and slide into Rack Position 2, select Air Fry, set temperature to 350ºF (180ºC) and set time to 5 minutes.
6. Flip the knots halfway through the cooking time.
7. When done, the knots should be golden brown. Remove from the oven and serve immediately.

541.Easy Corn And Bell Pepper Casserole

Servings:4
Cooking Time: 20 Minutes
Ingredients:
- 1 cup corn kernels
- ¼ cup bell pepper, finely chopped
- ½ cup low-fat milk
- 1 large egg, beaten
- ½ cup yellow cornmeal
- ½ cup all-purpose flour
- ½ teaspoon baking powder
- 2 tablespoons melted unsalted butter
- 1 tablespoon granulated sugar
- Pinch of cayenne pepper
- ¼ teaspoon kosher salt

- Cooking spray

Directions:
1. Spritz the baking pan with cooking spray.
2. Combine all the ingredients in a large bowl. Stir to mix well. Pour the mixture into the baking pan.
3. Slide the baking pan into Rack Position 1, select Convection Bake, set temperature to 330ºF (166ºC) and set time to 20 minutes.
4. When cooking is complete, the casserole should be lightly browned and set.
5. Remove from the oven and serve immediately.

542.Chicken Ham Casserole

Servings:4 To 6
Cooking Time: 15 Minutes
Ingredients:
- 2 cups diced cooked chicken
- 1 cup diced ham
- ¼ teaspoon ground nutmeg
- ½ cup half-and-half
- ½ teaspoon ground black pepper
- 6 slices Swiss cheese
- Cooking spray

Directions:
1. Spritz the baking pan with cooking spray.
2. Combine the chicken, ham, nutmeg, half-and-half, and ground black pepper in a large bowl. Stir to mix well.
3. Pour half of the mixture into the baking pan, then top the mixture with 3 slices of Swiss cheese, then pour in the remaining mixture and top with remaining cheese slices.
4. Slide the baking pan into Rack Position 1, select Convection Bake, set temperature to 350ºF (180ºC) and set time to 15 minutes.
5. When cooking is complete, the egg should be set and the cheese should be melted.
6. Serve immediately.

543.Lemony Shishito Peppers

Servings:4
Cooking Time: 5 Minutes
Ingredients:
- ½ pound (227 g) shishito peppers (about 24)
- 1 tablespoon olive oil
- Coarse sea salt, to taste
- Lemon wedges, for serving
- Cooking spray

Directions:
1. Spritz the air fryer basket with cooking spray.
2. Toss the peppers with olive oil in a large bowl to coat well.
3. Arrange the peppers in the basket.
4. Put the air fryer basket on the baking pan and slide into Rack Position 2, select Air Fry, set temperature to 400ºF (205ºC) and set time to 5 minutes.
5. Flip the peppers and sprinkle the peppers with salt halfway through the cooking time.

6. When cooked, the peppers should be blistered and lightly charred. Transfer the peppers onto a plate and squeeze the lemon wedges on top before serving.

544.Kale Salad Sushi Rolls With Sriracha Mayonnaise

Servings:12
Cooking Time: 10 Minutes
Ingredients:
- Kale Salad:
- 1½ cups chopped kale
- 1 tablespoon sesame seeds
- ¾ teaspoon soy sauce
- ¾ teaspoon toasted sesame oil
- ½ teaspoon rice vinegar
- ¼ teaspoon ginger
- ⅛ teaspoon garlic powder
- Sushi Rolls:
- 3 sheets sushi nori
- 1 batch cauliflower rice
- ½ avocado, sliced
- Sriracha Mayonnaise:
- ¼ cup Sriracha sauce
- ¼ cup vegan mayonnaise
- Coating:
- ½ cup panko bread crumbs

Directions:
1. In a medium bowl, toss all the ingredients for the salad together until well coated and set aside.
2. Place a sheet of nori on a clean work surface and spread the cauliflower rice in an even layer on the nori. Scoop 2 to 3 tablespoon of kale salad on the rice and spread over. Place 1 or 2 avocado slices on top. Roll up the sushi, pressing gently to get a nice, tight roll. Repeat to make the remaining 2 rolls.
3. In a bowl, stir together the Sriracha sauce and mayonnaise until smooth. Add bread crumbs to a separate bowl.
4. Dredge the sushi rolls in Sriracha Mayonnaise, then roll in bread crumbs till well coated.
5. Place the coated sushi rolls in the air fryer basket.
6. Put the air fryer basket on the baking pan and slide into Rack Position 2, select Air Fry, set temperature to 390ºF (199ºC) and set time to 10 minutes.
7. Flip the sushi rolls halfway through the cooking time.
8. When cooking is complete, the sushi rolls will be golden brown and crispy. .
9. Transfer to a platter and rest for 5 minutes before slicing each roll into 8 pieces. Serve warm.

545.Sweet And Sour Peanuts

Servings:9
Cooking Time: 5 Minutes
Ingredients:
- 3 cups shelled raw peanuts
- 1 tablespoon hot red pepper sauce
- 3 tablespoons granulated white sugar

Directions:
1. Put the peanuts in a large bowl, then drizzle with hot red pepper sauce and sprinkle with sugar. Toss to coat well.
2. Pour the peanuts in the air fryer basket.
3. Put the air fryer basket on the baking pan and slide into Rack Position 2, select Air Fry, set temperature to 400ºF (205ºC) and set time to 5 minutes.
4. Stir the peanuts halfway through the cooking time.
5. When cooking is complete, the peanuts will be crispy and browned. Remove from the oven and serve immediately.

546.Caesar Salad Dressing

Servings: About ²/₃ Cup
Cooking Time: 0 Minutes
Ingredients:
- ½ cup extra-virgin olive oil
- 2 tablespoons freshly squeezed lemon juice
- 1 teaspoon anchovy paste
- ¼ teaspoon kosher salt or ⅛ teaspoon fine salt
- ¼ teaspoon minced or pressed garlic
- 1 egg, beaten
- Add all the ingredients to a tall, narrow container.

Directions:
1. Purée the mixture with an immersion blender until smooth.
2. Use immediately.

547.Chorizo, Corn, And Potato Frittata

Servings:4
Cooking Time: 12 Minutes
Ingredients:
- 2 tablespoons olive oil
- 1 chorizo, sliced
- 4 eggs
- ½ cup corn
- 1 large potato, boiled and cubed
- 1 tablespoon chopped parsley
- ½ cup feta cheese, crumbled
- Salt and ground black pepper, to taste

Directions:
1. Heat the olive oil in a nonstick skillet over medium heat until shimmering.
2. Add the chorizo and cook for 4 minutes or until golden brown.
3. Whisk the eggs in a bowl, then sprinkle with salt and ground black pepper.
4. Mix the remaining ingredients in the egg mixture, then pour the chorizo and its fat into the baking pan. Pour in the egg mixture.
5. Slide the baking pan into Rack Position 1, select Convection Bake, set temperature to 330ºF (166ºC) and set time to 8 minutes.
6. Stir the mixture halfway through.

7. When cooking is complete, the eggs should be set.
8. Serve immediately.

548. Chocolate And Coconut Macaroons

Servings: 24 Macaroons
Cooking Time: 8 Minutes
Ingredients:
- 3 large egg whites, at room temperature
- ¼ teaspoon salt
- ¾ cup granulated white sugar
- 4½ tablespoons unsweetened cocoa powder
- 2¼ cups unsweetened shredded coconut

Directions:
1. Line the air fryer basket with parchment paper.
2. Whisk the egg whites with salt in a large bowl with a hand mixer on high speed until stiff peaks form.
3. Whisk in the sugar with the hand mixer on high speed until the mixture is thick. Mix in the cocoa powder and coconut.
4. Scoop 2 tablespoons of the mixture and shape the mixture in a ball. Repeat with remaining mixture to make 24 balls in total.
5. Arrange the balls in a single layer in the basket and leave a little space between each two balls.
6. Put the air fryer basket on the baking pan and slide into Rack Position 2, select Air Fry, set temperature to 375ºF (190ºC) and set time to 8 minutes.
7. When cooking is complete, the balls should be golden brown.
8. Serve immediately.

549. Goat Cheese And Asparagus Frittata

Servings:2 To 4
Cooking Time: 25 Minutes
Ingredients:
- 1 cup asparagus spears, cut into 1-inch pieces
- 1 teaspoon vegetable oil
- 1 tablespoon milk
- 6 eggs, beaten
- 2 ounces (57 g) goat cheese, crumbled
- 1 tablespoon minced chives, optional
- Kosher salt and pepper, to taste
- Add the asparagus spears to a small bowl and drizzle with the vegetable oil. Toss until well coated and transfer to the air fryer basket.

Directions:
1. Put the air fryer basket on the baking pan and slide into Rack Position 2, select Air Fry,

set temperature to 400ºF (205ºC) and set time to 5 minutes.
2. Flip the asparagus halfway through.
3. When cooking is complete, the asparagus should be tender and slightly wilted.
4. Remove from the oven to the baking pan.
5. Stir together the milk and eggs in a medium bowl. Pour the mixture over the asparagus in the pan. Sprinkle with the goat cheese and the chives (if using) over the eggs. Season with salt and pepper.
6. Slide the baking pan into Rack Position 1, select Convection Bake, set temperature to 320ºF (160ºC) and set time to 20 minutes.
7. When cooking is complete, the top should be golden and the eggs should be set.
8. Transfer to a serving dish. Slice and serve.

550. Roasted Mushrooms

Servings: About 1½ Cups
Cooking Time: 30 Minutes
Ingredients:
- 1 pound (454 g) button or cremini mushrooms, washed, stems trimmed, and cut into quarters or thick slices
- ¼ cup water
- 1 teaspoon kosher salt or ½ teaspoon fine salt
- 3 tablespoons unsalted butter, cut into pieces, or extra-virgin olive oil

Directions:
1. Place a large piece of aluminum foil on the sheet pan. Place the mushroom pieces in the middle of the foil. Spread them out into an even layer. Pour the water over them, season with the salt, and add the butter. Wrap the mushrooms in the foil.
2. Select Roast, set the temperature to 325ºF (163ºC), and set the time for 15 minutes. Select Start to begin preheating.
3. Once the unit has preheated, place the pan in the oven.
4. After 15 minutes, remove the pan from the oven. Transfer the foil packet to a cutting board and carefully unwrap it. Pour the mushrooms and cooking liquid from the foil onto the sheet pan.
5. Select Roast, set the temperature to 350ºF (180ºC), and set the time for 15 minutes. Return the pan to the oven. Select Start to begin.
6. After about 10 minutes, remove the pan from the oven and stir the mushrooms. Return the pan to the oven and continue cooking for anywhere from 5 to 15 more minutes, or until the liquid is mostly gone and the mushrooms start to brown.
7. Serve immediately.